Evaluating Research for Evidence-Based Nursing Practice

Jacqueline Fawcett, PhD, FAAN

Joan Garity, EdD, RN

College of Nursing and Health Sciences
University of Massachusetts, Boston

D0179974

F. A. DAVIS COMPANY • Philadelphia

F. A. Davis Company
1915 Arch Street
Philadelphia, PA 19103
www.fadavis.com

Printed in the United States of America

Last digit indicates print number: 10 9 8 7 6 5 4 3 2 1

Publisher, Nursing: Joanne Patzek DaCunha, RN, MSN
Director of Content Development: Darlene D. Pedersen
Project Editor: Padraic J. Maroney
Design and Illustrations Manager: Carolyn O'Brien

As new scientific information becomes available through basic and clinical research, recommended treatments and drug therapies undergo changes. The author(s) and publisher have done everything possible to make this book accurate, up-to-date, and in accord with accepted standards at the time of publication. The author(s), editors, and publisher are not responsible for errors or omissions or for consequences from application of the book and make no warranty, expressed or implied, in regard to the contents of the book. Any practice described in this book should be applied by the reader in accordance with professional standards of care used in regard to the unique circumstances that may apply in each situation. The reader is advised always to check product information (package inserts) for changes and new information regarding dose and contraindications before administering any drug. Caution is especially urged when using new or infrequently ordered drugs.

Library of Congress Cataloging-in-Publication Data

Library of Congress Cataloging-in-Publication Data

Fawcett, Jacqueline.
Evaluating research for evidence-based nursing practice/Jacqueline Fawcett, Joan Garity.
     p.; cm.
Includes bibliographical references and index.
ISBN-13: 978-0-8036-1489-5 (alk. paper)
1. Nursing—Research—Evaluation. 2. Evidence-based nursing. I. Garity, Joan. II. Title.
[DNLM: 1. Nursing Research—methods. 2. Evaluation Studies as Topic. 3. Evidence-Based Medicine. WY 20.5 F278e 2009]
RT81.5.F39 2009
610.73—dc22

                                                                                            2008016804

Dedication

To my husband, John S. Fawcett,
for his love and his willingness to support
my passion for writing about the conceptual,
theoretical, and empirical components
of nursing research.

Jacqueline Fawcett

In memory of my parents, my first teachers,
who encouraged me to be a lifelong seeker of
knowledge and teaching-learning opportunities.

Joan Garity

Preface

Nursing research is conducted to generate or test middle-range theories, which provide the evidence used for all phases of the nursing practice process, including assessment, planning, intervention, and evaluation. Although a considerable amount of research that is relevant for nursing practice already exists, students and practicing nurses do not yet routinely evaluate that research. We believe that the lack of attention to existing research stems from lack of understanding of the criteria used to evaluate reports of research in a systematic manner.

This book presents a comprehensive framework of criteria for the evaluation of reports of nursing research. The framework incorporates the components of conceptual-theoretical-empirical (C-T-E) structures for nursing research, with emphasis on the middle-range theories that are the product of all types of qualitative and quantitative research designs. We have placed middle-range theories within the context of their parent conceptual models of nursing and the empirical research methods used to generate and test the theories.

Although written specifically as a text for a baccalaureate-program nursing research course, this book is appropriate for all nursing students and practicing nurses who want to learn how to evaluate reports of nursing research for evidence-based practice. The book contents are the result of our many discussions while revising and co-teaching an undergraduate nursing research course at the University of Massachusetts, Boston. We wanted to demystify the research process and infuse our students with a lifelong learning approach to evaluating and utilizing nursing research. Demystifying research for undergraduate students, as many faculty have discovered, is a major challenge. Students express their concerns about nursing research with comments such as: "I get anxious just thinking about research." "I'm not very good at math, so I'm worried about how I will do with the statistics." "Reading a research article hurts my head." "Will I really use this material in my nursing practice?"

Throughout the book, we have focused exclusively on the evaluation, rather than the conduct, of research. In doing so, we have found that the book contents eliminated many of our students' concerns about nursing research and facilitated their ability to understand and evaluate the conceptual, theoretical, and empirical components of published research reports.

We recommend that the book be read in the order in which the content is presented. The book is divided into five parts. Part One introduces the reader to our view of the world of nursing research, including the ideas that:

- research is equivalent to theory development,
- theory is equivalent to evidence, and
- practice is equivalent to research.

In Chapter 1, we provide definitions of research, theory, evidence, and evidence-based practice, and we explain why research is conducted, the links between research and theory and theory and evidence, and the link between the nursing practice process and the nursing research process. In addition, we discuss various sources of knowledge, various types of theories, and the type of evidence that each source of knowledge and each type of theory provides. In Chapter 2, we introduce the idea of C-T-E structures for theory-generating research and theory-testing nursing research. In Chapter 3, we describe the contents of typical research reports and explain where to find each component of the C-T-E structure in them. In Chapter 4, we present our comprehensive framework of criteria for evaluation of C-T-E structures for nursing research.

Part Two focuses on the conceptual and theoretical components of C-T-E structures for nursing research. In Chapter 5, we introduce readers to the criteria to evaluate the conceptual model used by the researcher to guide a theory-generating or theory-testing study. In Chapter 6, we identify and describe the criteria used to evaluate the middle-range theory that was generated or tested. Tables containing summaries of several conceptual models of nursing and nursing grand theories, as well as research focus guidelines and research methods guidelines for those conceptual models and grand theories are in the Chapter 5 files on the CD that comes with this book. Tables containing lists of middle-range theories developed by nurses and members of other disciplines are in the Chapter 6 files on the CD.

Part Three addresses the empirical research methods component of C-T-E structures for nursing research. The six chapters address the criterion for evaluation of the five elements of empirical research methods: research design (Chapter 7), samples (Chapter 8), research instruments and experimental conditions (Chapter 9), procedures for data collection and protection of research participants (Chapters 10 and 11, respectively), and data analysis techniques (Chapter 12). A special feature of Part Three is the discussion of both qualitative and quantitative research in each chapter and the categorization of research as descriptive, correlational, or experimental. Due to our special concerns about the ethical aspects of research, Chapter 11 highlights the parallels between the research-relevant content of the American Nurses' Association Code of Ethics and research ethics codes, including the Nuremberg Code, the Declaration of Helsinki, and the Belmont Report, as well as the research implications of the Patient's Bill of Rights.

Part Four returns attention to the theoretical and conceptual components of C-T-E structures and completes discussion of the framework for evaluation of C-T-E structures. In Chapter 13, we discuss the criterion used to evaluate research findings. In Chapter 14, we present the criterion used to evaluate the utility of the middle-range theory for practice. A highlight of Chapter 14 is a decision tree that illustrates the options for use of a theory in practice, including whether the middle-range theory requires additional study, should be used in practice, could be tried in practice, or should not be used. In Chapter 15, we identify the criterion used to evaluate the utility and soundness of the conceptual model that guided the research.

The single chapter in Part Five of the book focuses on integration of research and practice. Specifically, in Chapter 16 we discuss strategies that all nurses can use to bring evidence-based practice to life by integrating nursing research and nursing practice.

Throughout the book, we emphasize three questions about information contained in published research reports:

Where is the information?
What is the information?
How good is the information?

We provide numerous examples drawn from existing research reports to facilitate readers' understanding of the *where, what,* and *how good* of information. The examples we selected encompass a large number of qualitative and quantitative research designs. Many of these examples are given in the chapters, and additional examples are given in detailed tables that are found on the CD that comes with this book. The tables for Chapters 8 through 15 provide information on every research design introduced in Chapter 7. Other files found on the CD include an example of a complete research report (Chapter 3), directories for research instruments (Chapter 9), templates for evidence-based practice papers for practice tools and intervention protocols (Chapter 14), and a searchable bibliography of nursing conceptual model-based research with instructions for searching that literature. In addition, the CD includes a complete list of all references cited in the book. The reference list is also printed at the end of the book.

In addition, the CD includes learning activities, practice examination questions, and PowerPoint slides for each chapter. We designed learning activities and practice examination questions that should help readers to understand how to apply the content of each chapter in diverse ways. The PowerPoint slides for each chapter can be used as the basis for personal notes about chapter content.

We designed the book contents and the CD files to help the students, faculty, and practicing nurses who will use this book to better incorporate the evaluation of nursing research into their varied practice settings. We are mindful, given the present faculty shortage, that faculty with diverse educational backgrounds may be asked to teach nursing research to diverse students in a variety of settings. We have endeavored to include enough information so that faculty will be able to competently help students learn how to evaluate reports of nursing research using only this one book.

We hope that all readers of this book will embrace evaluating C-T-E structures for theory-generating and theory-testing research. We also hope that readers will become expert evaluators of research reports and, given the sound foundation provided by this book, be better prepared to pursue graduate education and learn how to conduct rigorous nursing conceptual model–based, theory-generating and theory-testing research that will enhance the health-related quality of life of all people who come to nurses for care.

The writing of this book was enlightening. Despite many years of experience conducting our own research, we learned a great deal about research as we wrote each chapter. Our passion for research and our conviction that research is conducted for the sake of theory development only increased as we wrote successive drafts of the chapters. A particular challenge was to convey our idea of C-T-E structures for research in a way that readers would understand. Our students' comments and their performance on course examinations indicate that we have been successful; we hope that all of our readers will agree.

The mountains depicted on the cover of this book symbolize nurses' efforts to understand and promote research and evidence-based practice, as well as our own efforts to write a book that can serve as a comprehensive reference for evaluation of C-T-E structures for research. We acknowledge the continuous support and encouragement that we received from many colleagues and friends from inception to completion of our book. We are indebted to our students and colleagues at the University of Massachusetts, Boston for their support, intellectual challenges, and constructive criticism. We would like to especially acknowledge the contributions to our thinking about nursing research offered by our colleague Susan DeSanto-Madeya, the contributions to our understanding of statistics by our colleagues Laura Milliken and Jie Chen, and the contributions to ways to teach nursing research offered by our colleague

Sheila Cannon. We gratefully acknowledge the opportunity given to us by Cynthia Aber, our Nursing Department Chairperson, to teach an undergraduate nursing research course. We also acknowledge the assistance of Amanda Hall of Waldoboro, Maine, who helped us compile the conceptual models of nursing bibliographies. We are indebted to Joanne P. DaCunha of F. A. Davis Company for her encouragement and the time spent discussing the content and design of this book, to Barbara Tchabovsky for her superb editing of every chapter, and to Padraic J. Maroney for all he did to facilitate production of the book.

Reviewers

Robert Atkins, PhD, MSN, BSN, BA
Assistant Professor
Rutgers University
Newark, New Jersey

Martha C. Baker, PhD, RN, APRN-BC
Director, BSN Program
Southwest Baptist University
Springfield, Missouri

Elizabeth W. Black, MSN, CSN
Assistant Professor
Gwynedd-Mercy College
Gwynedd Valley, Pennsylvania

Lucille C. Gambardella, PhD, RN, CS,
APRN-BC, CNE
Chair and Professor, Department of Nursing
Wesley College
Dover, Delaware

Nancy C. Goddard, RN, MN, PhD
Nursing Instructor
Red Deer College
Red Deer, Alberta, Canada
Adjunct Assistant Professor
University of Alberta
Alberta, Canada

Kristen Gulbransen, RN, BScN, MN
Nursing Educator
Red Deer College
Red Deer, Alberta, Canada

Susan M. Hinck, PhD, RN
Associate Professor
Missouri State University
Springfield, Missouri

Violet Malinski, BS, MA, PhD
Associate Professor and Graduate Program
  Director
Hunter Bellevue School of Nursing
New York, New York

Maryellen McBride, PhD(c), ARNP, BC,
CARN
Assistant Professor
Washburn University
Topeka, Kansas

Mary Ellen Mitchell-Rosen, BSN, MSN, RN
Assistant Professor
Nova Southeastern University
Fort Lauderdale, Florida

Mario R. Ortiz, RN, PhD, CNS
Assistant Professor
Purdue University
Westville, Indiana

Mary E. Partusch, PhD, RN
Professor
Nebraska Methodist College
Omaha, Nebraska

Christine E. Pilon-Kacir, PhD, RN
Professor
Winona State University
Rochester, Minnesota

Janice Putnam, RN, PhD
Associate Professor
University of Central Missouri
Warrensburg, Missouri

Debra L. Renna, MSN, CCRN
Instructor
Keiser University
Fort Lauderdale, Florida

Charlene M. Romer, RN, PhD
Associate Professor
Clayton State University
Morrow, Georgia

Michele J. Upvall, PhD, CRNP
  Professor, Associate Dean, and Director
    of the School of Nursing
  Carlow University
  Pittsburgh, Pennsylvania

Carolyn F. Waltz, RN, PhD, FAAN
  Professor and Director of International
    Activities
  University of Maryland
  Baltimore, Maryland

Patricia E. Zander, BSN, MSN, PhD, RN
  Nursing Professor and Assistant Dean
    of BSNC Program
  Viterbo University
  La Crosse, Wisconsin

Contents

CD CONTENTS

Part One

Introduction to Research

Chapter 1

Research and Evidence-Based Nursing Practice

Evidence for nursing practice comes from research and other sources. Evidence-based practice requires an understanding of how research findings and other evidence inform and guide practice. In this chapter, you will learn the importance of conducting nursing research and the connection between research and evidence-based nursing practice. We start by providing definitions for research and nursing research. We continue with a discussion of the reason research is conducted and add definitions for evidence and evidence-based practice. We also provide an overview of different sources of knowledge that are used as evidence, a definition of theory, and a discussion of the evidence provided by five different types of theories.

KEYWORDS

Aesthetic Nursing Theories	Explanatory Nursing Theories
Applied Research	Knowledge
A Priori	Metaparadigm
Authority	Metaparadigm of Nursing
Basic Research	Nursing Research
Clinical Research	Predictive Nursing Theories
Concepts	Propositions
Data	Research
Descriptive Nursing Theories	Sociopolitical Theories
Empirical Nursing Theories	Tenacity
Ethical Nursing Theories	Theories of Personal Knowing
Evidence	Theory
Evidence-Based Nursing Practice	Utilization of Research

WHAT IS RESEARCH?

Research can be defined in various ways. Some definitions of research found in the Oxford English Dictionary (OED) (2005) are:

- the act of searching (closely or carefully) for or after a specified thing or person

- a search or investigation directed to the discovery of some fact by careful consideration or study of a subject; a course of critical or scientific inquiry
- an investigation; an inquiry into things

The dictionary definitions draw our attention to research as a thorough search, an investigation, or a critical inquiry. The goal of the search, investigation, or inquiry is the discovery of something.

Definitions of research found in textbooks, such as the definitions listed below, underscore the thorough and critical nature of research and draw attention to the discovery or development of knowledge as the specific goal. The definitions indicate that research is:

- "A diligent, systemic inquiry or study that validates and refines existing knowledge and develops new knowledge" (Burns & Grove, 2007, p. 3)
- "Systematic inquiry that uses disciplined methods to answer questions or solve problems" (Polit & Beck, 2006, p. 4)
- "A rigorous process of inquiry designed to provide answers to questions about things of concern in an academic discipline or profession" (Anders, Daly, Thompson, Elliott, & Chang, 2005, p. 155)
- A formal, systematic, and rigorous process used to generate and test theories (Fawcett, 1999)

Although Polit and Beck (2006) refer to research as a way to solve problems, it is important to point out that research is not the same as problem-solving. Research focuses on developing knowledge to enhance understanding, whereas problem-solving focuses on using existing knowledge to resolve practical problems (Fain, 2004). More precisely, knowledge developed by means of research does not provide answers to problems but rather helps us to think differently about the problems we encounter in practice.

Knowledge, Theory, and Research

Fawcett (1999) mentions theories in her definition of research, whereas Burns and Grove (2007) mention knowledge, as did Hunt (1981), who also pointed out that "research increases the body of knowledge" (p. 190).

Knowledge is a very broad term that encompasses all that is known about something (OED, 2005). The spectrum of knowledge ranges from very broad statements to very precise statements.

A **theory** is regarded as knowledge that is at the relatively precise end of the knowledge spectrum. Theories are made up of one or more ideas and statements about those ideas. When discussing theories, ideas are referred to as **concepts**, and statements are referred to as **propositions**. Examples of theory concepts are functional status and physical energy. One type of proposition is a statement that defines a concept. An example is:

Functional status is defined as the performance of usual activities of daily living.

Another type of proposition is a statement about the association between two concepts. An example is:

Physical energy is related to functional status.

Our definition of theory given below identifies the number of concepts (one or more) and the type of concepts (concrete and specific), as well as the type of propositions (descriptions of concepts and associations between concepts) that make up a theory.

- A theory is made up of one or more relatively concrete and specific concepts, the propositions that narrowly describe those concepts, and the propositions that state relatively concrete and specific associations between two or more of the concepts.

Research is the process used to gather and convert words and numbers—which are referred to as **data**—into theories. The definition of research we prefer combines the idea that research is a rigorous and systematic type of inquiry with the idea that research is directed toward the development of knowledge through the generation and testing of theories.

- Research is a formal, systematic, and rigorous process of inquiry used to generate and test theories.

Unfortunately, in some cases, the theory that is generated or tested through the use of data is not always obvious, and the research appears to be what Chinn and Kramer (2004) called "theory-isolated" (p. 123). They explained that the contribution of research that is not explicitly directed toward theory development is very limited.

WHAT IS NURSING RESEARCH?

Nursing research "provides the scientific basis for the practice of the profession" (American Association of Colleges of Nursing, 2005, p. 1). Definitions of nursing research tend to be circular, requiring an understanding of the meaning of research and the meaning of nursing. For example, Nieswiadomy (2008) defined nursing research as "the systematic, objective process of analyzing phenomena of importance to nursing" (p. 54). Burns and Grove (2007) pointed out that the definition of nursing research requires an understanding of what knowledge is relevant for nursing, and specifically what knowledge is needed to improve nursing practice.

The meaning of nursing and the identification of categories of knowledge that are relevant for nursing practice are summarized in what is called the **metaparadigm of nursing**. A **metaparadigm** is a global statement that identifies the subject matter of each discipline or field of study (Fawcett, 2005b). The metaparadigm of nursing identifies human beings, the environment, health, and nursing as the subject matter of interest to nurses. The distinctive focus of the discipline of nursing is on nursing actions and processes directed toward human beings that take into account the environment in which human beings reside and in which nursing practice occurs.

We have already defined research. Based on that definition and the metaparadigm of nursing, we offer this definition of nursing research:

- Nursing research is a formal, systematic, and rigorous process of inquiry used to generate and test theories about the health-related experiences of human beings within their environments and about the actions and processes that nurses use in practice.

WHY CONDUCT RESEARCH?

We believe that one of the most compelling reasons to conduct research is to develop theories. Sometimes research is conducted to generate theories, while at other times research is conducted to test theories.

Basic, Applied, and Clinical Research

Research designed to generate or test theories is considered **basic research**. Tests of the limits of the applicability of theories in different situations with diverse populations are considered **applied research** (Donaldson & Crowley, 1978). Tests of theories about the effectiveness of interventions are considered **clinical research** (Donaldson & Crowley).

Research and Theory Development

The product of research is always theory. In Box 1–1, we deliberately use equal signs (=) to signify the equivalence of the terms. Thus, we believe that research does not lead to theory development but rather that research is the process of theory development. Similarly, theory does not lead to evidence but instead is the evidence. And practice does not lead to research, but rather practice and research are the same process. Appreciating the equivalence of practice and research highlights the practicing nurse's ability to be a "knowledge producer" as well as a "knowledge consumer or user" (Reed, 2006, p. 36).

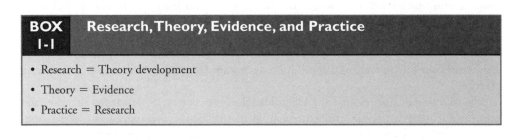

BOX 1-1	Research, Theory, Evidence, and Practice

- Research = Theory development
- Theory = Evidence
- Practice = Research

Theories as Evidence

Theories can be thought of as **evidence** (see Box 1–1), which is something that serves as proof (OED, 2005). When theories are used as evidence, the "proof" should be considered tentative or uncertain, because no theory is absolutely true and actually may be false (Popper, 1965). In other words, a theory can never be proved to be true, so it should never be considered final or absolute. It is always possible that additional tests of the theory will yield findings that would contradict it or that other theories will provide a better fit with the data (Hoyle, Harris, & Judd, 2002). In nursing, evidence in the form of theory is used to guide practice.

Practice and Research

When theories are thought of as evidence, it becomes clear that the evidence needed for practice actually is theory (Walker & Avant, 2005). It may not be surprising, therefore, to learn that practice and research are essentially the same process (see Box 1–1). This means that the nursing practice process and the nursing research process involve the same critical thinking skills and actions. When professional practice is as rigorous and systematic as we expect research to be, the nursing practice process "mirrors" the nursing research process (Cipriano, 2007, p. 27). In each process, a problem is identified and then a plan is developed, implemented, and evaluated.

As can be seen in Table 1–1, the results of assessment of a person's health-related experiences can be considered the statement of the research problem—that is, the purpose of the research. Sometimes, the results of the assessment are summarized with a label or diagnosis that specifies a health-related experience and influencing factors. The label or diagnosis used in practice becomes a more elaborate statement of the problem in research. Planning in nursing practice, or developing a plan of care for a person, a family, or a community, is the same as identification of the methods for research. Implementation in practice comprises the nursing interventions; in research, implementation refers to the actual conduct of research, including recruiting research participants and collecting and analyzing data. Evaluation in practice can be considered the same as the interpretation of research results. Written or computerized documentation of each step of the nursing process in practice is equivalent to the research report.

Table 1–1 The Parallel Between the Nursing Practice Process and the Nursing Research Process	
NURSING PRACTICE PROCESS	**NURSING RESEARCH PROCESS**
Assessment	Statement of the problem
Planning	Research methods
Implementation	Conduct of the research
Evaluation	Interpretation of results
Documentation	Research report

Adapted from Fawcett, J. (2005). *Contemporary nursing knowledge: Analysis and evaluation of nursing models and theories* (2nd ed., p. 595). Philadelphia: F. A. Davis, with permission.

WHAT IS EVIDENCE-BASED NURSING PRACTICE?

In recent years, a great deal of attention has been paid to the need to base practice on evidence. The term **evidence-based nursing practice** refers to the use of evidence to guide nursing practice. Some discussions of evidence-based nursing practice reflect an atheoretical, biomedically dominated, empirical perspective in which the randomized clinical trial—a very rigorous type of experimental research—is the only legitimate source of evidence. Along with Fawcett and colleagues (2001) and Ingersoll (2000), we believe that such a narrow viewpoint detracts from thinking about theories as the evidence for practice. A broader viewpoint, but one that does not explicitly include theory, was given by Pearson, Wiechula, Court, and Lockwood (2007), who are associated with the Joanna Briggs Institute, an Australian organization devoted to advancement of evidence-based nursing care. They stated, "The Joanna Briggs Institute (JBI) model of evidence-based healthcare conceptualizes evidence-based practice as clinical decision-making that considers the best available evidence, the context in which the care is delivered, client preference, and the professional judgment of the health professional" (p. 85). Similarly, Porter-O'Grady (2006) defined evidence-based practice as "simply the integration of the best possible research . . . evidence with clinical expertise and with patient needs" (p. 1).

The definitions of evidence-based practice given here highlight theory as central. These definitions assert that evidence-based practice is:

- "Conscientious, explicit, and judicious use of theory-derived, research-based information in making decisions about care delivery to individuals or groups of patients and in consideration of individual needs and preferences" (Ingersoll, 2000, p. 152)
- "Conscious and intentful use of research- and theory-based information to make decisions about patient care delivery" (Macnee, 2004, p. 5)
- "Explicit and judicious decision making about health care delivery for individuals or groups of patients based on the consensus of the most relevant and supported evidence derived from theory-derived research and data-based information to respond to consumers' preferences and societal expectations" (Driever, 2002, p. 593)

Our definition of evidence-based nursing practice draws from those definitions, as well as from our emphasis on research as theory development, theory as evidence, and practice as research (see Box 1–1).

- Evidence-based nursing practice is the deliberate and critical use of theories about human beings' health-related experiences to guide actions associated with each step of the nursing process.

At times, evidence-based practice is equated with **research utilization** (Hasseler, 2006), which has been the focus of a great deal of literature and many projects during the past 30 years. At other times, evidence-based practice is regarded as different from or broader than research utilization. Stetler (2001b) viewed evidence-based practice and research utilization as different but acknowledged that the connection between them "is somewhat murky in the literature" (p. 272). She pointed out that research utilization "provides the requisite preparatory steps for research-related actions that, when implemented and sustained, result in [evidence-based practice]" (p. 272). Polit and Beck (2006) regard evidence-based practice as broader than research utilization, claiming that evidence-based practice involves basing nursing care decisions on the best available evidence, whereas research utilization involves the translation of the results of research into the real world of practice. Brown (1999) referred to "research-based practice," which can be thought of as a bridge between research utilization and evidence-based practice. She defined research-based practice as "healthcare practitioners' use of research findings and collective research evidence to shape general approaches to care, specific courses of action, and recommendations made to individual patients" (p. 4). In this book, we focus on evidence-based practice.

WHAT ARE THE SOURCES OF KNOWLEDGE USED AS EVIDENCE FOR PRACTICE?

We believe that theory is the very best source of knowledge used as evidence for nursing practice. We acknowledge, however, that other sources of knowledge exist and sometimes are evidence for practice. For example, knowledge that serves as evidence for practice may come from medical record data, quality improvement and infection control reports, healthcare professionals' clinical expertise and judgment, and patient preferences based on values and culture (Driever, 2002; Macnee & McCabe, 2008; Pearson et al., 2007).

Other sources of knowledge are various methods of knowing. The philosopher Charles Sanders Peirce (1839–1914) identified **four methods of knowing**—tenacity, authority, *a priori*, and science—as sources of knowledge that sometimes are used as evidence for practice (Cohen & Nagel, 1934; Kerlinger & Lee, 2000). We have substituted "theory" for "science" because "[t]he basic aim of science is theory" (Kerlinger & Lee, p. 11). Understanding the meaning and the limitations of each method of knowing can help increase our commitment to develop the theories that are needed to guide nursing practice (Table 1–2).

Tenacity

One method of knowing is **tenacity**, which has also been called **tradition** (Dzurec, 1998; Polit & Beck, 2006). Tenacity refers to persistent, unsubstantiated, personal opinions about things in the world. Tenacious opinions are those that people believe to be true because they know that they are true on the basis of their always having known that they are true (Kerlinger & Lee, 2000). In practice, tenacity guides us to do certain things in a certain way just because we have always done them that way. Tenacity is evident in the many habits, rituals, and customs we find in practice. For example, it is customary to bathe a patient from head to toe.

A major limitation of tenacity is that any opinion that contradicts the tenaciously held opinion is ignored as unworthy of attention or regarded as disloyal. Another limitation is that there is no way for a person to decide which one of various conflicting opinions might be best. Still another limitation is that reliance on tenacity as evidence "sometimes [leads] to unanticipated outcomes" that may be harmful (Thompson, McCaughan, Cullum, Sheldon, & Reynor, 2005, p. 438).

Authority

Another method of knowing is **authority**. This method, which is similar to faith, involves appeal to a highly respected source—the authority—for evidence. The authority might be a

Table 1–2	Description and Limitations of Four Methods of Knowing Used as Evidence	
DESCRIPTION	**LIMITATIONS**
Tenacity	
"We've always done it that way; it's the custom."	Ignores contradictory evidence and opinions.
"It's the traditional way to do it here."	There is no way to decide between conflicting opinions.
	There are unanticipated negative outcomes.
Authority	
"The textbook tells us to do it that way."	Authoritative sources are not infallible.
"My teacher told me to do it this way."	There is no way to decide which authoritative source is correct.
A Priori	
"It seems reasonable."	One person's idea of reasonable is not the same as another's.
	There is no way to decide whether reasonableness depends on the current way of thinking or previous education.
Theory	
"The theory guides me to do it."	Must be developed through rigorous inquiry.
	Theories can be false.

book, a journal article, a governmental agency, or a person who is considered an expert. The words written in the book, article, or agency report or uttered by the person are accepted as the truth because the book, article, report, or person is highly respected. Authority is evident in the laws, rules, and procedures of daily life and practice. Authority, in the form of the opinions of people regarded by their peers as experts, also is evident in organizational or national standards for practice that are not based on theory (Panfil & Wurster, as cited in Hasseler, 2006).

Use of authority as evidence may be justified because authorities may be correct or because people do not have the time or adequate knowledge and skills to find the evidence themselves. Reliance on authoritative sources may, however, ignore the potential fallibility of written or spoken words. For example, errors may be found in a textbook; a teacher may present evidence that has been discredited by new research results; or a nurse manager may hold atheoretical opinions. And because some authorities sometimes rely on other persons who also are thought to be authorities or on their own tenacious opinions, their words cannot always be regarded as accurate evidence. A teacher, for example, may not notice an error on a particular page in a textbook before referring students to that page.

A Priori

Still another method of knowing is *a priori*—that is, "the use of reason alone, without experimental evidence" (Payton, 1994, p. 11). This method, which is also referred to as **intuition** or **common sense**, involves reliance on the obviously true or self-evident nature of the evidence. The evidence may agree with reason, although it may not agree with experience. The *a priori* method often involves trial and error or "isolated and unsystematic clinical experiences" (Stetler, 2001a, p. 186) that are never formalized as procedures, although a procedure that seems to be effective may be passed from one practitioner to others. For example, one nurse may tell other nurses that all patients experience good outcomes when they walk a short distance on the first postoperative day.

A limitation of the *a priori* method is that what one person regards as reasonable may not be the same as what another person regards as reasonable. Another limitation is that the self-evident nature of something may reflect a way of thinking that is popular at a particular time or that was learned at an earlier time.

Theory

The best method of knowing used for evidence is **theory**. Others have identified science or research, which is the method of science, as the best way to acquire evidence in the form of theory because it is much more reliable and self-corrective than the tenacity, authority, and *a priori* methods (Cohen & Nagel, 1934; Kerlinger & Lee, 2000). We agree with Polit and Beck (2006) that research "is the most sophisticated method of acquiring evidence that humans have developed" (p. 13). Research can be regarded as sophisticated because it requires the researcher to consider alternatives. Researchers, as Cohen and Nagel pointed out, are "never too certain about [their] results" (p. 195). Consequently, as the product of research, theory is not regarded as the truth but rather as the best currently available evidence. A theory that represents the best available evidence may, for example, indicate that words of encouragement from nurses and family members hasten patients' recovery from surgery.

A limitation of theory as evidence is that it must be developed through careful and systematic research, which typically takes a long time. Thus, a theory may not yet be available to guide a particular practice action. Another limitation is that a theory may be false (Popper, 1965). The geocentric theory, which asserts that the planet Earth is the center of our solar system, is an example of a theory about the physical world that currently is regarded as false.

WHAT TYPES OF THEORIES ARE USED AS EVIDENCE FOR NURSING PRACTICE?

Many nursing actions are very complex and "are based to a very large degree on interaction, communication, and human care, [which] cannot be measured at all, nor can they be standardized or shown to be effective" (Hasseler, 2006, p. 227). Nursing actions may also be based on "clinical expertise, patient choices, and critical evaluation of the literature" (Cumulative

Index of Nursing and Allied Health Literature, 2005). Consequently, our thinking about theory as evidence for evidence-based nursing practice has to account for all of the complex human care actions performed by nurses.

Five types of theories can be used as evidence for evidence-based nursing practice—empirical, aesthetic, ethical, personal knowing, and sociopolitical (Carper, 1978; Chinn & Kramer, 2004; White, 1995). Each type of theory is developed by means of a different type of inquiry, and each is a different type of evidence.

Empirical Theories

Empirical nursing theories are publicly verifiable factual descriptions, explanations, or predictions based on subjective or objective data about groups of people. The data used for empirical theories are summarized as group averages. Empirical theories make up the science of nursing (Table 1–3).

Chinn and Kramer (2004, p. 10) identified two critical questions that are answered by empirical theories:

- "What is this?"
- "How does it work?"

We add two other questions that are answered by empirical theories:

- How do I know what my own best practices are?
- How do I know how to get desired outcomes?

Three types of empirical theories are used as evidence for nursing practice—descriptive theories, explanatory theories, and predictive theories. Each type of empirical theory is developed by means of a particular type of **empirical research** (see Table 1–3).

Descriptive Nursing Theories

Descriptive nursing theories are detailed descriptions of people's health-related experiences; they are developed by means of **descriptive research**. Descriptive theories are the evidence needed to develop tools that nurses can use to assess people's health-related experiences. A theory about the concept of empathy, called the Theory of Personal System Empathy, is an example of a descriptive nursing theory (Alligood & May, 2000). This theory is a description of what nurses do when they feel empathy for a patient. Specifically, the theory "proposes that empathy organizes perceptions; facilitates awareness of self and others; increases sensitivity; promotes shared respect, mutual goals, and social awareness; cultivates understanding of individuals within a historical and social context; and affects learning" (p. 243). This theory is the evidence needed for development of a nursing practice tool to assess nurses' empathy for patients.

Explanatory Nursing Theories

Explanatory nursing theories are explanations of the relation between people's health-related experiences and environmental factors that influence those experiences; they are

Table 1–3	Types of Nursing Theories and Modes of Inquiry with Examples: Empirical Theories		
TYPE OF THEORY	**DESCRIPTION**	**MODE OF INQUIRY**	**EXAMPLES**
Empirical theories The science of nursing	Publicly verifiable factual descriptions, explanations, or predictions based on subjective or objective group data	Empirical research	Scientific data
Descriptive theories	Descriptions of people and situations	Descriptive research	Descriptions of people's health experiences
Explanatory theories	Explanations of environmental factors that influence people and situations	Correlational research	Explanations of factors that influence health experiences
Predictive theories	Predictions about the effects of some actions or processes on people and situations	Experimental research	Outcomes of nursing interventions

Adapted from Fawcett, J., Watson, J., Neuman, B., Hinton-Walker, P., & Fitzpatrick, J. J. (2001). On theories and evidence. *Journal of Nursing Scholarship*, 33, 115–119, with permission.

developed by means of **correlational research**. Explanatory theories are the evidence nurses need to link assessments of health-related experiences with assessments of environmental factors and to understand which environmental factors influence which aspects of health-related experiences. The Theory of Chronic Pain is an example of an explanatory nursing theory (Tsai, Tak, Moore, & Palencia, 2003). The theory indicates that pain, disability, and social support are related to daily stress and that daily stress is related to depression in older individuals with arthritis. This theory is the evidence needed to link assessments of pain, disability, and social support with assessment of daily stress and assessment of daily stress with assessment of depression in older people who have arthritis.

Predictive Nursing Theories

Predictive nursing theories are predictions about the effects of some nursing intervention on people's health-related experiences; they are developed by means of **experimental research**.

Predictive theories are the evidence needed to link nursing interventions to outcomes experienced by people with diverse health conditions. The Theory of Dependent Care is an example of a predictive nursing theory (Arndt & Horodynski, 2004). This theory predicts that group and individual education for parents about child development, feeding, food, nutrition, and parent mealtime practices will result in toddlers' self-regulation of feeding and mealtime interactions. The theory is the evidence needed for the development of group and individual educational programs for parents that are targeted to toddlers' feeding behaviors and interactions during meals.

Knowledge progresses from descriptive theories developed by means of descriptive research to explanatory theories developed by means of correlational research to predictive theories developed by means of experimental research. Although researchers sometimes are tempted to omit the crucial steps of descriptive and explanatory theory development in their haste to test predictive theories of the effects of interventions, we agree with Lobo (2005) that "[w]e must value and support the descriptive research that helps us understand individuals, families, and groups of people with specific needs. . . . We must encourage the logical development of nursing knowledge, starting with descriptive, foundational research that must be completed before specific interventions can be developed and tested" by means of experimental research (p. 6).

Aesthetic Nursing Theories

Aesthetic nursing theories focus on individuals, rather than groups. They emphasize the nurse's perception of what is significant in an individual's behavior. This type of theory highlights the nurse's ability to know what is happening to a particular patient in a subjective, intuitive way, without relying on objective information, such as vital signs. Aesthetic theories also address the "artful" performance of manual and technical skills. They make up the art of nursing (Table 1–4).

Chinn and Kramer (2004, p. 10) identified two critical questions that are answered by aesthetic theories:

- What does this mean?"
- "How is this significant?"

We add one other question:

- How do I know what each individual needs?

Aesthetic theories are developed by means of envisioning the possibilities about nursing practice with each individual and rehearsing the art and acts of nursing, with emphasis on developing an appreciation of aesthetic meanings in practice and inspiration for the development of the art of nursing. This type of theory is expressed in philosophical essays about nursing as an art, in aesthetic criticism of the performance of the art of nursing through manual and technical skills, and in works of art, such as paintings, drawings, sculpture, poetry, fiction and nonfiction, music, acting, and dance. An example of an aesthetic nursing theory is the Theory of Nursing Art (Chinn, 2001). This theory "offers a conceptual definition of the art of nursing—explanations as to how nursing art evolves as a distinct aspect of nursing practice and explanations of artistic validity in nursing" (p. 287). Chinn emphasized that the theory is

Table 1–4 Types of Nursing Theories and Modes of Inquiry with Examples: Aesthetic Theories			
TYPE OF THEORY	**DESCRIPTION**	**MODE OF INQUIRY**	**EXAMPLES**
Aesthetic theories The art and act of nursing	Expressions of the nurse's perception of what is significant in the individual patient's behavior	Envisioning the possibilities of practice with an individual	Philosophical essays Works of art
	Performance of nursing actions in an artful manner	Rehearsing nursing art and acts and observing or performing nursing art	Aesthetic criticism

Adapted from Fawcett, J., Watson, J., Neuman, B., Hinton-Walker, P., & Fitzpatrick, J. J. (2001). On theories and evidence. *Journal of Nursing Scholarship*, 33, 115–119, with permission.

not empirical and therefore "is not intended to be subjected to empirical testing but rather to be considered from a logical, philosophic, and aesthetic perspective" (p. 287). Another example of an aesthetic nursing theory is Masson's (2001) poem about her experiences with a sister who had breast cancer.

Ethical Theories

Ethical nursing theories, which are descriptions of obligations, values, and desired outcomes, also are used for practice. This type of theory is made up of concepts and propositions about nurses' personal beliefs and values and the collective values of the professional discipline of nursing. Ethical theories make up the ethics of nursing (Table 1–5).

Chinn and Kramer (2004, p. 10) identified two critical questions that are answered by ethical theories:

- "Is this right?"
- "Is this responsible?"

We add two other questions:

- How do I know what I *should* do?
- How do I know what the *right* things to do are?

Ethical theories are developed by means of ethical inquiries that focus on identification and analysis of the beliefs and values held by individuals and groups, dialogue about and

Table 1–5	Types of Nursing Theories and Modes of Inquiry with Examples: Ethical Theories		
TYPE OF THEORY	**DESCRIPTION**	**MODE OF INQUIRY**	**EXAMPLES**
Ethical theories The ethics of nursing	Descriptions of moral obligations, moral and non-moral values, and desired ends	Identification, analy-sis, and clarifica-tion of beliefs and values Dialogue about and justification of beliefs and values	Standards of practice Codes of ethics Philosophies of nursing

Adapted from Fawcett, J., Watson, J., Neuman, B., Hinton-Walker, P., & Fitzpatrick, J. J. (2001). On theories and evidence. *Journal of Nursing Scholarship, 33*, 115–119, with permission.

clarification of beliefs and values, and establishment of justification for beliefs and values. Sometimes, ethical inquiry and empirical research overlap. As Chinn and Kramer (2004) pointed out, descriptive ethics is an empirical endeavor, in that people are asked about their beliefs and values.

Codes of ethics, standards of practice, and philosophical essays about how nurses should behave can be considered ethical theories. An example is the American Nurses' Association (ANA) (2001) Code of Ethics. The Code of Ethics is a statement of professional goals and values that guide nurses' conduct (ANA's Code of Ethics Project Task Force, 2000).

Theories of Personal Knowing

Nursing theories of personal knowing are another type of theory used as evidence for prac-tice. This type of theory is concerned with the nurse's knowing, encountering, and actualizing the authentic self. This means that personal knowing theories focus on how each nurse knows how to be authentic in relationships with patients—that is, how he or she knows how to express concern and caring for another human being. Personal knowing is not "knowing one's self," but rather knowing how to be authentic with others, what can be thought of as know-ing one's own personal style of being with another person. Personal knowing is what we mean when we talk about therapeutic nurse/patient relationships and when we discuss the quality and authenticity of the interpersonal process between each nurse and each patient. Personal knowing theories are the interpersonal relationships of nursing (Table 1–6).

Chinn and Kramer (2004, p. 10) identified two critical questions that are answered by per-sonal knowing theories:

- "Do I know what I do?"
- "Do I do what I know?"

Table 1–6	Types of Nursing Theories and Modes of Inquiry with Examples: Theories of Personal Knowing		
TYPE OF THEORY	**DESCRIPTION**	**MODE OF INQUIRY**	**EXAMPLES**
Theories of personal knowledge The interpersonal relationships of nursing	Expressions of the quality and authenticity of the interpersonal process between each nurse and each patient	Opening, centering, thinking, listening, and reflecting	Essays Nurses' autobiographical stories

Adapted from Fawcett, J., Watson, J., Neuman, B., Hinton-Walker, P., & Fitzpatrick, J. J. (2001). On theories and evidence. *Journal of Nursing Scholarship,* 33, 115–119, with permission.

We add two other questions:

- How do I know how to be with people who come to me for nursing?
- How do I know how to be therapeutic?

Personal knowing theories are developed as nurses open and center themselves in their work with patients, as they think about how they are or can be authentic, and as they listen to responses from others and reflect on those responses. This type of theory requires the nurse to draw on "personal qualities . . . [such as] self-awareness, sensitivity, warmth, and a positive non-blaming attitude" to develop effective and authentic relationships with patients (Hewitt & Coffey, 2005, p. 563). Theories of personal knowing are found in nurses' autobiographical stories about the genuine, authentic self, as well as in essays about personal knowing. Diers' (2005) description of her work as a nurse is an example of a nursing theory of personal knowing presented as a short autobiographical story. Meisenhelder's (2006) discussion of personal knowledge of spirituality is an example of a personal knowing nursing theory presented as an essay. The theory proposes that nurses' personal self-knowledge of spirituality is required to address patients' spiritual needs.

Sociopolitical Theories

Sociopolitical nursing theories help nurses to understand the context of nursing practice and facilitate acceptance of multiple perspectives of a situation. This type of theory provides the context or cultural location for nurse/patient interactions and the broader context in which nursing and health care take place. They focus on exposing and exploring alternate constructions of reality (Table 1–7).

The question we think is relevant for sociopolitical knowing is:

- How do I know what is "real" in practice situations?

Sociopolitical theories are generated and tested by means of critiques of situations and of alternate constructions of reality, as well as by hearing and attending to the voices of all who are concerned with a particular situation, the stakeholders. Henderson (2005) pointed out that a combination of methods, including description of "the 'stage' upon which practice occurs, . . . shared implicit meanings within an interaction, . . . and . . . beliefs and values ascribed to symbolic acts and objects inherent in the hospital" or other health-care organization, can be used to describe the context of health care (p. 555). This type of theory is found in documents and statements that indicate that the many voices involved in nursing practice are heard and acknowledged. For example, a sociopolitical theory is evident in Browne's (2001) discussion of the influence of liberal political ideology on nursing science. Browne proposed that the development of empirical nursing theories is strongly influenced by the beliefs and values of liberal political philosophy, including individualism, egalitarianism, individual freedom and tolerance, neutrality, and a free-market economy. Her theory is a critique of nursing's "implicit political allegiances" and the implications of those allegiances on nursing knowledge development that "help us to understand whether our science disrupts or inadvertently helps to maintain social inequities" (Browne, p. 129). Daiski's (2004) response to Browne brings other viewpoints and voices to our attention. She cited Carper's (1978) and White's (1995) contributions to our understanding of nonempirical nursing theories, as well as Silva and Rothbart's (1984) discussion of historicism as a strong influence on nursing theory development. Historicism, Daiski explained, is "concerned with whole persons and their experiences . . . [and acknowledges] multiple realities" (p. 117). Browne (2004) later acknowledged that "a diversity of paradigms, theories and perspectives are required to inform knowledge development in nursing" (p. 123). She also pointed out, "Studies of health and illness are not neutral scholarly activities; they are loaded with social, political and economic consequences for individuals and society" (p. 123).

Table 1–7	Types of Nursing Theories and Modes of Inquiry with Examples: Sociopolitical Theories		
TYPE OF THEORY	**DESCRIPTION**	**MODE OF INQUIRY**	**EXAMPLES**
Sociopolitical theories The politics and policies of nursing	Descriptions and expressions of the context or cultural location for nurse/patient interactions and the broader context in which nursing and health care take place	Critique of situations Critique of alternate constructions of reality Hearing and attending to all relevant views	Written or oral criticism Written or oral criticism Written or oral documentation of voices heard and acknowledged

Adapted from Fawcett, J., Watson, J., Neuman, B., Hinton-Walker, P., & Fitzpatrick, J. J. (2001). On theories and evidence. *Journal of Nursing Scholarship, 33,* 115–119, with permission.

HOW ARE NURSING THEORIES USED IN NURSING PRACTICE?

Nursing's distinctive body of knowledge includes empirical, aesthetic, ethical, personal knowing, and sociopolitical theories. Each type of theory is an essential component of the integrated knowledge base for evidence-based nursing practice, so no one type of theory should be used in isolation from the others. As Carper (1978) pointed out, "Nursing [practice] depends on the scientific knowledge of human behavior in health and in illness, the aesthetic perception of significant human experiences, a personal understanding of the unique individuality of the self and the capacity to make choices within concrete situations involving particular moral judgments" (p. 22). White (1995) added that sociopolitical theories are "essential to an understanding of all the [other types of theories]" (p. 83). Furthermore, Hallberg (2003) mentioned the need for theories about clinical expertise and patient choices, as well as empirical theories, for evidence-based nursing practice. Aesthetic theories and theories of personal knowing address clinical expertise, and ethical and sociopolitical theories address patient choices.

No one type of theory should be regarded as superior or inferior to another. Rather, each type of theory is useful for understanding particular aspects of nursing practice. When nurses integrate specific empirical, aesthetic, ethical, personal knowing, and sociopolitical theories, they combine them to form a new, interactive, and unified base of knowledge for practice (Westra & Rodgers, 1991). Nurses then use the unified knowledge to help people attain their health-related goals. An example of the integration of multiple types of theories is Schwartz's (2001) commentary about the presence of family members when a patient is receiving invasive procedures or is being resuscitated. Pointing out that nurses frequently know when a patient's family members should be present and when they should not be present, Schwartz stated, "Nursing will always entail the balance of art [aesthetic theory] and science [empirical theory]" (p. 11), as well as ethical, personal knowing, and sociopolitical theories.

Another example is Andrews and Waterman's (2005) description of the knowledge nurses use to report patients' physiological deterioration to physicians. They developed an Early Warning Score (EWS), which "packages" the nurse's objective (empirical) and subjective (aesthetic, ethical, personal, and sociopolitical) knowledge about a patient's deteriorating physiological condition. The EWS "gives nurses a precise, concise, and unambiguous means of communicating deterioration" (p. 473) to physicians.

Conclusion

In this chapter, you have learned how research, theory, evidence, and evidence-based practice are defined. You also have learned why research is conducted and the links between research and theory and theory and evidence, as well as the link between the nursing practice process and the nursing research process. And you have learned about various sources of knowledge used as evidence for practice, various types of theories, and the type of evidence that each source of evidence and each type of theory provides.

The remainder of this book focuses on how empirical research provides the evidence needed for evidence-based nursing practice. Although we recognize and value the contributions of all

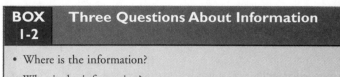

BOX 1-2   Three Questions About Information

- Where is the information?
- What is the information?
- How good is the information?

five types of theories—empirical, aesthetic, ethical, personal knowing, and sociopolitical—as evidence, we will focus on empirical theories and empirical research throughout the rest of the book.

Three questions about information contained in published research reports provide the organizing framework for the remaining chapters in this book (Box 1–2).

You will be able to answer the question, "Where is the information?" when you learn how to identify where in research reports you can find each component of conceptual-theoretical-empirical (C-T-E) structures for research. We introduce C-T-E structures in Chapter 2 and discuss where to find the information about each of the components in research reports in Chapter 3. We then discuss each component in detail in Chapters 5 through 15.

You will be able to answer the question, "What is the information?" when you learn how to identify what the information is. In Chapter 3, we explain not only where to find the information but also what information is contained in each section of a research report. We discuss that information in much more detail in subsequent chapters.

Finally, you will be able to answer the question, "How good is the information?" when you learn how to determine whether the information meets certain criteria. We identify those criteria in Chapter 4 and discuss them in more detail in Chapters 5 through 15.

References

Full citations for all references cited in this chapter are provided in the Reference section at the end of the book.

Learning Activities

Activities to supplement what you have learned in this chapter, along with practice examination questions, are provided on the CD that comes with this book.

Chapter 2

Conceptual-Theoretical-Empirical Structures for Research

Recall from Chapter 1 that we define research as a formal, systematic, and rigorous process of inquiry used to generate and test theories. Also recall that we pointed out that theories are the best source of evidence for practice, and we identified five types of theories—empirical, aesthetic, ethical, personal knowing, and sociopolitical. Each of these types of theories provides a different type of evidence for nursing practice. Although we place equal value on each type of theory, in this and all remaining chapters of this book, we will focus on the contents of reports of completed empirical research that was designed either to generate or to test empirical theories.

We believe that empirical research is always based on a conceptual model, always focuses on generation or testing of an empirical theory, and is always conducted using empirical methods. Accordingly, in this chapter, you will learn about the three components of conceptual-theoretical-empirical (C-T-E) structures for empirical research. Specifically, you will learn about the conceptual model (C) on which the research is based, the middle-range theory (T) that is generated or tested, and the empirical research methods (E) that are used to conduct the research. We start by providing a definition for each component of a C-T-E structure and a description of its function. Then, we describe two types of C-T-E structures—one for theory-generating research and another for theory-testing research.

KEYWORDS

Category

Conceptual Model

Conceptual-Theoretical-Empirical
(C-T-E) Structures

Constitutive Definition

Control Treatment

Data Analysis Techniques

Dependent Variable

Empirical Indicators

Empirical Research Methods

Experimental Conditions

Experimental Treatment

Grand Theory

Hypothesis

Independent Variable

Middle-Range Theory

Operational Definition

Relational Propositions

Research Design

Research Focus Guidelines

Research Instruments

Research Methods Guidelines

Research Procedures

Sample

Theme

Theory

Theory-Generating Research

Theory-Testing Research

Variable

WHAT ARE CONCEPTUAL-THEORETICAL-EMPIRICAL STRUCTURES?

Reports of empirical research *should* always include information about the three components that make up **conceptual-theoretical-empirical (C-T-E) structures** for research—the **conceptual model (C)**, the **theory (T)**, and the **empirical research methods (E)** (Box 2–1). We acknowledge, however, that all three components of C-T-E structures for research are not found in all research reports. Many reports do not include any content about the conceptual model on which the research was based. Similarly, many reports do not include a name or label for the theory that was generated or tested. However, virtually all research reports include content about the empirical methods used to conduct the research. In later chapters we will explain where to find and evaluate the C (conceptual model), T (middle-range theory), and E (empirical research methods) components of a C-T-E structure if they are not explicitly identified or given in the research report.

BOX 2-1	Three Components of C-T-E Structures for Research
• C = conceptual model • T = theory • E = empirical research methods	

WHAT IS A CONCEPTUAL MODEL?

The C component of a C-T-E structure for research is the **conceptual model**, which also may be referred to as a conceptual framework, a conceptual system, or a paradigm. Sometimes, the conceptual model is inaccurately referred to as the theory or the theoretical framework. It is inaccurate to refer to a conceptual model as a theory or a theoretical framework because conceptual models and theories are not the same. A conceptual model is a relatively broad—or abstract and general—kind of knowledge that is much less concrete and specific than a theory. Our definition of a conceptual model indicates that it is the most abstract and general component of a C-T-E structure.

- A conceptual model . . . is a set of relatively abstract and general concepts that address the [things that are] of central interest to a discipline, the propositions that broadly describe those concepts, and the propositions that state relatively abstract and general [associations] between two or more of the concepts. (Fawcett, 2005b, p. 16)

Recall from Chapter 1 that a **concept** is a word or phrase that summarizes some idea, and that a **proposition** is a statement about one concept or about the association between two or more concepts. Propositions that are statements about a single concept are called **constitutive definitions**. Sometimes referred to as a **theoretical definition**, a constitutive definition is similar to a definition found in a dictionary; it describes and provides meaning for the concept. Propositions that are statements about two or more concepts are called **relational propositions**. They assert the association between the concepts. The association may be a relation—or correlation—between concepts or the effect of one concept on another concept. Examples of concepts and propositions from two conceptual models of nursing—King's Conceptual System and Roy's Adaptation Model—are given in Box 2–2.

BOX 2-2	Examples of Conceptual Model Concepts and Propositions

King's Conceptual System

• One concept of this conceptual model is personal system.

• A proposition that broadly describes this concept is: A personal system is defined as "a unified, complex whole self who perceives, thinks, desires, imagines, decides, identifies goals, and selects means to achieve them" (King, 1981, p. 27). This proposition is a constitutive definition.

• A proposition that states the association between a personal and an interpersonal system, which is another concept of King's Conceptual System, is: The personal system and the interpersonal system are interrelated. This is a relational proposition that asserts the relation between the two concepts.

Roy's Adaptation Model

• One concept of Roy's conceptual model is stimuli.

• A proposition that broadly describes that concept is: Stimuli are defined as environmental factors that "provoke a response" (Roy & Andrews, 1999, p. 32). This proposition is a constitutive definition.

• A proposition that states the association between stimuli and coping processes, which is another concept of Roy's Adaptation Model, is: Stimuli affect coping processes. This is a relational proposition that asserts the effect of one concept on another.

Conceptual Models and Research

We believe that a conceptual model is always the starting point for research. The relatively abstract and general concepts and propositions that make up a conceptual model, however, cannot be directly tested. The function of the C component of C-T-E structures is to guide research by providing a distinctive frame of reference, "a horizon of expectations" (Popper, 1965, p. 47), or a broad lens through which to view the research.

The conceptual model (C) acts as an umbrella for the theory (T) and the empirical research methods (E) components of the C-T-E structure. It helps the researcher to "ask the right questions" (Glanz, 2002, p. 556) when beginning a research project. More specifically, the conceptual model helps the researcher to determine "what should be studied, what questions should be asked, how they should be asked, and what rules should be followed in interpreting the answers obtained" (Ritzer, 1980, p. 7).

The content of conceptual models is obvious in the **research guidelines** that are associated with each one. Seven general guidelines for research, which were adapted by Fawcett (2005b) from earlier works by Laudan (1981) and Schlotfeldt (1975), are listed here. Specific guidelines associated with several conceptual models of nursing are given in Chapter 5. The seven general guidelines identify:

1. The purposes of the research
2. The health-related experiences to be studied
3. The nature of problems to be studied
4. The nature of contributions that the research will make to the advancement of nursing knowledge
5. The source of data and the settings in which data are to be gathered
6. The research designs, instruments, and data collection procedures to be used
7. The methods to be used to analyze the data

Guidelines 1, 2, 3, and 4 provide a focus for research within the context of each conceptual model; they are called **research focus guidelines**. Guidelines 5, 6, and 7 specify methods to be used when conducting research within the context of each conceptual model; they are called **research methods guidelines**.

WHAT IS A THEORY?

The T component of a C-T-E structure for research is the **theory**, which also may be referred to as a theoretical framework. Recall from Chapter 1 that we defined a theory as one or more relatively concrete and specific concepts, the propositions that narrowly describe those concepts, and the propositions that state relatively concrete and specific associations between two or more of the concepts. Here, we provide a slightly more elaborate definition of theory that reflects the close connection between theories and conceptual models.

• A theory is defined as one or more relatively concrete and specific concepts that are derived from a conceptual model, the propositions that narrowly describe those concepts, and the propositions that state relatively concrete and specific [associations] between two or more of the concepts. (Fawcett, 2005b, p. 18)

We already defined concepts and propositions earlier in this chapter and in Chapter 1. The only difference between conceptual model concepts and propositions and theory concepts and propositions is the level of abstraction—theory concepts and propositions are less abstract than conceptual model concepts and propositions. Box 2–3 gives examples of concepts and propositions from the Theory of Goal Attainment, which was derived from King's Conceptual System, and from the Theory of Adaptation During Childbearing, which was derived from Roy's Adaptation Model.

Middle-Range Theories

Both of the theories mentioned in Box 2–3 are **middle-range theories**, the kind of theory that is the T component of C-T-E structures. The idea of middle-range theory was put forth by Merton (1968), who called for increased emphasis on the development of theories of the middle range. Merton pointed out that middle-range theories are narrower in scope than

BOX 2-3	Examples of Theory Concepts and Propositions

Theory of Goal Attainment (King, 1981)

• Derived from King's Conceptual System

• One concept is perception.

• A proposition that narrowly defines perception is "each person's representation of reality . . . an awareness of persons, objects, and events" (King, 1981, p. 146). This proposition is a constitutive definition.

• A proposition that states a relation between perception and transaction, another concept of the theory, is: If perception is accurate, transactions in nurse-client interactions will occur. This is a relational proposition that asserts a relation between the two concepts.

Theory of Adaptation During Childbearing (Tulman & Fawcett, 2003)

• Derived from Roy's Adaptation Model

• One concept is functional status.

• A proposition that narrowly defines functional status is: Performance of usual household, social and community, personal care, child care, occupational, and educational activities. This proposition is a constitutive definition.

• A proposition that states an association between functional status and physical symptoms, which is another concept of the theory, is: There is a negative relation between physical symptoms and functional status, such that as physical symptoms increase, functional status decreases. This is a relational proposition that asserts a relation between the two concepts.

much broader conceptual models but broader than hunches about what is observed in day-to-day life and professional practice.

A middle-range theory is regarded as a "basic, usable structure of ideas" that is "focused on a limited dimension of reality" (Smith & Liehr, 2003, pp. xi, 8). There is general agreement in the nursing literature that middle-range theories are relatively narrow in scope, are made up of fewer concepts and propositions than conceptual models, can be empirically tested, and can be applied in practice (Peterson & Bredow, 2004).

One function of the T component of C-T-E structures is to provide a more concrete and specific version of some of the conceptual model concepts and propositions. Another function is to help us to better understand previously puzzling or confusing ideas and observations (Bengtson, Acock, Allen, Dilworth-Anderson, & Klein, 2005). However, the major function of the T component is to guide research in a very specific way.

Whereas a conceptual model provides a broad frame of reference and guidelines for research, a middle-range theory is the basis for the specific aims for the research. If research is designed to generate a nursing middle-range theory, the specific aim might be to generate a theory about people's responses to or perceptions of a particular health-related experience. For example, the specific aim of Knipp's (2006) research was to generate a theory of teens' perceptions about attention deficit/hyperactivity disorder (ADHD) and medications. If research is designed to test a theory, the specific aim is to test that theory. For example, after the theory of teens' perceptions about ADHD and medications is generated, the specific aim of a study could be to test a theory of the relation between age at diagnosis and teens' perceptions about ADHD and medications, or between parental support and teens' perceptions about ADHD and medications. Middle-range theories are discussed in detail in Chapter 6.

Grand Theories

Grand theories are another kind of theory mentioned in the nursing literature. A grand theory is not as broad as a conceptual model but broader than a middle-range theory. As we will explain in Chapter 5, grand theories are sometimes used in place of conceptual models for the C component of C-T-E structures for research.

WHAT ARE THE EMPIRICAL RESEARCH METHODS?

The E component of a C-T-E structure for research—the empirical research methods—is the most concrete and specific component. Its function is to identify ways to gather information and to provide the analytical techniques needed to make sense of the information and to draw a conclusion about the theory that was generated or tested.

The information gathered and analyzed as part of theory-generating research or theory-testing research is in the form of words and numbers, which typically are referred to as **data** (see Chapter 1). Words are most frequently associated with theory-generating research, whereas numbers are most frequently associated with theory-testing research. However, both word and number data can be gathered for either type of research. An example of data that are words are the responses people give to a question such as, "How do you feel about the medications you take for attention deficit/hyperactivity disorder?" An example of data that are numbers are the responses people give to a question such as, "On a scale of 1 = very negative to 10 = very positive, how do you feel about the medications you take for attention deficit/hyperactivity disorder?"

Elements of Empirical Research Methods

Empirical research methods encompass five elements that are listed and discussed briefly here. These elements are discussed in detail in Chapters 7-12.

1. The specific research design
2. The sample
3. The instruments and experimental conditions that serve as very concrete and specific real-world substitutes, or proxies, for theory concepts
4. The procedures used to gather data and protect research participants from harm
5. The techniques used to analyze the data

Research Design

The research design is the specific way in which the research is conducted. There are three broad types of research designs—descriptive research designs, correlational research designs, and experimental research designs. Descriptive research designs are used to generate and test descriptive theories, correlational designs are used to test explanatory theories, and experimental designs are used to test predictive theories (see Table 1–3 in Chapter 1 and Table 2–1).

Table 2–1	Theory-Generating and Theory-Testing Research: Types of Middle-Range Theories and Research Designs	
TYPE OF RESEARCH	**TYPE OF MIDDLE-RANGE THEORY**	**TYPE OF RESEARCH DESIGN**
Theory generating	Descriptive theories	Descriptive research
Theory testing	Descriptive theories	Descriptive research
	Explanatory theories	Correlational research
	Predictive theories	Experimental research

Sample

The **sample** is the source of the data. Samples may be made up of people, animals, organizations, or documents. For example, Saburi, Mapanga, and Mapanga (2006) recruited a sample of 66 adults who had epilepsy to participate in the research they conducted to test their Theory of the Relation Between Perceived Family Reactions and Quality of Life. When people make up the sample, they may be referred to as research participants, study participants, subjects, informants, or respondents.

Research Instruments and Experimental Conditions

The **research instruments or experimental conditions**, which sometimes are called **empirical indicators**, specify how the data were collected. An example of an empirical indicator that is an instrument is the Quality of Life in Epilepsy-89 Patient Inventory, which Saburi et al. (2006) adapted to measure quality of life. Another example is the Perceived Family Reactions Instrument, which Saburi et al. developed to measure overprotection, secrecy, concealment, and acceptance strategies used by families and individuals to manage epilepsy. Research instruments are used for descriptive, correlational, and experimental research.

Experimental conditions, which are used only for experimental research, encompass one or more experimental treatments and one or more control treatments. An **experimental treatment** usually is a new intervention that is being tested to determine whether it is more effective than the current intervention, which is considered the **control treatment**. An example of an empirical indicator that is an experimental condition is: The experimental treatment consisted of a combination of telephone social support and education, and the control treatment consisted of education only (Coleman et al., 2005).

Research Procedures

The **research procedures**, which include an explanation of when, where, and by whom the data were collected, as well as an explanation of how research participants were protected from harm, are usually simply called the **procedures**. Saburi et al. (2006), for example, explained that the data were collected by the first author at five city health clinics in Harare, Zimbabwe, at the time of the research participants' follow-up appointments. They also indicated that the research instruments were administered orally during an interview and that a signed consent form was obtained from each participant.

Data Analysis Techniques

The **data analysis techniques** may be some method of coding data that are words or statistical procedures applied to data that are numbers. For example, Knipp (2006) used a technique called **content analysis** to analyze the word data obtained from interviews of teens with ADHD. Saburi et al. (2006) used various **statistical techniques** to analyze the number data obtained from the research participants' responses to the Quality of Life in Epilepsy-89 Patient Inventory and the Perceived Family Reactions Instrument.

The Language of Empirical Research Methods

Concepts and propositions are the special language of conceptual models and theories. When translated into the language of empirical research methods, concepts become **themes**, **categories**, **constants**, or **variables**, and propositions become **operational definitions** and **hypotheses**.

Concepts, Themes, Categories, Constants, and Variables

As previously explained, a **concept** is a word or phrase that summarizes a thing or an idea. Concepts may be referred to as themes or categories, especially when the research is theory generating. A **theme** or **category** is the label given to recurring ideas found in data that are words. For example, in her theory-generating study of family members who cared for a loved one with Alzheimer's disease, Garity (2006) identified four themes—significant interaction, role disruption, guilt, and uncertainty about the future—in the words family members used to describe their feelings after the loved one went to a nursing home. Each theme can be considered a concept.

Concepts may also be considered constants or variables, especially when the research is theory testing and the data are numbers. **Constants** are concepts that do not have any variation and therefore are considered nonvariables. Constants have only one form. When the constant is measured, there can be just one score. For example, if all research participants are female, the concept can be labeled "female," classified as a constant, and scored as "1."

Variables are concepts that have some variation and therefore have more than one form. When the variable is measured, there can be more than one score. Variables are classified as categorical or continuous. A **categorical variable** has various distinct categories of variation. For example, if some research participants are female and some are male, the concept can be labeled "gender," classified as a categorical variable, and scored as "1" for females and "2" for males. A categorical variable that can take only two scores—such as "1" and "2"—is sometimes referred to as a **dichotomous variable**. A **continuous variable** has a continuum of variation. For example, the actual age of the research participants is a concept that is classified as a continuous variable; the scores could be 20, 21, 22, 25, 27, 30, or whatever the actual age of each research participant is.

Variables are also classified as independent and dependent. The **independent variable**, typically labeled x, is a concept that influences another concept. The independent variable, then, is the presumed antecedent to or cause of another concept. The **dependent variable**, typically labeled y, is a concept that is influenced by another concept. The dependent variable therefore is the presumed consequence, effect, or outcome of another concept.

Descriptive research usually deals with only one concept. Therefore, when the concept is a variable, it is neither independent nor dependent. Independent and dependent variables are, however, relevant for correlational research and experimental research. In correlational research, both independent variables and dependent variables can be either categorical or continuous. The number of physical symptoms, for example, is a continuous independent variable, x, and the extent of functional status is a continuous dependent variable, y. Alternatively, the presence or absence of a certain symptom is a categorical independent variable, and functional status, if scored as adequate or inadequate, is a categorical dependent variable.

In experimental research, the independent variable, x, comprises the experimental conditions—the experimental and control treatments—and therefore typically is categorical. The dependent variable, y, in experimental research may be categorical or continuous. For example, an experimental physical activity intervention and a control usual activity intervention make up a categorical independent variable, and the extent of functional status is a continuous dependent variable. Functional status, if scored as adequate or inadequate, is a categorical dependent variable.

Propositions, Operational Definitions, and Hypotheses

As previously explained, a **proposition** is a statement about a concept or a statement about the association between two or more concepts. When used in the E component of C-T-E structures for research, propositions take the form of operational definitions of concepts and hypotheses.

An **operational definition** is a very precise proposition that states exactly how a concept is measured by identifying the name of the research instrument or experimental conditions used to measure the concept. "The beauty of an operational definition," according to Hoyle, Harris, and Judd (2002), "is that it specifies precisely how to measure a variable in such a concrete and specific manner that anyone else could repeat the steps and obtain the same measurements" (p. 76).

An example of an operational definition that identifies the name of the research instrument is: Physical symptoms were measured by the Symptom Checklist. An example of an operational definition that identifies experimental conditions is: The experimental physical activity treatment is defined as walking 20 minutes every day for 4 weeks. The control usual activity treatment is defined as walking approximately 10 minutes every other day for 4 weeks.

A **hypothesis** is a special type of proposition that is a conjecture or tentative statement about one concept or the association between two or more concepts (Kerlinger & Lee, 2000; Popper, 1965). More specifically, hypotheses are statements that substitute research-instrument or experimental-condition labels for the concepts identified in the theory propositions (Fawcett, 1999). Hypotheses are found only in theory-testing descriptive, correlational, and experimental research. Hypotheses are not part of theory-generating research because the theory concepts about which conjectures can be made are not known prior to the completion of the research.

A hypothesis about one concept can be a conjecture that uses the label of the instrument that measures the concept. An example of a proposition about one concept as stated in a theory tested by descriptive research is: Functional status is defined as performance of household activities, child care activities, social and community activities, personal care activities, occupational activities, and educational activities. Substituting the research-instrument label for the concept, the hypothesis is: Items on the Inventory of Functional Status-Antepartum Period are grouped into six subscales—household activities, child care activities, social and community activities, personal care activities, occupational activities, and educational activities (Tulman et al., 1991).

A hypothesis about a relational proposition—a statement of an association between two or more concepts—is a conjecture that uses the label for instruments or experimental conditions that measure the concepts. An example of a relational proposition as stated in a theory tested by correlational research is: Physical symptoms and functional status are related. Using the labels for the instruments that measure physical symptoms and functional status, the hypothesis is: As scores on the Symptom Checklist increase, scores on the Inventory of Functional Status-Antepartum Period will decrease. An example of a relational proposition as stated in a theory tested by experimental research is: Physical activity has an effect on physical energy. Using the labels for the experimental conditions and an instrument, the hypothesis is: "A group of women who walk 20 minutes every day for 4 weeks (experimental treatment) will have higher scores on the Physical Energy Scale than a group of women who walk approximately 10 minutes every other day for 4 weeks (control treatment)."

WHAT ARE THE TWO TYPES OF C-T-E STRUCTURES FOR RESEARCH?

There are two general types of C-T-E structures for research (Fawcett, 1999). One type of C-T-E structure depicts research that is designed to generate middle-range theories; the other type of C-T-E structure depicts research that is designed to test middle-range theories.

C-T-E Structures for Theory-Generating Research

Theory-generating research, which usually is descriptive research, is designed to discover a new middle-range theory. The newly discovered theory is usually a descriptive theory (see Table 2–1).

Each conceptual model guides the generation of a middle-range theory through application of its research guidelines. As we explained earlier in this chapter, the guidelines draw attention to certain concepts and propositions and to particular empirical research methods to use for the discovery of new middle-range theories. As can be seen in Figure 2–1, theory-generating research proceeds directly from the conceptual model to the empirical research methods (══). The data collected are analyzed, and a new middle-range theory emerges from the data (........). An example of a theory-generating C-T-E structure is illustrated in Figure 2–2. The diagram indicates that the conceptual model guiding the study was King's Conceptual System and that a descriptive research design was used, content analysis was applied to responses to a Caregiver Rewards Interview Guide from caregivers of family members with Alzheimer's disease, and a middle-range Theory of Rewards of Caregiving was generated from the data.

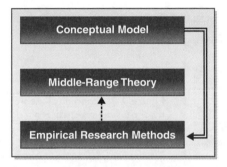

Figure 2-1. Conceptual-theoretical-empirical structure for theory-generating research: From conceptual model to empirical research methods to middle-range theory. *From Fawcett, J. (1999). The relationship of theory and research (3rd ed., p.11). Philadelphia: F. A. Davis, with permission.*

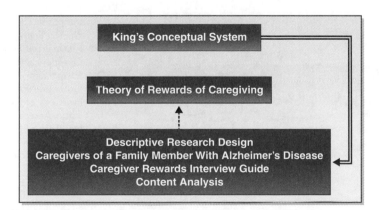

Figure 2-2. Conceptual-theoretical-empirical structure for study of responses to caring for a family member with Alzheimer's disease.

C-T-E Structures for Theory-Testing Research

Theory-testing research is designed to test a middle-range theory. Theory-testing research may be descriptive, correlational, or experimental, so the theory that is tested may be a descriptive theory, an explanatory theory, or a predictive theory (see Table 2–1).

Each conceptual model guides the test of a middle-range theory through application of its research guidelines. First, the concepts and propositions of the middle-range theory are linked with the concepts and propositions of the conceptual model. Then, the middle-range theory is tested by using the empirical research methods that are identified in the research guidelines. As can be seen in Figure 2–3, theory testing proceeds from the conceptual model to the theory (===), and from the theory to the empirical research methods (........). An example of a theory-testing C-T-E structure is displayed in Figure 2–4. The diagram

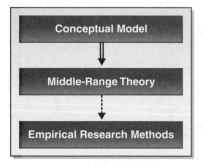

Figure 2-3. Conceptual-theoretical-empirical structure for theory-testing research: From conceptual model to middle-range theory to empirical research methods. *From Fawcett, J. (1999). The relationship of theory and research (3rd ed., p. 13). Philadelphia: F. A. Davis, with permission.*

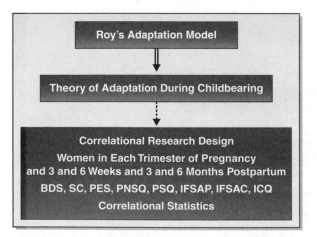

Figure 2-4. Conceptual-theoretical-empirical structure for study of women's adaptation during child-bearing.

BDS   Background Data Sheet
SC   Symptoms Checklist
PES   Physical Energy Scale
PNSQ   Prenatal Self-Evaluation Questionnaire
PSQ   Postpartum Self-Evaluation Questionnaire
IFSAP   Inventory of Functional Status-Antepartum Period
IFSAC   Inventory of Functional Status After Childbirth
ICQ   Infant Characteristics Questionaire

indicates that the conceptual model guiding the study was Roy's Adaptation Model and that a middle-range Theory of Adaptation During Childbearing was derived from Roy's model, the theory was tested, using a correlational research design, with women in each trimester of pregnancy and at four times during the postpartum using several questionnaires, and correlational statistical techniques were used to analyze the data.

Conclusion

In this chapter, you learned what the components of C-T-E structures for research are. You also learned that there are two types of C-T-E structures—one for theory-generating research and another for theory-testing research. And you learned that although conceptual models are the starting points for both theory-generating and theory-testing research, theory-generating research proceeds from the conceptual model to the empirical research methods and then to the middle-range theory, whereas theory-testing research proceeds from the conceptual model to the middle-range theory and then to the empirical research methods. In Chapter 3, you will learn where to locate each component of a C-T-E structure.

References

Full citations for all references cited in this chapter are provided in the Reference section at the end of the book.

Learning Activities

Activities to supplement what you have learned in this chapter, along with practice examination questions, are provided on the CD that comes with this book.

The Contents of Research Reports

Recall that in Chapter 2, we identified the three components of conceptual-theoretical-empirical (C-T-E) structures for research—the conceptual model on which the research is based (C), the middle-range theory that is generated or tested (T), and the empirical research methods that are used to conduct the research (E). In this chapter, you will learn how to answer the question, "Where is the information?" as you find out *where* to find the information about C-T-E structures that is contained in research reports. In addition, you will learn how to answer the question, "What is the information?" as you find out *what* information you can expect to find in each section and subsection of a research report. We start by defining what we mean by a research report. Then, we describe the contents of a typical research report and explain where to find each component of the C-T-E structure for the research. We have included an example of a research report on the CD that comes with this book, with labels corresponding to the sections and subsections identified in this chapter.

KEYWORDS

Abstract	Method
Attrition Rate	Procedures
Background	Research Design
Control Treatment	Research Findings
Data Analysis Techniques	Research Problem
Discussion	Research Report
Exclusion Criteria	Response Rate
Experimental Conditions	Results
Experimental Treatment	Sample
Inclusion Criteria	Social Significance
Instruments	Theoretical Significance
Introduction	

WHAT IS A RESEARCH REPORT?

A **research report** is a document that contains the elements of what typically is called a **study** or a **research project**. In other words, a research report is a description of a study that includes

---

*Portions of this chapter are adapted from Fawcett, J. (1999). *The relationship of theory and research* (3rd ed., pp. 144–198). Philadelphia: F. A. Davis, with permission.

why the study was conducted, how it was conducted, what the results of the study were, and what the results mean. In this and the remaining chapters of this book, we will use the terms research and study interchangeably.

Research reports may be published as journal articles, book chapters, or even entire books. Reports of research also may be published as part of the proceedings of a conference, either as full reports of studies or in summary form as abstracts. Citations for many reports of nursing research guided by nursing conceptual models are given in the searchable bibliography on the CD included with this book.

WHAT ARE THE CONTENTS OF RESEARCH REPORTS?

A full report of completed research usually includes five sections—the abstract, an introduction to the research problem, the method, the results, and the discussion of results. In addition, each section may be separated into subsections. For example, the introduction may be separated into subsections for an overview of the research problem and the specific aims of the research, the conceptual framework, and the literature review; the methods may be separated into subsections for the research design, the sample, the instruments, the data collection procedures and the procedures for protecting participants from harm, and data analysis techniques; and the discussion may be separated into subsections for discussion of results, study limitations, and implications for future research and practice. The actual label for each section and subsection may vary, according to the publisher's preference. For example, the introduction may be labeled the "background," the sample may be labeled "research participants" or "study participants," and the results may be labeled the "findings." Each section of a research report contains information about one or more of the components of the C-T-E structure for the study. You will begin to be able to answer the questions, Where is the information? and What is the information? when you know what information is found in each section of a typical research report. The contents of a research report are summarized in Table 3–1 at the end of this chapter.

The Abstract

Most research reports include an **abstract,** which is a concise summary of the contents of the full report. The exact format of an abstract usually is specified by the publisher to whom the research report was submitted. Some publishers require a structured abstract with specific headings, whereas others specify an unstructured format. Virtually all publishers place an upper limit on the number of words to be contained in an abstract, such as 100, 250, or 300 words, which is why an abstract is so brief.

Abstracts typically include a statement of the purpose of the research. Some abstracts also include the name of the conceptual model that guided the research and the name of the middle-range theory that was generated or tested. As we pointed out in Chapter 2, not all studies are guided by an explicit conceptual model, so the conceptual model (C) component of the C-T-E structure may not be mentioned in the abstract. We also pointed out in Chapter 2 that inasmuch as the concepts of a middle-range theory are sometimes referred to as themes or variables, the name of the middle-range theory that was generated or tested may not be given. Instead, a list of themes may be provided for theory-generating research, or a list of study variables may be provided for theory-testing research.

The abstract usually also includes one or more sentences that provide a reason—or rationale—for the study or establish the need for the study. In addition, the abstract typically includes a brief description of the empirical research methods, including the type of research design, the number and particularly important characteristics of the sample, and, if space permits, the label for each instrument, the procedures used to collect the data, and the data analysis techniques used. In addition, the abstract includes a concise summary and interpretation of the results. In abstracts of theory-generating research, the result is the middle-range theory that emerged from the analysis of the data. In abstracts of theory-testing research, the results are the findings of statistical tests of hypotheses.

The Introduction

The **introduction** section of a research report provides an overview of the topic that was studied, with emphasis on information about the conceptual model (C) and theory (T) components of the C-T-E structure. This section includes an explanation of the need for the research and provides a description of the frame of reference for the study. The introduction has three major subsections: a brief description of a topic that required investigation, a statement of the purpose of the study, and the background literature.

Description of the Research Topic

The **research topic** usually is referred to as the **research problem**. Use of the term "problem" does not, however, mean that research is the same as problem-solving (see Chapter 1). The research problem subsection should present a compelling rationale for the study by explaining the social significance and theoretical significance of the middle-range theory that was generated or tested. The **social significance** of the middle-range nursing theory can be justified by identifying the magnitude of a problem, which frequently is done by citing statistics for the number of people who have a certain health condition, undergo a certain medical procedure, or receive a certain nursing intervention. Social significance also can be justified by an explanation of how the middle-range theory addresses a health policy issue or a research priority set by a practice specialty organization or a funding agency. The **theoretical significance** of the middle-range theory can be justified by an explanation of what already is known about the problem and how the current study is needed to extend or fill gaps in existing middle-range theories about a health-related experience.

Statement of the Purpose of the Study

The subsection containing the **statement of the study purpose** might come at the end of the introduction, or it could be the very first sentence in the introduction, or it could be located at the beginning of the method section. The purpose is stated precisely and concisely. In reports of theory-generating research, the study purpose typically is stated as the topic that was studied. In reports of theory-testing research, the statement of the study purpose typically includes the names of the main concepts, or study variables, and propositions, or hypotheses, of the theory. The purpose of the study may be stated as a narrative statement, a list of specific aims, or a list of research questions. The statement of the study purpose may also include the type of research—descriptive, correlational, or experimental—that was conducted.

The Background and Literature Review

The **background** subsection includes an overview of the conceptual model that guided the research, as well as a critical and integrative review of relevant theoretical and empirical literature. The literature review subsection may not include all that is known about the research problem and related methodology; a comprehensive literature review may instead be presented in a separate publication, sometimes referred to as a "state of the science" paper. In that case, this subsection may be limited to a critical review of only the most relevant literature needed to provide a rationale for the type of research conducted and any hypotheses proposed.

In reports of theory-generating research, the background subsection may be quite brief. In that case, the conceptual model that guided the study is summarized and linked to the research problem and empirical research methods. The typical literature review is a critical discussion of previous theoretical and empirical works that clearly emphasizes a lack of knowledge, which supports the need for a theory-generating study.

In reports of theory-testing research, a concise summary of the conceptual model is presented, and linkages between the conceptual model concepts and propositions and the concepts and propositions of the middle-range theory that was tested are explained. The literature review includes statements of the theory propositions and a critical discussion of the rationale for each proposition. Constitutive definitions for the theory concepts may be given as each concept is introduced. Alternatively, constitutive definitions may be given when the empirical indicators are described in the method section. The literature review may conclude with a statement of the research hypotheses. A diagram of the C-T-E structure for the study may be presented in the background subsection, or the concepts and propositions of the theory may be depicted in a diagram. We explain how conceptual models guide theory-generating and theory-testing research in detail in Chapter 5.

The Method

The **method** section contains information about the empirical research methods (E) component of the C-T-E structure. This section of a research report has several subsections—research design, sample, instruments and any experimental conditions, procedures for data collection and for protection of participants from harm, and data analysis techniques.

Research Design

The **research design** subsection typically is made up of one or two sentences that identify the specific research design used. We discuss many different research designs in Chapter 7.

Sample

The **sample** subsection presents a description of the sample size, a rationale or justification for the size of the sample, how people were recruited for the study, or how other sources of data—such as animals, organizations, or documents—were obtained, and the inclusion and exclusion criteria. **Inclusion criteria** refer to characteristics that the source of data must have to be included in the sample. **Exclusion criteria** refer to the characteristics that exclude certain people or other sources of data from the sample. Examples of inclusion and exclusion criteria for people are age range, language spoken, reading ability, level of education, and health condition.

The sample subsection also may include the **response rate**, or the number of invited people who actually agreed to participate in the study, as well as the **attrition rate**, or the number of people who did not complete the study. Usually, this subsection also includes a summary of the demographic and health-related characteristics of the sample, which may be augmented by data presented in a table. Sometimes, however, the summary of sample characteristics is found at the beginning of the results section. In addition, the sample subsection may include the informed-consent procedure; alternatively, that information may be found in the procedures subsection. We discuss sample selection in detail in Chapter 8.

Instruments and Experimental Conditions

The **instruments** subsection contains a description of each instrument, including the label for each instrument used to collect the word or number data, as well as the name of the concept measured by each instrument. If the instrument is used to collect word data, the description may be limited to the questions asked. If the instrument is used to collect number data, the instrument description usually includes the number and some examples of questions, the scale used to rate questions, the range of possible scores, and an explanation of the interpretation of the scores. Information about the quality of data collected by each instrument also is reported. The quality of word data is estimated by dependability and credibility, whereas the quality of number data is estimated by reliability and validity. We discuss different types of instruments and criteria used to estimate their quality in detail in Chapter 9.

If experimental research has been conducted, the instruments subsection also may include a description of the **experimental conditions**, or that information may be in a separate subsection of the methods section, or it may even be part of the procedures subsection. The experimental conditions encompass the experimental treatment and the control treatment. The **experimental treatment** frequently is a new intervention that is being tested to determine if it leads to a more beneficial outcome than the usual intervention. The usual intervention typically is referred to as the **control treatment**. The description of the experimental and control treatments may be referred to as a **protocol**. We discuss experimental conditions in detail in Chapter 9.

Procedures

The **procedures** subsection provides a concise but detailed description of the procedures used to collect the data and protect participants from harm. It may be subdivided by one heading for data collection procedures and another for protection of participants, or both topics may be discussed under the general subsection heading.

The procedure used to recruit the sample may be explained in the procedures subsection, if it is not noted in the sample subsection. In addition, the people who collected the data may be identified, and any special training required for data collection may be explained. The setting for data collection also may be identified, and if more than one instrument is used, the order in which the instruments are used may be noted. If the research involves collection of data more than one time, the number of times each instrument was administered and the rationale for the time intervals may be stated. The time required for data collection also may be noted. We discuss data collection procedures in detail in Chapter 10.

The information about participant protection, which may be labeled "ethical considerations," should include a statement indicating approval of the study by an institutional review board or ethics committee, as well as an explanation of the procedure used to obtain informed consent. Any financial or other incentives given to members of the sample also may be noted. We discuss procedures for protecting research participants in Chapter 11.

Data Analysis Techniques

A subsection for **data analysis techniques** may be included in the research report, especially if those techniques are unusual. If the techniques used are well known, they may be named only in the results section. If more detail is required, the techniques may be explained in the procedures subsection or in a separate data analysis techniques subsection. A data analysis subsection in which the specific techniques used to analyze and interpret word data are described is often included in reports of theory-generating research. When a data analysis subsection is included in reports of theory-testing research, the way in which a particular statistical technique was used to analyze number data is explained. We discuss data analysis techniques for theory-generating research and theory-testing research in Chapter 12.

The Results

The **results** section, which is structured according to the specific aims, research questions, or hypotheses of the study, presents the theory component of the C-T-E in the form of the **research findings**—that is, the results of the data analysis.

The results section of theory-generating research reports contains a description of the theory that was generated—that is, the concepts and propositions that emerged from the data analysis, frequently in the form of themes or categories. Definitions or descriptions of the themes or categories and quotations from participants that reflect each theme or category also are given.

In theory-testing research, the results section usually starts with descriptive statistics that summarize the scores for the major concepts of the theory. Statistical procedures used to test each hypothesis or analyze the data related to each specific aim or research question may be identified if a separate data analysis technique subsection is not included in the report. The result for each statistical test is presented, and a conclusion is drawn with regard to the support or lack of support for each hypothesis that was tested. Tables and figures can be used to supplement the narrative description of the research results. We discuss evaluation of the adequacy of research findings in Chapter 13.

The Discussion

The **discussion** section, which also is structured according to specific aims, research questions, or hypotheses, presents an interpretation of the research results within the context of the C-T-E structure. Results usually are not repeated in the discussion section, although they may be summarized to enhance clarity of the discussion. In theory-generating research, a comparison of the theory that was generated with any similar existing theories may be included. In theory-testing research, the results may be compared with those of previous research.

This section also may include various methodological and/or theoretical explanations for the research findings. In addition, the discussion section may include a conclusion regarding the adequacy of the middle-range theory and the utility and soundness of the conceptual model. We discuss the adequacy of the middle-range theory in Chapter 13 and the utility and soundness of the conceptual model in Chapter 15.

The discussion section also usually includes the limitations of the research, such as any flaws in the data collection procedures and the extent to which the findings may be applicable to various other people or other settings. The discussion section frequently ends with the investigator's recommendations for future research about the research problem. In addition, the discussion section may include recommendations for practical uses of the theory that was generated or tested, such as a guide for development of an assessment tool, an intervention protocol, practice guidelines, or health policies. We discuss recommendations for practical uses of theories in detail in Chapter 14.

Conclusion

In this chapter, you learned where to locate content about each component of a C-T-E structure in research reports. In Chapter 4, you will learn what criteria are used to evaluate each of the three components of C-T-E structures for research.

Learning Activities

Activities to supplement what you have learned in this chapter, along with practice examination questions, are provided on the CD that comes with this book.

Table 3–1 Contents of Research Reports

ABSTRACT

The abstract presents a concise summary of the conceptual-theoretical-empirical structure.

- Look for a statement of the purpose of the research.
- Look for the name of the conceptual model that guided the research.
- Look for the name of the theory that was generated or tested.
- Look for a rationale for the research.
- Look for a description of the empirical research methods.
- Look for a summary and interpretation of the research results.

INTRODUCTION

The introduction establishes the need for theory-generating research or theory-testing research to investigate a particular health-related experience and identifies the frame of reference for the research. This section includes information about the conceptual model and theory components of the conceptual-theoretical-empirical structure.

- Look for an explanation of how the theory that was generated or tested addresses a topic that is important to society—that is, the social significance of the topic.
- Look for an explanation of how the theory that was generated or tested extends or fills gaps in existing knowledge about a health-related experience—that is, the theoretical significance of the topic.
- Look for a statement of the purpose or specific aims of the study.
- Look for an overview of the conceptual model that guided the study.
- Look for a description of the linkages between the conceptual model, the middle-range theory concepts and propositions, and the empirical research methods.
- Look for a critical review of relevant theoretical and empirical literature.

For theory-testing research,

- Look for a description of the middle-range theory that was tested, constitutive definitions for the concepts of the theory, and support from the literature for theory propositions, as well as a statement of the research hypotheses.

METHOD

The method section presents the empirical research methods component of the conceptual-theoretical-empirical structure, including identification of the research design, a description of the sample, a description of research instruments and any experimental conditions, an explanation of the procedures, and a description of the data analysis techniques.

Research Design

- Look for a statement that identifies the research design.

Table 3–1	Contents of Research Reports—*cont'd*

Sample

- Look for a description of the sample, including the source of the data, such as individuals, animals, organizations, or documents; the size of the sample; and a justification for the sample size.
- Look for an explanation of how the sample was recruited.
- Look for an explanation of sample inclusion and exclusion criteria.
- Look for the response rate and the attrition rate.
- Look for a description of the demographic and other relevant characteristics of the sample.

Instruments and Experimental Conditions

- Look for the label for each research instrument used and the name of the middle-range theory concept measured by each instrument.
- For instruments yielding word data, look for a description of the questions asked.
- For instruments yielding number data, look for a description of the items on each instrument and the scale used to rate the items, as well as an explanation of the range of possible scores and how the scores are interpreted.
- Look for a description of the quality of data collected by each instrument, including dependability and credibility for word data and reliability and validity for number data.
- For experimental research, look for a description of the experimental and control treatment protocols.

Procedures

- Look for a description of the data collection procedures, including when the data were collected, where the data were collected, who collected the data, the number of times and the order in which the research instruments were administered, and the length of time required to collect data from each study participant.
- Look for a statement regarding protection of human or animal study participants, such as an explanation of how informed consent from human beings was obtained, as well as a statement indicating approval of the study by an institutional review board or ethics committee, and any financial or other incentives offered to participants.

Data Analysis Techniques

- Look for a description of the techniques used to analyze the data.

Continued

Table 3–1	Contents of Research Reports—*cont'd*

RESULTS

The results section presents the theoretical component of the conceptual-theoretical-empirical structure in the form of the study findings. Expect this section to be structured according to specific aims, research questions, or hypotheses.

- Look for a description of the results of the data analysis.

- For theory-generating research, look for names and descriptions of the concepts and propositions of the middle-range theory that emerged from the analysis of data.

- For theory-testing research, look for statistics that summarize scores for variables and the results of statistical tests of hypotheses.

- For theory-testing research, look for a definitive conclusion regarding support or lack of support for each hypothesis.

DISCUSSION

The discussion section presents an interpretation of the research results within the context of the conceptual-theoretical-empirical structure for the research. Expect this section also to be structured according to specific aims, research questions, or hypotheses.

- Look for an explanation and interpretation of the results.

- Look for alternative methodological and theoretical explanations.

- Look for conclusions about the adequacy of the middle-range theory.

- Look for conclusions about the soundness and utility of the conceptual model.

- Look for implications for future research.

- Look for implications for practice guidelines and public policies.

Adapted from Fawcett, J. (1999). *The relationship of theory and research* (3rd ed., pp. 144–145). Philadelphia: F. A. Davis, with permission.

Chapter 4*

A Framework for Evaluating Conceptual-Theoretical-Empirical Structures for Research

In Chapter 2, you learned about the three components of conceptual-theoretical-empirical (C-T-E) structures for research—the conceptual model on which the research is based (C), the middle-range theory that is generated or tested (T), and the empirical research methods that are used to conduct the research (E). In Chapter 3, you learned *where* to find information about each component of a C-T-E structure in a typical research report and *what* information about the components you can expect to find in each section and subsection of the research report.

In this chapter, you will begin to learn how to answer the question "How good is the information?" Here, we identify a framework for evaluating C-T-E structures for research that is made up of criteria that focus on one or more of the three components. We present an overview of the criteria in this chapter; much more detail about each criterion and examples will be given in Chapters 5 through 15.

Evaluation of C-T-E structures for research involves thinking critically and making judgments about the extent to which the information about each component of the C-T-E structure included in a research report satisfies the criteria we identify in this chapter. The ability to evaluate C-T-E structures for theory-generating research and theory-testing research is a basic cognitive skill that needs to be mastered as part of educational preparation for professional nursing practice (Anders, Daly, Thompson, Elliott, & Chang, 2005).

KEYWORDS

Empirical Adequacy	Parsimony
Internal Consistency	Significance
Legitimacy	Specification Adequacy
Linkage Adequacy	Pragmatic Adequacy
Operational Adequacy	Testability

---

*Portions of this chapter are adapted from Fawcett, J. (1999). *The relationship of theory and research* (3rd ed., pp. 85–113). Philadelphia: F. A. Davis, with permission.

HOW ARE CONCEPTUAL-THEORETICAL-EMPIRICAL STRUCTURES FOR RESEARCH EVALUATED?

The publication of a research report does not mean the research was perfect—it is virtually impossible to conduct perfect research. Instead, publication usually signifies that the research addressed an important topic, that there were no "fatal flaws" in the conceptual model, theory, or empirical research methods components of the C-T-E structure, and that the written report clearly conveys what was done, why it was done, what was found, and what the research and practice implications of what was found are.

We recognize that not all research reports include information about each component of the C-T-E structure, especially the C component or even the T component. We have, however, developed a framework for evaluation of C-T-E structures for research that allows the reader of research reports to determine the extent to which each component is included. The framework sensitizes the reader of research reports to the need for and value of information about all three components. We believe that the exclusion of any of the components limits the reader's understanding of the contribution of the research to the advancement of knowledge about a particular topic.

Various criteria for the evaluation of middle-range theories and empirical research methods are available in the literature of many disciplines, including nursing (e.g., Alligood, 2006; Barnum, 1998; Duffy & Muhlenkamp, 1974; Ellis, 1968; Parse, 2005; Whall, 2005). Our review of those criteria led us to conclude that there is general agreement about how to determine how good middle-range theories are and, especially, how good empirical research methods are. Very few criteria, however, focus on the connection between a middle-range theory and the empirical research methods used to generate or test that theory. Furthermore, although the authors of some other nursing research textbooks include brief discussions of conceptual models (e.g., Burns & Grove, 2007; Fain, 2004; Nieswiadomy, 2008; Polit & Beck, 2006), hardly any attention has been given to specific criteria that can be used to determine how good conceptual models are as guides for research, or to criteria addressing the connection of conceptual models to middle-range theories and to empirical research methods. The evaluation criteria that we present in this chapter focus your attention on the essential connections between the three components of C-T-E structures for research.

WHAT ARE THE SIX STEPS OF C-T-E STRUCTURE EVALUATION?

We selected criteria that can be used to evaluate C-T-E structures for both theory-generating research and theory-testing research, and we arranged those criteria in a framework made up of six steps. We present a summary of the framework steps and criteria, along with where to find information about each criterion, in Table 4–1 at the end of this chapter. Examples of the application of the criteria are given in Chapters 5 through 15.

Step One: Evaluation of the Conceptual Component of C-T-E Structures

The first step in evaluation of C-T-E structures for theory-generating research and theory-testing research focuses on the conceptual model (C) component. We call the criteria *specification adequacy* and *linkage adequacy.*

Specification Adequacy

Specification adequacy refers to the amount of information about the conceptual model that is given in a research report. The criterion of specification adequacy requires that the conceptual model that guided the research be identified explicitly. The criterion also requires the content of the conceptual model to be described clearly and concisely. In addition, this criterion requires the connection between the conceptual model and the research topic to be explained.

The information needed to evaluate specification adequacy is usually found in the background or conceptual framework subsection of the introduction section of a research report. Examples of application of the specification adequacy criterion are given in Chapter 5. In addition, tables for Chapter 5 that are on the CD that comes with this book include overviews of several nursing conceptual models to help you understand how the content of a conceptual model can be described clearly and concisely, along with examples of the application of the criterion of specification adequacy.

Linkage Adequacy

Linkage adequacy refers to the amount of information about the connections between the conceptual model, the middle-range theory, and the empirical research methods that is given in a research report. The criterion of linkage adequacy requires those connections to be stated explicitly and completely. This criterion also requires the empirical research methods to be consistent with the conceptual model.

The information needed to evaluate linkage adequacy is usually found in the background or conceptual framework subsection of the introduction section of a research report. Examples of application of the criterion of linkage adequacy are given in Chapter 5.

Step Two: Evaluation of the Middle-Range Theory Component of C-T-E Structures

The second step in evaluation of C-T-E structures for theory-generating research and theory-testing research focuses on the theory (T) component. Four criteria—*significance, internal consistency, parsimony, and testability*—are used to evaluate middle-range theories. Examples of each criterion are given in Chapter 6.

Significance of the Middle-Range Theory

Significance refers to the extent to which the middle-range theory is socially and theoretically important. The criterion of significance requires that the theory deal with a topic that society currently regards as practically important. The criterion also requires that the theory offer new, compelling, and nontrivial insights into the topic.

A summary of the information needed to evaluate theory significance is usually found at the beginning of the introduction section of a research report; more detailed information may be given in the background or literature review subsection.

Internal Consistency of the Middle-Range Theory

Internal consistency refers to the extent to which the concepts and propositions of the middle-range theory are comprehensible. The criterion of internal consistency requires the theory concepts to be explicitly identified and clearly defined. The criterion also requires that the same term be used for each concept throughout the research report and the same definition be used for each term. The criterion of internal consistency additionally requires the propositions of the theory to be reasonable.

The information needed to evaluate internal consistency is usually found in the background or literature review subsection of the introduction section of a research report, or even throughout the entire report.

Parsimony of the Middle-Range Theory

Parsimony refers to the extent to which the content of the middle-range theory is stated as concisely as possible. The criterion of parsimony requires the theory to be made up of as few concepts and propositions as necessary to clearly convey the meaning of each.

The information needed to evaluate parsimony usually is found in the background or literature review subsection of the introduction section of the research report. Additional information may be found in the results or discussion section.

Testability of the Middle-Range Theory

Testability refers to the extent to which the theory can be empirically tested. The criterion of testability requires each concept of the middle-range theory to be empirically measurable either directly—typically by actually seeing or hearing something—or through use of some type of research instrument. The criterion also requires each assertion made by the middle-range theory propositions to be testable through some data analysis technique.

The information needed to evaluate testability usually is found in the method and results sections of a research report.

Step Three: Evaluation of the Empirical Research Methods of C-T-E Structures

The third step in evaluation of C-T-E structures for theory-generating research and theory-testing research focuses on the empirical research methods (E) component. We call the criterion *operational adequacy.*

Operational adequacy refers to the amount of information about each element of the empirical research methods that is given in a research report, as well as to the appropriateness of methods used. The criterion of operational adequacy requires every element of the empirical research methods—the research design, the sample, the instruments and any experimental conditions, the procedures for collection of data and protection of research participants from harm, and the data analysis techniques—to be clearly described and to be an appropriate way to conduct research about a particular health-related experience. Specifically, the operational adequacy criterion requires that the research design be an appropriate way to obtain "adequate and proper data" (McCall, as cited in Campbell & Stanley, 1963, p. 1), based on what already is known and what needs to be known about the health-related experience. The criterion also requires that the sample be an appropriate source of data for the theory that is being generated or tested. In addition, the criterion requires that the instruments and any experimental conditions be appropriate ways to measure the theory concepts and that the procedure be a methodologically and ethically appropriate way to collect the data. Finally, the criterion of operational adequacy requires that the data analysis techniques be appropriate for the type and amount of data collected.

The information needed to evaluate operational adequacy typically is found in the method section of a research report; additional information may be found in the results section. Sometimes, information about the research design may even be found in the introduction, as part of the statement of the purpose of the research. Examples of the application of the different elements of the criterion of operational adequacy are given in Chapters 7 through 12.

Step Four: Evaluation of the Research Findings

The fourth step in evaluation of C-T-E structures for theory-generating research and theory-testing research returns the focus to the theory (T) component. We call the criterion *empirical adequacy*.

Empirical adequacy refers to the extent to which the research results—the data—agree with the concepts and propositions as specified in the theory. The criterion of empirical adequacy requires that the theoretical claims as stipulated by the middle-range theory concepts and propositions be completely congruent with the data that were collected. If the data are not completely congruent with theoretical claims, the theory cannot be regarded as empirically adequate. This does not necessarily mean that the theory is worthless. Rather, it may mean that the content of the theory needs to be modified by eliminating or adding one or more concepts and propositions. Or it could mean that the theory is indeed worthless and should be discarded.

The information needed to evaluate empirical adequacy is typically found in the results and discussion sections of a research report. Examples of the application of the criterion of empirical adequacy are given in Chapter 13.

Step Five: Evaluation of the Utility of the Theory for Practice

The fifth step in evaluation of C-T-E structures for theory-generating research and theory-testing research also focuses on the theory (T) component. We call the criterion *pragmatic adequacy*.

Pragmatic adequacy refers to the usefulness of the theory for nursing practice. The criterion of pragmatic adequacy requires that the theory be used as evidence for development of assessment tools, interventional protocols, and practice guidelines that are socially meaningful; that it be appropriate for use within a particular practice setting, feasible in the real world of practice, and consistent with the public's expectations; and that practitioners have legal control over use of the theory in practice (Fawcett, 1999; Pearson, Wiechula, Court, & Lockwood, 2007). The criterion also requires that the theory be used as evidence for development of an organizational, professional association or governmental policy that influences nursing practice and the delivery of nursing services.

The information needed to evaluate pragmatic adequacy typically is found in the discussion section of a research report, perhaps in a practice implications subsection. Examples of application of the criterion of pragmatic adequacy are given in Chapter 14.

Step Six: Evaluation of the Utility and Soundness of the Conceptual Model

The sixth and final step in evaluation of C-T-E structures for theory-generating research and theory-testing research returns the focus to the conceptual model (C) component. We call the criterion *legitimacy*.

Legitimacy, which in the past was called credibility (Fawcett, 1999, 2005b), refers to the extent to which the research findings support the usefulness of the conceptual model as a guide for the research, as well as to the soundness of its content. The criterion of legitimacy requires the conceptual model to have been a useful guide for the research. The criterion also requires that the research design and findings reveal that the conceptual model concepts and propositions are sound and believable, that is, that no major flaws in the concepts or propositions were uncovered in the conduct of the theory-generating research or theory-testing research. If flaws are identified, the conceptual model cannot be considered legitimate. Identification of flaws may mean that the content of the conceptual model needs to be modified. Or the flaws may indicate that the conceptual model is indeed worthless and should no longer be used to guide research.

Information about legitimacy may be found in the discussion section of a research report. Examples of application of the criterion of legitimacy are given in Chapter 15.

Conclusion

In this chapter, you began to learn about criteria that can be used to evaluate each component of C-T-E structures for research. The merit of research frequently is said to be based on the consistency of the connections among the theoretical, design, and analysis components of a study. The criteria for evaluation of C-T-E structures that we presented in this chapter direct your attention to those aspects of research, as well as to the conceptual model that guided the study. Each criterion will be considered in much greater detail in Chapters 5 through 15, where we convert the requirements for each criterion to questions you can ask and answer about the contents of reports of theory-generating research and theory-testing research.

References

Full citations for all references cited in this chapter are provided in the Reference section at the end of the book.

Learning Activities

Activities to supplement what you have learned in this chapter, along with practice examination questions, are provided on the CD that comes with this book.

Table 4–1	Steps in the Evaluation of Conceptual-Theoretical-Empirical Structures for Research

STEP ONE: EVALUATION OF THE CONCEPTUAL MODEL COMPONENT OF C-T-E STRUCTURES

Specification adequacy is evident (see Chapter 5).

- Refers to the amount of information about the conceptual model given in the research report.
- The conceptual model that guided the research is explicitly identified.
- A clear and concise overview of the content of the conceptual model is given.
- The connection between the conceptual model and the research topic is explained.

Look in the background or conceptual framework subsection of the introduction section of the research report for the information needed to evaluate specification adequacy.

Linkage adequacy is evident (see Chapter 5).

- Refers to the amount of information about the connections between the conceptual model, the middle-range theory, and the empirical research methods given in the research report.
- The connections between the conceptual model, middle-range theory, and empirical research methods are stated explicitly.
- The connections between the conceptual model, middle-range theory, and empirical research methods are complete.
- The empirical research methods are congruent with the conceptual model.

Look in the background or conceptual framework subsection of the introduction section of the research report for the information needed to evaluate linkage adequacy.

STEP TWO: EVALUATION OF THE MIDDLE-RANGE THEORY COMPONENT OF C-T-E STRUCTURES

The theory is **significant** (see Chapter 6).

- Refers to the extent of social and theoretical importance of the theory
- The theory should address a topic that is of practical importance to society.
- The theory should offer new insights into the topic.

Look in the introduction section of the research report for the information needed to evaluate significance.

Continued

Table 4–1	Steps in the Evaluation of Conceptual-Theoretical-Empirical Structures for Research—cont'd

The theory is **internally consistent** (see Chapter 6).

- Refers to the extent to which the theory is comprehensible.
- The concepts should be explicitly identified and clearly defined.
- The same term and definition should be used for each concept throughout the research report.
- The propositions should be reasonable.

Look in all sections of the research report for the information needed to evaluate internal consistency.

The theory is **parsimonious** (see Chapter 6).

- Refers to the extent to which the theory is stated as concisely as possible
- The theory should be made up of as few concepts and propositions as necessary to convey its meaning.

Look in the introduction, results, and discussion sections of the research report for the information needed to evaluate parsimony.

The theory is **testable** (see Chapter 6).

- Refers to the extent to which the theory can be tested empirically.
- All concepts should be measured.
- All assertions should be testable through some data analysis technique.

Look in the method and results sections for the information needed to evaluate testability.

STEP THREE: EVALUATION OF THE EMPIRICAL RESEARCH METHODS COMPONENT OF C-T-E STRUCTURES

Operational adequacy is evident (see Chapters 7–12).

- Refers to the amount of information about the empirical research methods given in the research report and to the appropriateness of the methods used.
- The methods used to conduct the research—research design, sample, instruments and any experimental conditions, procedures for data collection and protection of participants from harm, data analysis techniques—should be appropriate and clearly described.

Look in the method and results sections of the research report for the information needed to evaluate operational adequacy.

STEP FOUR: EVALUATION OF THE RESEARCH FINDINGS

Information regarding the **empirical adequacy** of the middle-range theory is given (see Chapter 13).

- Refers to the extent to which the data agree with the theory.
- The concepts and propositions of the theory should be congruent with the research findings.

Look in the results and discussion sections of the research report for the information needed to evaluate empirical adequacy.

Table 4–1	Steps in the Evaluation of Conceptual-Theoretical-Empirical Structures for Research—*cont'd*

STEP FIVE: EVALUATION OF THE UTILITY OF THE THEORY FOR PRACTICE

Information regarding the **pragmatic adequacy** of the theory is given (see Chapter 14).

- Refers to the extent to which the theory should serve as a basis for practical activities.
- Use of the theory should be meaningful to society.
- The theory should be appropriate for use in a specific practice situation.
- Use of the theory should be feasible in a particular practice setting.
- Use of the theory should be consistent with the public's expectations.
- Practitioners should have legal control of use of the theory in practice.

Look in the discussion section of the research report for the information needed to evaluate pragmatic adequacy.

STEP SIX: EVALUATION OF THE UTILITY AND SOUNDNESS OF THE CONCEPTUAL MODEL

Information regarding the **legitimacy** of the conceptual model is given (see Chapter 15).

- Refers to the extent to which the research supports the usefulness and soundness of the conceptual model.
- The conceptual model should be a useful guide for research.
- The research design and findings should reveal that the content of the conceptual model is sound and believable.

Look in the discussion section of the research report for the information needed to evaluate legitimacy.

Part Two

Evaluation of Conceptual Models and Theories

Chapter 5

Evaluation of Conceptual-Theoretical-Empirical Linkages

This chapter focuses primarily on the conceptual model (C) component of conceptual-theoretical-empirical (C-T-E) structures for research and how the C component is linked to the theory (T) and empirical research methods (E) components.

KEYWORDS

Linkage Adequacy

Research Guidelines

Research Focus Guidelines

Research Method Guidelines

Specification Adequacy

   Recall from Chapter 2 that the C component of a C-T-E structure is the conceptual model that guides the research. In that chapter, we defined a conceptual model as a set of relatively abstract and general concepts and propositions, and we pointed out that a conceptual model is always the starting point for research. We also mentioned that specific research guidelines are associated with each conceptual model. In Chapter 3, we explained *where* to look for information about the conceptual model in research reports (Box 5–1) and *what* information you could expect to find (Box 5–2).

   Recall also that in Chapter 4, you began to learn how to determine *how good* the available information about the conceptual model that guided the research is, and we presented a framework for evaluating C-T-E structures for theory-generating research and theory-testing research.

BOX 5-1	Evaluation of Conceptual-Theoretical-Empirical Linkages: *Where Is the Information?*

Content about the conceptual-theoretical-empirical linkages typically is found in the background or conceptual framework subsection of the introduction section of the research report.

BOX 5-2	Evaluation of Conceptual-Theoretical-Empirical Linkages: *What Is the Information?*

Look for the name and an overview of the conceptual model in the research report, as well as an explanation about the connection between the conceptual model and the research topic.

In this chapter, we help you learn more about how to determine *how good* the information about the C component of C-T-E structures for theory-generating research and theory-testing research is. To help you learn about how a conceptual model guides research, we summarize the content of seven conceptual models of nursing and identify guidelines for research associated with each of them. We also discuss in detail the two criteria for evaluating the C component of the C-T-E structure that we identified in Chapter 4—namely, specification adequacy and linkage adequacy—and provide examples that should help you better understand how to apply the criteria as you read research reports. Application of the criteria will facilitate your evaluation of *how good* the information about the conceptual model and its connections to the middle-range theory and empirical research methods is.

DO CONCEPTUAL MODELS GUIDE RESEARCH?

Although the conceptual model that guided the research is not always mentioned in the report of the research, some frame of reference *always* guides researchers to select a particular topic, to review certain literature, and to conduct theory-generating research or theory-testing research in a certain way. Popper (1965), a philosopher of science, stated that in as much as researchers always conduct studies within the context of a preconceived "horizon of expectations" (p. 47), the belief held by some researchers that theories are developed without guidance from a conceptual model is "absurd" (p. 46). And Serlin (1987), a psychologist, deemed the selection of research methods not guided by conceptual models to be "hobbies" (p. 371).

The challenge, then, is to determine what information about the C component of the C-T-E structure is given in a research report and how that information is connected to the T and E components. You can evaluate how well the information is explained in a research report by applying the criteria of specification adequacy and linkage adequacy.

HOW IS THE CRITERION OF SPECIFICATION ADEQUACY APPLIED?

Specification adequacy draws attention to the C component of the C-T-E structure. Application of the criterion of specification adequacy helps you determine whether enough information about the C component is given in a research report. Enough information means that you can understand how the conceptual model served as the basis for the theory-generating research or theory-testing research. Application of the criterion of specification adequacy is especially important because some researchers do little more than cite the name of a particular conceptual model in the research report (Fawcett, 1996; Silva, 1987). The same level of detail about the conceptual model should be included in reports of both theory-generating research and theory-testing research.

The criterion of specification adequacy is met when you can answer yes to three questions:

- Is the name of the conceptual model given in the research report?
- Is an overview of the conceptual model provided?
- Is the connection between the conceptual model and the research topic explained?

Is the Name of the Conceptual Model Given?

The criterion of specification adequacy requires the conceptual model that guided the theory-generating research or theory-testing research to be identified explicitly. In other words, the name of the conceptual model should be given (Box 5–3).

BOX 5-3	Applying the Criterion of Specification Adequacy

Is the name of the conceptual model given in the research report?

Examples:

This study was based on King's Conceptual System.

King's Conceptual System guided the design of this study.

Is an overview of the conceptual model provided?

Example: King's Conceptual System focuses on the continuing ability of individuals to meet their basic needs so that they may function in their socially defined roles. Environmental stressors are thought to contribute to problems in the individual's ability to function optimally in social roles.
     This conceptual model of nursing also focuses on three open, dynamic, interacting systems. The three systems are the personal system, the interpersonal system, and the social system. Personal systems are individuals, such as patients or nurses. Interpersonal systems are two or three individuals or a small group of people who are interacting in a specific situation, such as a patient and a nurse; a patient, a nurse, and a physical therapist; or a patient, the patient's family members, and a nurse. Social systems are groups that form for specific purposes, such as a family, a school system, a hospital, or a church. Each system is made up of several dimensions that can be studied. Personal systems dimensions are perception, self, growth and development, body image, time, personal space, and learning. Interpersonal system dimensions are verbal and nonverbal communication, transaction, role, stress, and coping. Social system dimensions are interaction, organization, authority, power, status, decision making, and control.

Is the connection between the conceptual model and the research topic explained?

Example: King's personal system dimension of perception was of particular interest in this study of the individual caregiver's awareness of the rewards he or she experienced while caring for a family member with Alzheimer's disease.

Conceptual Models Widely Used by Nurse Researchers

Several different **conceptual models** are used by nurse researchers. Seven nursing conceptual models, developed as broad frames of reference for nursing practice and research, are used by nurse researchers in many countries. The seven nursing conceptual models and relevant recent citations are:

1. Johnson's Behavioral System Model (Holaday, 2006)
2. King's Conceptual System (King, 2006; Sieloff, 2006)

3.   Levine's Conservation Model (Schaefer & Pond, 1991)
4.   Neuman's Systems Model (Neuman & Fawcett, 2002)
5.   Orem's Self-Care Framework (Orem, 2001)
6.   Rogers' Science of Unitary Human Beings (Malinski, 2006)
7.   Roy's Adaptation Model (Roy & Andrews, 1999)

Brief summaries of the seven nursing conceptual models are given in Table 5–1, which is on the CD that comes with this book. The content of each model is organized according to the concepts of the metaparadigm of nursing (see Chapter 1)—human beings, environment, health, and nursing.

Use of Conceptual Models for a Specialty Practice or From Another Discipline

Some nurse researchers use conceptual models that were developed for a particular practice specialty area of nursing. For example, the Synergy Model (Hardin & Kaplow, 2005) was developed by members of the American Association of Critical Care Nurses to guide practice with and research about critically ill patients. Research guided by the Synergy Model focuses attention on the match between certain characteristics of patients and certain competencies of nurses. According to the model, when nurse competencies are a good match with patient characteristics, the likelihood of attaining optimal patient outcomes is increased. Rex-Smith (2007) used the Synergy Model to guide her study of nurses' own spirituality and their assessment of the spiritual care needs of critically ill patients.

In addition, nurse researchers sometimes use conceptual models from disciplines other than nursing. For example, the Health Belief Model (Becker, 1974; Janz, Champion, & Strecher, 2002), which was developed within the discipline of psychology, is sometimes used by nurses who want to study how people's beliefs about their susceptibility to a health problem, the seriousness of the health problem, and the benefits of and barriers to taking action influence actions taken to reduce the threat of contracting the health problem. Van Horn (2005) used the Health Belief Model to guide her study of adults' beliefs about their risk of recurrent injury, the factors they thought were associated with use of injury prevention actions, and the barriers to prevention of injuries they identified.

Nursing Grand Theories

Sometimes, nurse researchers inaccurately refer to the conceptual model as a theory or a theoretical framework. For example, researchers may inaccurately write, "Roy's theory of adaptation guided the study" when they should have written, "Roy's Adaptation Model guided the study." At other times, nurse researchers use what we consider grand theories for the C component of the C-T-E structure. Recall from Chapter 2 that a **grand theory** is less abstract than a conceptual model but not as concrete as a middle-range theory (Fawcett, 2005b). Three nursing grand theories that are used extensively as guides for nursing research are:

1.   Leininger's Theory of Culture Care Diversity and Universality (Leininger & McFarlane, 2006)

2. Newman's Theory of Health as Expanded Consciousness (Newman, 1994)
3. Parse's Theory of Human Becoming (Parse, 1998)

Brief summaries of the three grand theories and relevant citations are given in Table 5–2, which is on the CD that comes with this book. As can be seen in the table, each grand theory addresses just three of the four concepts of nursing metaparadigm—human beings, environment, and health. All four concepts are not addressed because grand theories are not as broad as conceptual models, which do address all four nursing metaparadigm concepts (see Table 5–1).

More detailed overviews of the seven conceptual models of models of nursing mentioned earlier and of the three grand theories can be found in *Taber's Cyclopedic Medical Dictionary* (Fawcett, 2005a) and the *Encyclopedia of Nursing Research* (Fitzpatrick & Wallace, 2006). Comprehensive discussions of one or more of the conceptual models and grand theories can be found in several books (Fawcett, 2005b; Fitzpatrick & Whall, 2005; George, 2002; Marriner Tomy & Alligood, 2006; Parker, 2006; Sitzman & Eichelberger, 2004).

Is an Overview of the Conceptual Model Provided?

Although the criterion of specification adequacy requires that a report of theory-generating research or theory-testing research includes the name of the conceptual model that guided the study, simply naming the conceptual model is not sufficient. The criterion of specification adequacy also requires that the research report include a clear and concise overview of the conceptual model (see Box 5–3). The overview may be a brief description of the entire conceptual model or may highlight only the content that is essential for understanding why that model was selected to guide the research.

Is the Connection Between the Conceptual Model and the Research Topic Explained?

In addition, the criterion of specification adequacy requires that the connection between the conceptual model and the research topic be explained clearly (see Box 5–3). This aspect of the criterion of specification adequacy is crucial. If the connection between the conceptual model and the research topic is not clear, any mention of the conceptual model in the research report will seem unnecessary to the reader.

Research Focus Guidelines

The connection between the conceptual model and the research topic should not only be stated clearly but also reflect the content of the conceptual model as stated in those research guidelines that specify the focus of research based on that model. The **research focus guidelines** associated with each conceptual model identify the reason why research is conducted, provide direction for the selection of a health-related experience to study within the context of that conceptual model, shape the way in which the specific research problem is stated, and identify the contribution of research findings to the advancement of knowledge. In other words, the research focus guidelines emphasize the connection between the C and T components of the C-T-E structure. The research focus guidelines for seven nursing conceptual models we identified earlier in this chapter are given in Table 5–3, which is on the CD.

Research focus guidelines for other conceptual models of nursing, such as the Synergy Model, have not yet been developed. Research guidelines for conceptual models from other disciplines, such as the Health Belief Model, are not always stated explicitly but may be extracted from books and articles about the use of the model as a guide for research or from analysis of the way in which research based on the model was conducted. Research focus guidelines for the three nursing grand theories we identified earlier are given in Table 5–4, which is on the CD.

HOW IS THE CRITERION OF LINKAGE ADEQUACY APPLIED?

Linkage adequacy draws attention to the connections between all three components of C-T-E structures. Application of the criterion of linkage adequacy helps you determine whether enough information about the connections among the C, T, and E components of the C-T-E structure was given in a research report. Enough information for this criterion means that you can understand exactly which conceptual model concepts and propositions guided the theory-generating research or theory-testing research, how those concepts and propositions were connected to the middle-range theory concepts and propositions, how the middle-range theory concepts and propositions were connected to the empirical research methods, and how the conceptual model influenced the selection of empirical research methods.

The criterion of linkage adequacy is met when you can answer yes to three questions:

• Are the C-T-E linkages stated explicitly in the research report?
• Are the linkages complete?
• Are the empirical research methods congruent with the conceptual model?

Are the C-T-E Linkages Explicit and Complete?

The criterion of linkage adequacy requires the links or connections between the C, T, and E components of the C-T-E structure to be stated explicitly. In other words, the research report should include statements describing exactly how one or more conceptual model concepts and propositions guided the research.

The criterion of linkage adequacy also requires the connections between the C, T, and E components to be complete. Although the research report should contain narrative statements expressing complete C-T-E linkages, evaluation of linkage adequacy may be easier if the C-T-E structure is illustrated in a diagram. If a diagram is not included, you can try to draw a diagram of the C-T-E structure based on the statements about the C-T-E linkages you find in the research report.

Recall from Chapter 2 that the flow of connections among the C, T, and E components differs for theory-generating research and theory-testing research.

C-T-E Linkages for Theory-Generating Research

In **theory-generating research**, the connections flow from the C component of the C-T-E structure to the E component and then to the T component.

The explanation of linkages given in theory-generating research reports usually starts with a statement of the connection between a particular conceptual model concept and a particular research instrument. The explanation of linkages may expand to encompass all elements of the empirical research methods, including the research design, the sample, the instruments and any experimental conditions, the procedures used to collect data, and the techniques used to analyze the data. The example in Box 5–4 includes statements that completely link a conceptual model concept to four elements of empirical research methods—research design, sample, instrument, and data analysis technique. The example also includes a statement linking the empirical research methods to the middle-range theory concept that was discovered in the data. The narrative linkage statements in Box 5–4 are illustrated in Figure 5–1; the diagram illustrates complete C-T-E linkages.

The linkage of a conceptual model concept and a research instrument may be explicitly stated in various ways. Three examples are given here:

- The personal system dimensions of perception, growth and development, and self-guided development of the *Caregiver Rewards Interview Guide* (see Box 5–4).
- Development of the *Caregiver Rewards Interview Guide* was based on the perception, growth and development, and self dimensions of the personal system.
- The items on the Caregiver Rewards Interview Guide reflect the personal system dimensions of perception, growth and development, and self.

Each example illustrates the linkage of three dimensions of a concept of King's Conceptual System—perception, which are dimensions of the concept of the personal system—to a research instrument called the *Caregiver Rewards Interview Guide.*

Conceptual model propositions provide some guidance for theory-generating research. In particular, propositions that are definitions of conceptual model concepts may influence the selection of study participants and development of research instruments. For example, in King's Conceptual System, the personal system is defined as individuals, and the dimension of perception is defined as "an awareness of persons, objects, and events" (King, 1981, p. 146). Therefore, research guided by King's concept of the personal system and her definition of perception would have to include individuals, rather than groups, as research participants, and a research instrument should contain items dealing with the individual's awareness of other people, objects in the environment, and relevant events.

C-T-E Linkages for Theory-Testing Research

In **theory-testing research**, the connections flow from the C component of the C-T-E structure to the T component and then to the E component.

BOX 5-4	Applying the Criterion of Linkage Adequacy for Theory-Generating Research

Are the C-T-E linkages explicit and complete?

King's personal system dimensions of perception, growth and development, and self-guided development of the *Caregiver Rewards Interview Guide,* used in descriptive qualitative theory-generating research to identify caregivers' awareness of rewards they experienced while caring for a family member with Alzheimer's disease. Content analysis of caregivers' responses to the *Caregiver Rewards Interview Guide* yielded the Theory of Awareness of Rewards of Caring for a Family Member With Alzheimer's Disease.

(In this example, a concept [personal system] from King's Conceptual System [the conceptual model], and three of the concept dimensions [perception, growth and development, and self] are linked to the research design [descriptive qualitative], the sample [caregivers of family members with Alzheimer's disease], the research instrument [*Caregiver Rewards Interview Guide*], and the data analysis technique [content analysis]. The example also indicates that content analysis of the data obtained from the interview guide led to development of the middle-range theory.)

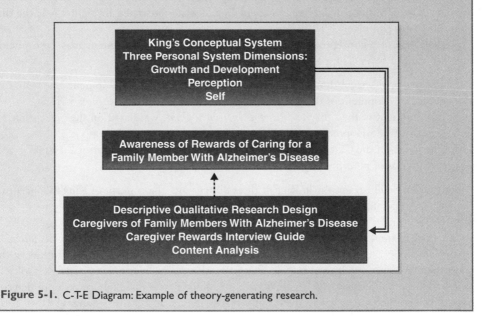

Figure 5-1. C-T-E Diagram: Example of theory-generating research.

The explanation of linkages given in theory-testing research reports usually starts with a statement of the connection between particular conceptual model concepts and particular middle-range theory concepts. The explanation expands to include the connection between each middle-range theory concept and particular elements of the empirical research methods, especially the research instruments. The example in Box 5–5 includes statements that completely link one conceptual model concept with one middle-range theory concept and then link the middle-range theory concept with one research instrument. Narrative linkage statements for an entire study of adaptation to motherhood, which are not included in Box 5–5 in the interest of brevity are illustrated in Figure 5–2; the diagram illustrates complete C-T-E linkages.

BOX 5-5	Applying the Criterion of Linkage Adequacy for Theory-Testing Research: Example of Concept Linkage

Are the C-T-E linkages explicit and complete?

Roy and Andrews (1999) explained that the overall adaptation level "represents the condition of the life processes" (p. 30). They identified three levels of adaptation: integrated, compensatory, and compromised. The integrated life process is the level of adaptation "at which the structures and functions of a life process are working as a whole to meet human needs" (p. 31). The compensatory life process is the level "at which the [coping mechanisms] have been activated by a challenge to the integrated life processes" (p. 31). The compromised life process is the level "resulting from inadequate integrated and compensatory life process" (p. 31) and signals a problem in adaptation. Adaptation level is represented in this study by adjustment to motherhood and is measured by the score for Question 11 on the Adaptation to Motherhood Interview Schedule.

(In this example, a concept [adaptation level] of Roy's Adaptation Model [the conceptual model] is linked to a middle-range theory concept [adjustment to motherhood], and that concept is linked to a research instrument [Adaptation to Motherhood Interview Schedule].)

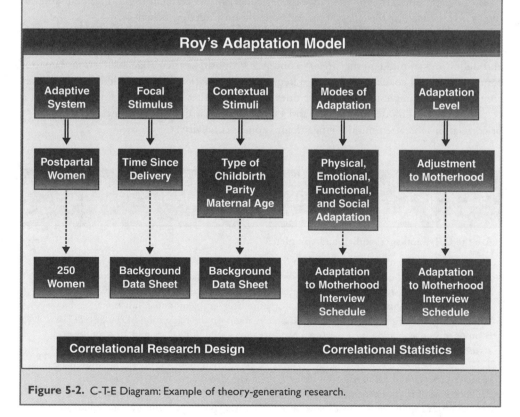

Figure 5-2. C-T-E Diagram: Example of theory-generating research.

Linkages between conceptual model concepts and middle-range theory concepts may be explicitly stated in various ways; three examples are:

- In this study, adaptation level was viewed as adjustment to motherhood.
- Adaptation level is represented by adjustment to motherhood.
- Adjustment to motherhood represents adaptation level.

These three examples are different ways to express the linkage between Roy's Adaptation Model concept, adaptation level, and the middle-range theory concept, adjustment to motherhood.

Linkages between middle-range theory concepts and research instruments also may be stated explicitly in various ways; two examples are given here:

- Adjustment to motherhood was measured by the score for Question 11 of the Adaptation to Motherhood Interview Schedule.
- The score for Question 11 of the Adaptation to Motherhood Interview Schedule was used to measure adjustment to motherhood.

In these examples, the middle-range theory concept is adjustment to motherhood, and the research instrument is the Adaptation to Motherhood Interview Schedule.

Conceptual model propositions guide the way that middle-range theory propositions are stated. Propositions that are definitions of conceptual model concepts influence the selection and definitions of middle-range theory concepts. Propositions that state associations between conceptual model concepts influence statements of association between middle-range theory concepts. The example in Box 5–6 includes a statement that expresses the linkage between a certain conceptual model proposition and a certain research aim that addresses the relations— or correlations—between middle-range theory concepts.brevity

---

BOX 5-6	Applying the Criterion of Linkage Adequacy for Theory-Testing Research: Example of Concept and Proposition Linkages

Are the C-T-E linkages explicit and complete?

A major proposition of the Roy Adaptation Model asserts that stimuli are related to adaptation. Accordingly, the aim of the present study was to examine the relation of variables representing the focal stimulus (time since delivery) and contextual stimuli (type of childbirth; parity, maternal age) to variables representing the four modes of adaptation (physical, emotional, functional, and social). Variables representing the stimuli were measured by items on the Background Data Sheet. The components of adaptation were measured by Questions 1 (physical), 2, 5, and 10 (emotional), 3 (functional), and 4 (social) on the Adaptation to Motherhood Interview Schedule.

(In this example, a Roy Adaptation Model [the conceptual model] proposition [stimuli are related to adaptation] is linked to a middle-range theory proposition [the relation of time since delivery, type of childbirth; parity, and maternal age to physical, emotional, functional, and social adaptation]. In addition, the links between the conceptual model concepts and the middle-range theory concepts can be identified; the middle-range theory concepts are referred to as variables and are named explicitly in the parentheses.)

Are the Empirical Research Methods Congruent With the Conceptual Model?

The criterion of linkage adequacy also requires that the empirical research methods be congruent with the conceptual model. You can determine whether this requirement was met in theory-generating research or theory-testing research by comparing the methods used with the research methods guidelines associated with the conceptual model that guided the study. The methods actually used should agree with the guidelines; an example is given in Box 5–7.

Research Methods Guidelines

The connections between the C, T, and E components of C-T-E structures should not only be stated explicitly and completely but also reflect the focus of the conceptual model as stated in research guidelines. We discussed the research focus guidelines, which draw attention to the connection between the C and T components, in the specification adequacy section of this chapter, and we list the research focus guidelines for seven conceptual models of nursing in Table 5–3, on the CD.

BOX 5-7   Applying the Criterion of Linkage Adequacy

Are the empirical research methods congruent with the conceptual model?

The sample for this Roy's Adaptation Model–guided correlational study was women who had given birth to a full-term infant three weeks prior to data collection. The open-ended items on the Adaptation to Motherhood Interview Schedule reflect the four Roy model modes of adaptation. Data were collected in the woman's home during the third postpartum week. Women's responses to the Adaptation to Motherhood Interview Schedule were categorized using content analysis, and an adaptation score was calculated for Questions 1, 2, 3, and 4 by dividing the total number of adaptive responses to the four questions by the total number of responses (adaptive and ineffective responses) to the four questions and multiplying by 100. The potential range of adaptation scores is 0 to 100, with higher scores indicating greater adaptation to motherhood. The relations between variables representing the focal and contextual stimuli (see Box 5–6) and adaptation to motherhood were tested using correlational statistics.

(This example extends information given in Boxes 5–5 and 5–6 and is based on the research methods guidelines for Roy's Adaptation Model found in Table 5–5 on the CD. The correlational study design is congruent with designs that are appropriate for research guided by Roy's Adaptation Model. The sample and the setting for data collection are congruent with the research methods guideline indicating that individuals can be research participants and that data can be collected in any health-care setting. The research instrument was directly derived from the modes-of-adaptation concept of Roy's model. The instrument yielded both qualitative data from open-ended questions and quantitative data from the adaptation score. The data analysis technique of content analysis is consistent with the research methods guidelines for Roy's model, as are correlational statistics. There is, however, no evidence that the statistical techniques took reciprocal relations between variables representing the four adaptive modes into account.)

Research methods guidelines deal with the empirical research methods, including who should be asked to participate in research; where research should take place; which research design, instruments, and procedures should be used; and how data should be analyzed. In other words, the research methods guidelines draw attention to the connection between the C and E components of C-T-E structures.

The research methods guidelines for seven nursing conceptual models we identified earlier in this chapter are given in Table 5–5, which is on the CD that comes with this book. Research methods guidelines for other conceptual models of nursing, such as the Synergy Model, and for conceptual models from other disciplines, such as the Health Belief Model, may not be stated explicitly, although they may be identified by reviewing the way researchers have conducted studies based on each model. Research methods guidelines for the three nursing grand theories we identified earlier are given in Table 5–6 on the CD.

WHAT IS THE CONCEPTUAL MODEL USAGE RATING SCALE?

Application of the criteria of specification adequacy and linkage adequacy helps you to understand exactly how the conceptual model or grand theory guided the theory-generating research or theory-testing research. Evaluation of the two criteria can be summarized by applying the **Conceptual Model Usage Rating Scale** (Box 5–8). This rating scale can be used with either conceptual model– or grand theory–guided research.

BOX 5-8	Conceptual Model Usage Rating Scale

Directions: Read a research report. Circle the number that best describes the extent to which the research report contains information about the conceptual model and its linkage to the middle-range theory and empirical research methods.

Rating Scale

0 = Missing
   The conceptual model is not named.
1 = Insufficient Use
   The conceptual model is named.
2 = Minimal Use
   The conceptual model is named and briefly summarized.
3 = Moderate Use
   The conceptual model is named and briefly summarized. The linkages of the conceptual model concepts and propositions with the middle-range theory concepts and propositions and the empirical research methods are evident.
4 = Adequate Use
   The conceptual model is named and summarized clearly and concisely. The linkages of the conceptual model concepts and propositions with the middle-range theory concepts and propositions and the empirical research methods are clearly stated and are complete.

Adapted from Fawcett, J. (1999). *The relationship of theory and research* (3rd ed., p. 88). Philadelphia: F. A. Davis, with permission.

The Conceptual Model Usage Rating Scale permits assignment of a number and a descriptive term to signify the extent to which the conceptual model is identified and described in the research report, as well as the extent to which the conceptual model concepts and propositions are linked explicitly with the middle-range theory concepts and propositions and with the empirical research methods. The rating scale points are 0 = Missing, 1 = Insufficient Use, 2 = Minimal Use, 3 = Moderate Use, and 4 = Adequate Use. Examples of the rating scale points are given in Boxes 5–9 to 5–13. The examples are for a fictitious theory-generating study of stressors experienced by chronically ill home health-care clients that was guided by Neuman's Systems Model (see Table 5–1 on the CD).

BOX 5-9	Application of the Conceptual Model Usage Rating Scale

0 = Missing
 The purpose of this descriptive study was to identify stressors experienced by chronically ill home health-care clients.

BOX 5-10	Application of the Conceptual Model Usage Rating Scale

1 = Insufficient Use
 The purpose of this Neuman's Systems Model–based descriptive study was to identify stressors experienced by chronically ill home health-care clients.

BOX 5-11	Application of the Conceptual Model Usage Rating Scale

2 = Minimal Use
 The purpose of this Neuman's Systems Model–based descriptive study was to identify stressors experienced by chronically ill home health-care clients. Neuman's conceptual model focuses on clients' reactions to three types of stressors—intrapersonal, interpersonal, and extrapersonal.

BOX 5-12	Application of the Conceptual Model Usage Rating Scale

3 = Moderate Use
 The purpose of this Neuman's Systems Model–based descriptive study was to identify stressors experienced by chronically ill home health-care clients. Neuman's conceptual model focuses on clients' reactions to three types of stressors—intrapersonal, interpersonal, and extrapersonal—as perceived by clients and their nurses. The Stressor Inventory, which was administered to pairs of home health-care clients and nurses, was used to identify specific stressors. The Theory of Chronic Illness Stressors was generated from content analysis of responses to the Stressor Inventory, which revealed that clients and nurses identified all three types of stressors.

BOX 5-13	Application of the Conceptual Model Usage Rating Scale

4 = Adequate Use

The purpose of this Neuman's Systems Model–based descriptive study was to identify stressors experienced by chronically ill home health-care clients. Neuman's conceptual model focuses on clients' reactions to three types of stressors—intrapersonal, interpersonal, and extrapersonal. Intrapersonal stressors occur within the client; interpersonal stressors occur in interactions between the client and other persons; and extrapersonal stressors occur between the client and the community. Neuman's Systems Model takes both the client's and the nurse's perceptions of stressors into account. The Stressor Inventory, which was administered to pairs of home health-care clients and nurses, contains open-ended questions about each type of stressor. The Theory of Chronic Illness Stressors was generated from content analysis of clients' and nurses' responses to the Stressor Inventory, using the three types of stressors as pre-existing categories. Both clients and nurses identified lack of knowledge about chronic illness as the intrapersonal stressor, conflicts with family members about lifestyle behaviors as the interpersonal stressor, and transportation difficulties as the extrapersonal stressor. The conceptual-theoretical-empirical structure for the study is illustrated in Figure 5–3.

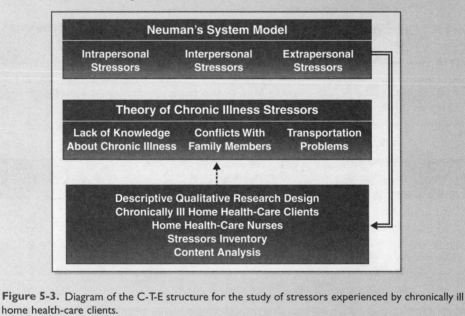

Figure 5-3. Diagram of the C-T-E structure for the study of stressors experienced by chronically ill home health-care clients.

Conclusion

In this chapter, you learned more about how to determine how good evidence given in reports of research is. Specifically, you learned how to evaluate the C component of C-T-E structures for theory-generating research and theory-testing research using the criterion of specification adequacy, and the connections between the C, T, and E components of C-T-E structures using the criterion of linkage adequacy. The questions to ask and answer as you evaluate the C-T-E linkages are listed in Box 5–14. The learning activities for this chapter will help you increase your understanding of the two criteria and their application to the contents of research reports.

BOX 5-14   Evaluation of Conceptual-Theoretical-Empirical Linkages: *How Good* Is the Information?

Specification adequacy

- Is the name of the conceptual model given in the research report?
- Is an overview of the conceptual model provided?
- Is the connection between the conceptual model and the research topic explained?

Linkage adequacy

- Are the C-T-E linkages stated explicitly in the research report?
- Are the linkages complete?
- Are the empirical research methods congruent with the conceptual model?

References

Full citations for all references cited in this chapter are provided in the Reference section at the end of the book.

Learning Activities

Activities to supplement what you have learned in this chapter, along with practice examination questions, are provided on the CD that comes with this book.

Chapter 6

Evaluation of Middle-Range Theories

This chapter focuses on the theory (T) component of conceptual-theoretical-empirical (C-T-E) structures for research.

KEYWORDS

Axiom	Premise
Deductive Reasoning	Reasoning
Explicit Middle-Range Theory	Semantic Clarity
Hypothesis	Semantic Consistency
Implicit Middle-Range Theory	Significance
Inductive Reasoning	Social Significance
Internal Consistency	Structural Consistency
Middle-Range Theory	Testability
Parsimony	Theorem
Postulate	Theoretical Significance

Recall from Chapter 2 that the T component of a C-T-E structure is the middle-range theory that was generated or tested by research. In that chapter, we defined a theory as a set of relatively concrete and specific concepts and propositions that are derived from the concepts and propositions of a conceptual model. We also pointed out that a middle-range theory guides research by providing the focus for the specific aims for the research. In Chapter 3 you began to learn *where* to look for information about the middle-range theory in research reports (Box 6–1) and *what* information you could expect to find (Box 6–2).

BOX 6-1	Evaluation of Middle-Range Theories: *Where Is* the Information?
Content about the middle-range theory may be found in every section of the research report.

BOX 6-2	Evaluation of Middle-Range Theories: *What Is* the Information?
The name of the middle-range theory

In Chapter 4, you began to learn how to determine *how good* the available information about the theory is. More specifically, in Chapter 4 we presented a framework for evaluation of the different components of C-T-E structures for theory-generating research and theory-testing research.

In this chapter, you will learn more about what middle-range theories are and how to evaluate them to determine *how good* the information about the T component for theory-generating research and theory-testing research is. After explaining how to identify a middle-range theory, we discuss in detail the four criteria in the framework identified in Chapter 4 for evaluating the T component of C-T-E structures—significance, internal consistency, parsimony, and testability—and provide examples that should help you better understand how to apply the criteria as you read research reports. Application of the criteria will facilitate your evaluation of *how good* the information about the middle-range theory provided in the research report is.

HOW IS THE MIDDLE-RANGE THEORY IDENTIFIED?

We believe that generating or testing a middle-range theory is the main reason for research. Consequently, a vast number of **middle-range theories** exist. Sometimes, the name of the middle-range theory is stated explicitly in the research report, but sometimes the middle-range theory is not stated explicitly and is only implied.

Explicit Middle-Range Theories

A review of research guided by seven different nursing conceptual models yielded more than 50 explicitly named middle-range theories that were directly derived from the conceptual models. The theories and the conceptual models from which they were derived are listed in Table 6–1 on the CD that comes with this book.

The conceptual frames of reference for three other explicit middle-range nursing theories were extracted from publications about the theories (Fawcett, 2005b). Although none of the theories were derived from a nursing conceptual model, statements reflecting some of the nursing metaparadigm concepts—human beings, environment, health, and nursing—were identified. The theories and relevant citations are:

1. Orlando's Theory of the Deliberative Nursing Process (Orlando, 1961; Schmieding, 2006)
2. Peplau's Theory of Interpersonal Relations (Peplau, 1952, 1997)
3. Watson's Theory of Human Caring (Watson, 1985, 2006)

The conceptual origins of many other explicitly named middle-range nursing theories are not yet clear; examples are listed in Table 6–2, which is included on the CD that comes with this book. Some explicitly named middle-range theories that are tested by nurse researchers come from other disciplines; examples are given in Table 6–3 on the CD. Additional information about the theories listed in Tables 6–2 and 6–3 can be found in Marriner Tomey and Alligood (2006), Peterson and Bredow (2004), Smith and Liehr (2003), and/or Ziegler (2005).

Although the conceptual frame of reference for the theories listed in Table 6–3 typically is not mentioned in the published research report, one such theory—the Theory of Planned Behavior (TPB)—was linked with Neuman's Systems Model and with Orem's Self-Care Framework by Villarruel and her colleagues (2001). They explained that the linkage placed the TPB within a nursing context and provided direction for a program of nursing research that could progress from "an explanation of the antecedents of behavioral actions to a prediction of the effects of nursing interventions on behavioral actions that are directed toward health promotion and disease prevention" (p. 160). They also explained that linkage of the TPB to a nursing conceptual model is needed if effects of interventions are to be studied, because interventions are not part of the TPB.

Implicit Middle-Range Theories

When the middle-range theory is implicit—that is, when it is not explicitly named—you may want to make up a name to increase your understanding of the theory. Finding the information

BOX 6-3	Naming an Implicit Middle-Range Theory

Example from a Theory-Generating Research Report

Study purpose

The purpose of this descriptive study was to identify patients' perceptions of fatigue during chemotherapy for Hodgkin's disease.

Results

Analysis of the patients' responses to an open-ended questionnaire revealed three categories of fatigue—exhausted, sleepy, and tired.

Possible names for the middle-range theory

• Perceptions of Fatigue Theory

• Theory of Categories of Chemotherapy Fatigue

Example from a Theory-Testing Research Report

Study purpose

The purpose of this experimental study was to determine the effect of exercise on chemotherapy-related fatigue.

Hypothesis

An increase in exercise will decrease chemotherapy-related fatigue.

Possible names for the middle-range theory

• Theory of the Effects of Exercise on Fatigue

• Exercise and Fatigue Theory

in a research report that may be used to identify a name for the theory can be challenging or even frustrating. Sometimes, the statement of the study purpose or aims can be used as the basis for the name of the theory. Or, you may have to rely on the categories or themes and their definitions in reports of theory-generating research and the study variables, definitions of variables, and hypotheses in reports of theory-testing research. Examples from fictitious studies are given in Box 6–3. (Recall that we discussed categories, themes, variables, definitions, and hypotheses in Chapter 2, and we identified where to look for the content of the T component in Chapters 3 and 4.)

HOW IS THE CRITERION OF SIGNIFICANCE OF A MIDDLE-RANGE THEORY APPLIED?

The criterion of **significance** of a middle-range theory draws attention to the importance of the theory to society and to the advancement of knowledge within a discipline. We call the importance of the theory to society its **social significance**, and the importance of the theory to advancement of knowledge its **theoretical significance**.

Application of the criterion of significance helps you determine whether enough information about social significance and theoretical significance is given in the research report. Enough information means that you can understand just how important the theory is to society and how the theory has filled a gap in or extended existing knowledge. The same amount of information about social significance and theoretical significance should be included in reports of both theory-generating research and theory-testing research.

The criterion of significance is met when you can answer yes to two questions:

- Is the middle-range theory socially significant?
- Is the middle-range theory theoretically significant?

Is the Middle-Range Theory Socially Significant?

The criterion of significance requires the middle-range theory to be socially significant. That means the theory is about people experiencing a health condition that currently is regarded as having some practical importance by the general public and members of one or more disciplines. The social significance of a middle-range theory is obvious when the theory focuses on a health condition, such as cancer, heart disease, or diabetes, that is experienced by a relatively large number of people. Social significance is also obvious when the theory focuses on a health condition that is experienced by a relatively small number of people but has a large impact on the quality of people's lives, such as spinal cord injury or mental illness. In other words, social significance is concerned with whether the health condition experienced by people is regarded as having a considerable actual or potential impact on desired lifestyle. The social significance of a middle-range theory typically is explained in a few sentences about the incidence of a particular health condition (Cowen, 2005). An example of social significance from Newman's (2005) study of correlates of functional status of caregivers of children in body casts is given in Box 6–4.

BOX 6-4	Example of Statement of Social Significance

The number of children who are placed in body casts each year is unknown. Observations in orthopedic clinics, however, indicate that a relatively small number of children are so treated. Mothers, fathers, and others who care for children in body casts face challenges that disrupt their usual pattern of daily living (Newman, 2005, p. 416).

(In this example, although a large number of children do not have a health condition requiring a body cast, their caregivers face considerable challenges.)

Is the Middle-Range Theory Theoretically Significant?

The criterion of significance also requires the middle-range theory to be theoretically significant. That means the theory offers new insights into the experiences of people who have a certain health condition. The theoretical significance of a nursing theory typically is explained in a concise summary of "what is known, what is not known, and how the results from [the research] advance . . . knowledge" (Cowen, 2005, p. 298). In other words, the information given in the research report about theoretical significance should tell you that the research focuses on the next meaningful step in the development of a theory about people with a certain health condition. Sometimes, a researcher will write that the research was conducted because nothing was known about the research topic. Such a statement does not meet the criterion of significance because it is possible that the topic is trivial and, therefore, the research is trivial. An example of an explanation of theoretical significance from Newman's study of correlates of functional status of caregivers of children in body casts is given in Box 6–5.

BOX 6-5	Example of Statement of Theoretical Significance

Developmental needs of the child, specific care requirements related to the body cast, and changes in parental functional status, health, psychological feelings, and family needs comprise typical challenges that must be faced by caregivers (Newman, 1997b; Newman & Fawcett, 1995). Previous studies of functional status during normal life transitions and serious illness have revealed that alterations in performance of usual role activities are influenced by demographic, health, psychological, and family variables (Tulman & Fawcett, 1996, 2003). This pilot study extended the investigation of correlates of functional status by examining the relation of personal health and self-esteem to functional status of caregivers of children in body casts [from] birth up to 3 years of age and [from] 3 to 12 years of age. The pilot study also provided data to determine the feasibility of a large-scale study. The long-term goal of the research is to assist caregivers to attain optimal functional status while caring for children in body casts (Newman, 2005, p. 416).

(In this example, the first two sentences tell you what is already known and include citations to previous research. The remaining three sentences tell you how the study extends knowledge, why it was conducted, and the long-term goal of the research.)

HOW IS THE CRITERION OF INTERNAL CONSISTENCY OF A MIDDLE-RANGE THEORY APPLIED?

Internal consistency draws attention to the comprehensibility of the middle-range theory. Application of the criterion of internal consistency helps determine whether enough information about the theory concepts and propositions is given in the research report. Enough information means that you can identify each concept and how the concepts are described and linked. The same amount of information about internal consistency should be included in reports of both theory-generating research and theory-testing research.

The criterion of internal consistency is met when you can answer yes to three questions:

- Is each concept of the middle-range theory explicitly identified and clearly defined?
- Are the same term and same definition used consistently for each concept?
- Are the propositions of the middle-range theory reasonable?

Is Each Middle-Range Theory Concept Explicitly Identified and Clearly Defined?

The criterion of internal consistency requires every concept of the theory to be explicitly identified and clearly defined. This requirement, which is called **semantic clarity** (Chinn & Kramer, 2004; Fawcett, 1999), is met when each concept can be identified and both theoretical and operational definitions for each concept are included in the research report. An example from Newman's (2005) study of correlates of functional status of caregivers of children in body casts is given in Box 6–6. (Recall from Chapter 2 that a constitutive definition provides meaning for a concept, and an operational definition indicates how the concept was measured.)

Semantic clarity requires that even concepts that are generally understood in everyday language must be clearly defined when used in theories. As Chinn and Kramer (2004) pointed out,

> Words like stress and coping have general common language meanings, and they also have specific theoretic meanings. . . . If words with multiple meanings are used in theory and not defined, a person's everyday meaning of the term, rather than what is meant in the theory, often is assumed; therefore, clarity is lost. (p. 110)

BOX 6-6	Example of Semantic Clarity of a Middle-Range Theory Concept

- **Concept:** Self-esteem
- **Constitutive definition:** Self-esteem "is defined as the caregiver's feelings of personal worth and value" (Newman, 2005, p. 417).
- **Operational definition:** Self-esteem was measured by Rosenberg's Self-Esteem Scale (Newman, 2005).

Are the Same Term and Same Definition Used Consistently for Each Middle-Range Theory Concept?

Semantic clarity is enhanced when the same term and same constitutive definition are used for each concept throughout the research report. The requirement for use of the same term and same constitutive definition is called **semantic consistency** (Chinn & Kramer, 2004; Fawcett, 1999). Although requiring use of the same term for the same concept may seem obvious, sometimes a researcher uses different labels for the same concept. For example, a researcher may reduce clarity by referring to both self-esteem and self-confidence in the same research report, although the theory focuses only on self-esteem. Chinn and Kramer (2004) explained,

> Normally, varying words to represent similar meanings is a writing skill that can be used to avoid overuse of a single term. But, in theory, if several similar concepts are used interchangeably when one would suffice, . . . the clarity of the [concept] is reduced rather than improved. (p. 110)

A researcher also may reduce clarity by using different constitutive definitions for the same concept. For example, if self-esteem is defined as "feelings of personal worth and value," that concept should not also be defined as "feelings of self-confidence" in the same research report. Different definitions of the same concept that are explicit are, as Chinn and Kramer (2004) noted, "fairly easy to uncover" (p. 111). In contrast, when a different definition is not explicit but only implied, the inconsistency may be more difficult to identify. Suppose, for example, that a researcher explicitly defined self-esteem as "feelings of personal worth and value" and then wrote about caregivers' feeling self-confident when bathing a child in a body cast. It would be difficult to know whether the researcher was referring to the caregivers' self-esteem or another concept when discussing feelings of self-confidence.

Sometimes a researcher may use more than one operational definition for the same concept. If all of the operational definitions identify instruments that measure the same constitutive definition of the concept, the requirement of semantic consistency is met. For example, using the constitutive definition given in Box 6–6, a researcher might operationally define self-esteem as measured by both Rosenberg's Self-Esteem Scale and a Personal Worth and Value Questionnaire that asks caregivers to rate their feelings of personal worth and value on a scale of 1 to 10, with 1 equivalent to feelings of very low personal worth and value and 10 equivalent to feelings of very high personal worth and value.

However, if the instruments identified in the operational definitions measure different constitutive definitions of the concept, the requirement of semantic consistency is not met. For example, again using the constitutive definition of self-esteem given in Box 6–6, a researcher might operationally define self-esteem as measured by the Personal Worth and Value Questionnaire, as well as a Self-Confidence Inventory, which measures self-esteem constitutively defined as "feelings of self-confidence."

Are the Middle-Range Theory Propositions Reasonable?

The criterion of internal consistency also requires the propositions of the theory to be reasonable. This requirement is called **structural consistency** (Chinn & Kramer, 2004;

Fawcett, 1999). Propositions are reasonable when they follow the rules of inductive or deductive reasoning. **Reasoning** is defined as "the processing and organizing of ideas in order to reach conclusions" (Burns & Grove, 2007, p. 16).

Inductive Reasoning

Inductive reasoning encompasses a set of particular observations and a general conclusion. This type of reasoning is "a process of starting with details of experience and moving to a general picture. Inductive reasoning involves the observation of a particular set of instances that belong to and can be identified as part of a larger set" (Liehr & Smith, 2006, p. 114). Inductive reasoning is most often found in reports of theory-generating research. Observations typically are quotations from study participants or are made by the researcher; the conclusion usually is referred to as a category or theme. The general form of inductive reasoning and an example from a fictitious study are given in Box 6–7.

Flaws in Inductive Reasoning

Flaws in inductive reasoning occur when a relevant observation is excluded (Kerlinger & Lee, 2000). For example, suppose that a researcher observed many white swans and concluded that all swans are white. The flaw would be discovered when another observation revealed a black swan. Or, suppose that a nurse observed that several people with a medical diagnosis of depression cried a lot and concluded that all people who cry are depressed. The flaw would be discovered when another observation revealed that people who were happy also cried. Consequently, when you evaluate the structural consistency of a middle-range theory in a theory-generating research report, consider whether the report includes a sufficient number and variety of observations to support each conclusion.

BOX 6-7	**Inductive Reasoning**

General form: Proceeds from the particular to the general
    Observation: A is an instance of x.
    Observation: B is an instance of x.
    Observation: C is an instance of x.
    Conclusion: A, B, and C make up x.
Example
    Observation: Doing household chores is a usual activity that is performed less frequently when a person is ill.
    Observation: Visiting friends is a usual activity that is performed less frequently when a person is ill.
    Observation: Exercising is a usual activity that is performed less frequently when a person is ill.
    Conclusion: All usual activities are performed less frequently when a person is ill.

Deductive Reasoning

Deductive reasoning encompasses a set of general propositions and a particular conclusion. This type of reasoning is "a process of starting with the general picture . . . and moving to a specific direction" (Liehr & Smith, 2006, p. 114). The general propositions of deductive reasoning typically are referred to as **premises**, **axioms**, or **postulates**; the particular conclusion is called a **theorem** or **hypothesis**. Premises, axioms, and postulates typically are drawn from literature reviews of previous research and are regarded as empirically adequate statements that do not have to be empirically tested again. A theorem or hypothesis, in contrast, must be tested by research. Deductive reasoning is most often found in reports of theory-testing research. The general form of deductive reasoning and an example constructed from Newman's (2005) study of correlates of functional status of caregivers of children in body casts are given in Box 6–8.

Flaws in Deductive Reasoning

Flaws in deductive reasoning occur when there is an error in a general proposition. Suppose, for example, that a researcher started with the premise that personal health status was related to functional status without providing any supporting research findings, added a premise that functional status was related to self-esteem, and then hypothesized that personal health status was related to self-esteem. The deduction in this example is flawed because the initial premise (personal health status is related to functional status) cannot be regarded as empirically adequate prior to testing the statement by conducting research. Although sets of deductive reasoning statements such as those seen in Box 6–8 are not usually found in research reports, the researcher should provide sufficient support for each hypothesis by citing relevant previous research as part of a critical review of the theoretical and empirical literature. Consequently, when you evaluate the structural consistency of a middle-range theory in a theory-testing research report, consider whether the report includes sufficient information to support any premises and each hypothesis.

BOX 6-8   Deductive Reasoning

General form: Proceeds from the general to the particular
    Premise: If x is related to y, and
    Premise: if y is related to z,
    Hypothesis: then x is related to z.
Example
    Premise: If personal health status is related to self-esteem, and
    Premise: if self-esteem is related to functional status,
    Hypothesis: then personal health status is related to functional status.

Example constructed from Newman (2005).

HOW IS THE CRITERION OF PARSIMONY OF THE MIDDLE-RANGE THEORY APPLIED?

Parsimony draws attention to the number of concepts and propositions that make up a middle-range theory. Application of the criterion of parsimony helps you determine whether the middle-range theory is stated as concisely as possible. The same standard of simplicity should be used to evaluate theories that were generated or tested.

The criterion of parsimony is met when you can answer yes to one question:

• Is the middle-range theory stated concisely?

Is the Middle-Range Theory Stated Concisely?

Parsimony requires that a middle-range theory be made up of as few concepts and propositions as necessary to clearly convey the meaning of the theory. Glanz (2002) referred to parsimony as "selective inclusion" of concepts (p. 546). Walker and Avant (2005) explained, "A parsimonious theory is one that is elegant in its simplicity even though it may be broad in its content" (p. 171).

The criterion of parsimony should not be confused with oversimplification of the content needed to convey the meaning of the theory. A theory should not be stated so simply that its meaning is lost. "Parsimony that does not capture the essential features of the [theory] is false economy" (Fawcett, 1999, p. 93). In other words, "A parsimonious theory explains a complex [thing] simply and briefly without sacrificing the theory's content, structure, or completeness" (Walker & Avant, 2005, p. 172).

A challenge in theory-generating research is to include all relevant data that were collected in one or just a few meaningful categories, rather than a large number of categories, subcategories, and sub-subcategories. For example, a researcher who regards household chores, visiting friends, and exercising as usual activities will present a much more parsimonious theory than a researcher who regards each of those activities as a separate category.

A challenge in theory-testing research is to determine whether the middle-range theory becomes more parsimonious as the result of testing. For example, Tulman and Fawcett (2003) found that several concepts and propositions of their Theory of Adaptation During Childbearing were not supported by their research. They concluded, "The collective quantitative results of our study revealed a somewhat more parsimonious version of the theory" (p. 151). Sometimes, a research report will include diagrams depicting the connections between the middle-range theory concepts before and after testing. Such diagrams can be helpful visual aids to evaluation of parsimony. Figure 6–1 depicts an example from a correlational study of the relations between type of cesarean birth and perception of the birth experience, perception of the birth experience and responses to cesarean birth, and type of childbirth and responses to cesarean birth (Fawcett et al., 2005).

As can be seen in the diagram, the middle-range theory before testing includes links between type of cesarean birth (unplanned and planned) and perception of the birth experience, perception of the birth experience and responses to cesarean birth, and type of cesarean birth and responses to cesarean birth (see Figure 6–1 part A). After testing, the theory includes

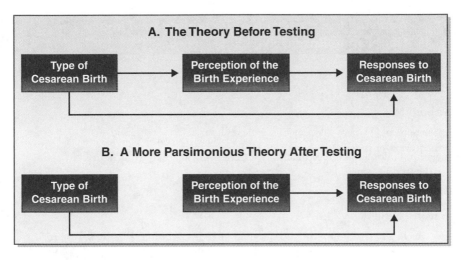

Figure 6-1. Diagrams of middle-range theory propositions before and after testing.

links only between perception of the birth experience and responses to cesarean birth, and type of cesarean birth and responses to cesarean birth (see Figure 6–1 part B). After testing, the theory is more parsimonious because no support was found for a link between type of cesarean birth and perception of the birth experience.

HOW IS THE CRITERION OF TESTABILITY OF THE MIDDLE-RANGE THEORY APPLIED?

Testability draws attention to whether the middle-range theory can be empirically tested. Application of the criterion of testability helps you determine whether enough information about the measurement of theory concepts is given in the research report. Enough information means that you can identify how each concept was operationally defined and how any associations between concepts were determined. The same amount of information about testability should be included in reports of both theory-generating research and theory-testing research.

The criterion of testability is met when you can answer yes to two questions:

• Was each concept measured?
• Were all assertions tested through some data analysis technique?

Was Each Concept Measured?

The criterion of testability requires each middle-range theory concept to be empirically observable—that is, measurable. The operational definition of the concept identifies the way in which it was measured. A diagram of the C-T-E structure for the research will help you to answer this question. If the research report does not include a C-T-E structure diagram, you can try to

BOX 6-9	Applying the Criterion of Testability for Theory-Generating Research

Conceptual Model

Roy's Adaptation Model

Conceptual Model Concept

Role function mode

Proposition Linking the Conceptual Model Concept to the Empirical Indicator

Development of the Usual Activities Interview Schedule was guided by the role function mode of adaptation.

Operational Definition

Content analysis of data from the Usual Activities Interview Schedule revealed one category, which was labeled "usual activities of ill people."

Middle-Range Theory Concept

Usual activities of ill people

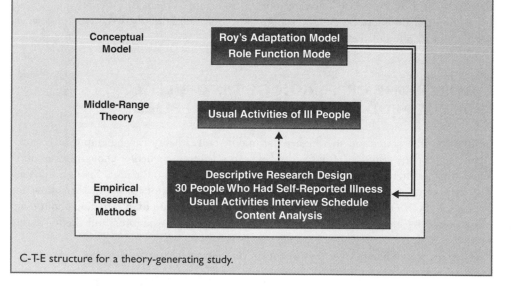

C-T-E structure for a theory-generating study.

draw one from the written information included in the report. The diagram will enable you to determine whether each concept is connected to an instrument or experimental conditions.

The example in Box 6–9 contains information from a fictitious theory-generating research report. The written information and the C-T-E diagram indicate that the criterion of testability was met. Suppose, however, that another category was mentioned in the report, such as special activities of ill people, and that no information about how the data used to generate the special activities category was given. In that instance, the diagram would not be complete and the criterion of testability would not have been met.

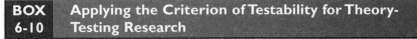

BOX 6-10 — **Applying the Criterion of Testability for Theory-Testing Research**

Conceptual Model

Roy's Adaptation Model

Conceptual Model Concepts

- Physiological mode
- Self-concept mode
- Role function mode

Propositions Linking the Conceptual Model and Middle-Range Theory Concepts

- The physiological mode was represented by personal health.
- The self-concept mode was represented by self-esteem.
- The role function mode was represented by functional status.

Middle-Range Theory Concepts

- Personal health
- Self-esteem
- Functional status

Operational Definitions

Personal health was measured by the Personal Health Questionnaire (PHQ). Self-esteem was measured by Rosenberg's Self-Esteem Scale (RSES). Functional status was measured by the Inventory of Functional Status–Caregiver of a Child in a Body Cast (IFSCCBC).

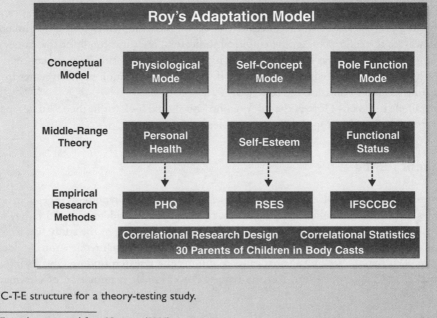

C-T-E structure for a theory-testing study.

Example constructed from Newman (2005).

The example in Box 6–10 contains information found in Newman's (2005) theory-testing research report. Although Newman did not include a C-T-E structure diagram, it was easily constructed from the written information in the conceptual framework and instruments subsections of the report. The written information and diagram reveal that the criterion of testability was met. Suppose, however, that Newman had not included an operational definition for one of the concepts. In that instance, the diagram would not be complete and the criterion of testability would not have been met.

Were All Assertions Tested Through Some Data Analysis Technique?

The criterion of testability requires each assertion made by the middle-range theory propositions to be measurable through some data analysis technique. Although most theory-generating research focuses on the description of a health-related experience in the form of one or a few concepts that are not connected to one another, some theory-generating research reports include propositions that state an association between two concepts. Suppose, for example, that a researcher generated a theory of usual activities of ill people from data collected from a group of chronically ill people and a group of acutely ill people. Suppose also that the researcher looked at the list of usual activities for each group, concluded that acutely ill people performed different usual activities than chronically ill people, and included a proposition stating that there is an association between the type of illness and the type of usual activities performed. In this example, a proposition stating an association between two concepts—type of illness and usual activities—was generated simply through visual inspection of the data.

Theory-testing research, in contrast, frequently involves use of statistical procedures to systematically test associations between two or more concepts. In theory-testing research, propositions stating associations between concepts, especially when the names of the instruments used to measure the concepts (i.e., the empirical indicators) are substituted for the names of the concepts, are referred to as hypotheses. Each hypothesized association between concepts is tested using a statistical procedure to determine if there is an association between scores from the instruments used to measure the concepts.

The example in Box 6–11 gives the information you should look for in the research report to determine whether the proposition was testable.

Hypothesis Testing

Theory-testing research involves tests of hypotheses. Sometimes, the hypothesis is explicit, and sometimes it is implicit. Explicit hypotheses are, of course, easy to identify because they are labeled as such. For example, a researcher may state that the purpose of the study was to test a particular hypothesis, or a few hypotheses will be listed in the research report. You can identify any implicit hypotheses by systematically examining the research findings and listing all the statistical procedures mentioned in the report. For example, examination of Newman's

BOX 6-11	Example of Testability of a Proposition Stating an Association Between Two Concepts

Middle-Range Theory Concepts

• Personal health

• Functional status

Proposition

There is a relation between personal health and functional status.

Operational Definitions

• Personal health was measured by the Personal Health Questionnaire (PHQ).

• Functional status was measured by the Inventory of Functional Status–Caregiver of a Child in a Body Cast (IFSCCBC).

Hypothesis

There is a relation between scores on the PHQ and scores on the IFSCCBC.

Statistical Procedure

A Pearson coefficient of correlation was used to determine the correlation between scores from the PHQ and the IFSCCBC.

Example constructed from Newman (2005).

(2005) research report revealed that she used a correlation coefficient to test the implicit hypothesis of a relation between scores on the Personal Health Questionnaire (PHQ) and scores on the Inventory of Functional Status–Caregiver of a Child in a Body Cast (IFSCCBC).

Hypotheses should be falsifiable (Popper, 1965; Schumacher & Gortner, 1992). That means that the way in which the hypothesis is stated should allow the researcher to conclude that the hypothesis was rejected if the data do not support the assertion made in the hypothesis. For example, suppose that a researcher hypothesized that all mothers and fathers have high, medium, or low scores on the IFSCCBC and high, medium, or low scores on the PHQ. The hypothesis cannot be falsified because it does not eliminate any logically or practically possible results. In contrast, the hypothesis that all mothers and fathers have medium scores on the PHQ and low scores on the IFSCCBC can be falsified because it asserts that the mothers and fathers will not have high or low scores on the PHQ and will not have high or medium scores on the IFSCCBC.

In addition, it is not correct to conclude that a hypothesis was partially supported. For example, suppose that a researcher hypothesized that both mothers' and fathers' scores on the PHQ were related to their scores on the IFSCCBC and that the results indicated that the hypothesis was supported only by the data from the mothers. It would not be correct to conclude that the hypothesis was partially supported because the mothers' data supported the hypothesis. Rather, the correct conclusion is that the hypothesis is rejected.

BOX 6-12	Evaluation of Middle-Range Theories: How Good Is the Information?

Significance

• Is the middle-range theory socially significant?

• Is the middle-range theory theoretically significant?

Internal Consistency

• Is each concept of the middle-range theory explicitly identified and clearly defined?

• Are the same term and same definition used consistently for each concept?

• Are the propositions of the middle-range theory reasonable?

Parsimony

• Is the middle-range theory stated concisely?

Testability

• Was each concept measured?

• Were all assertions tested through some data analysis technique?

Conclusion

In this chapter, you continued to learn about how to determine how good the information about a middle-range theory given in a research report is. Specifically, you learned how to evaluate the T component of C-T-E structures using the criteria of significance, internal consistency, parsimony, and testability. The questions to ask and answer as you evaluate the middle-range theory are listed in Box 6–12. Application of these four criteria should help you to better understand the link between the T and E components of C-T-E structures. The learning activities for this chapter will help you increase your understanding of the four criteria and their application to the contents of research reports.

References

Full citations for all references cited in this chapter are provided in the Reference section at the end of the book.

Learning Activities

Activities to supplement what you have learned in this chapter, along with practice examination questions, are provided on the CD that comes with this book.

Part Three

Evaluation of Empirical Research Methods

Chapter 7

Evaluation of Research Designs for Theory-Generating and Theory-Testing Research

This chapter and several of the following chapters focus on the empirical research methods, or E component, of conceptual-theoretical-empirical (C-T-E) structures for theory-generating and theory-testing research. Specifically, this chapter focuses on the research design element of the empirical research methods (E) component of C-T-E structures.

KEYWORDS

Action Research

Bivariate Research Design

Canonical Correlational Model

Case Study Research

Clinical Trial

Concept Analysis

Control Treatment

Correlational Research Design

Critical Emancipatory Paradigm

Crossover Design

Delphi Technique

Descriptive Theory

Descriptive Research Design

Ethnography

Ethnonursing Research Methodology

Evaluation Research

Experimental Treatment

Experimental Research Design

Explanatory Theory

Exploratory Research

Factorial Designs

Focus Group Research

Grounded Theory

Hermeneutics

Human Becoming Hermeneutic Method of Basic Research

Interrupted Time-Series Design

Instrument Development

Mixed Method Research

Model-Testing Designs

Multiple Regression

N-of-1 Randomized Controlled Trial

Naturalistic Paradigm

Nonequivalent Control Group Designs

Nonequivalent Control Group Pretest-Posttest Design

One-Group Pretest-Posttest Design

One-Group Posttest-Only Design

Operational Adequacy

Outcomes Research

Parse Basic Research Method

Continued

Recall from Chapter 2 that the E component of a C-T-E structure encompasses five major elements—the research design, the sample, the instruments and any experimental conditions, the procedures used to collect data and protect participants from harm, and the techniques used to analyze the data. This chapter presents an overview of one of these elements—research designs typically found in the literature of the health sciences, with an emphasis on nursing science. Recall from Chapters 3 and 4 that you began to learn *where* to look for information about the research design in research reports (Box 7–1) and *what* information you could expect to find (Box 7–2).

BOX 7-1	Evaluation of Research Design: *Where* Is the Information?

• Look in the method section of the research report
• May be a separate subsection for research design

BOX 7-2	Evaluation of Research Design: *What* Is the Information?

• The overall plan for conducting a study
• A blueprint
• A set of directions for the other elements of the E component of C-T-E structures

In Chapter 4, we presented a framework for evaluating C-T-E structures for research and explained how to determine *how good* the information about the research design is. In this chapter, we explain *what* research designs are used for theory-generating research and theory-testing research and more about how to determine *how good* the information about the research design is. More specifically, in this chapter we discuss in detail the criterion of **operational adequacy**, introduced in Chapter 4, as it applies to research design and provide examples that should help you better understand how to apply the criterion as you read research reports. Application of the criterion will facilitate your evaluation of *how good* the information about the research design provided in the research report is.

WHAT IS RESEARCH DESIGN?

Recall from Chapter 2 that theory-generating research focuses on discovery of middle-range theories and theory-testing research involves empirical tests of middle-range theories. **Research design**, whether for theory-generating research or theory-testing research, refers to the overall plan for conducting a study. The research design can be thought of as a blueprint or instructions for the way a study is conducted (Burns & Grove, 2007; Kerlinger & Lee, 2000; LoBiondo-Wood, 2006). Thus, the research design serves as a guide or set of directions for the other elements of the E component of a C-T-E structure—that is, the way in which the sample is selected, the type of instruments and any experimental conditions used, the procedures used to collect the data and protect participants from harm, and the techniques used to analyze the data. As we will explain later in this chapter, each of the three broad types of research we identified in Chapter 1—descriptive, correlational, and experimental—encompasses several specific research designs.

WHAT ARE THE PHILOSOPHICAL PARADIGMS ASSOCIATED WITH RESEARCH DESIGNS?

Research designs used to guide the study of human beings and human behavior were adapted from methods used by scholars in ancient times to think about and study the world, and more recently by 19th-century physicists and chemists to study the physical world (Babbie, 1990; Rolfe, 2006). Each research design reflects certain philosophical beliefs about how knowledge is developed—that is, how we learn about the world and how things can be known (Salsberry, 1994). Different sets of philosophical beliefs are referred to as **philosophical paradigms** or **worldviews**.

The three philosophical paradigms most often cited in connection with research designs are the naturalistic paradigm, the critical emancipatory paradigm, and the postpositivist paradigm (Ford-Gilboe, Campbell, & Berman, 1995; Giuliano, Tyer-Viola, & Lopez, 2005; Weaver & Olson, 2006). We agree with Weaver and Olson that each paradigm makes an equally valuable contribution to the development of knowledge and that knowledge gained from research conducted within the various paradigms is "sought and valued for its contributions in describing, interpreting, explaining and predicting the complexity of human health experiences and illness responses" (p. 467). The main features of each paradigm are listed in Box 7–3.

BOX 7-3	Philosophical Paradigms Associated With Research Designs

Naturalistic Paradigm

- Focuses attention on understanding the meaning of people's health-related experiences
- Emphasis is on disclosing meanings of health-related experiences.
- Goal is understanding.
- Typically associated with qualitative research designs

Critical Emancipatory Paradigm

- Focuses attention on how historical, cultural, gender, economic, social, and political factors influence people's perceptions and experiences of health
- Goal is emancipation.
- Typically associated with qualitative research designs

Postpositivist Paradigm

- Focuses attention on descriptions, explanations, and predictions about patterns and regularities in people's health-related experiences
- Emphasis is on constructing meanings of health-related experiences.
- Ultimate goal is prediction and control.
- Typically associated with quantitative research designs

Naturalistic Paradigm

The **naturalistic paradigm**, which is also referred to as the **interpretive paradigm** or the **humanistic paradigm**, draws attention to the subjectivity of human beings and their behavior. This means that research participants' descriptions of their own health-related experiences are central to research. The naturalistic paradigm is most closely associated with what some scholars call **human science** and what Rawnsley, a nurse scientist interviewed by Fawcett (2002), calls **human science 2**. Human science, Rawnsley explained, "can include anything that focuses on those characteristics specific to human beings . . . [and] human behavior" (Fawcett, p. 42). Human science 2 research focuses on the "understanding of life as it lived . . . [by] disclosing the meaning of [human beings'] experiences (Fawcett, p. 43). Moreover, human science 2 research is **value laden**, which means that what human beings believe to be true and good is an important aspect of the research.

The goal of naturalistic paradigm nursing research is to describe people's understanding of the meaning of some health-related experience (Ford-Gilboe et al., 1995; Weaver & Olson, 2006). For example, Bauer (2006) conducted a study within the context of the naturalistic paradigm. The study focused on Australian nursing home staff members' experiences of working with residents' families. Bauer noted that the naturalistic paradigm "acknowledges that all aspects of reality are interrelated and that reality cannot be separated from the world in which it is experienced. People's experiences of reality can, therefore, not be understood or described without reference to their interrelationships or contexts" (p. 46).

Critical Emancipatory Paradigm

The **critical emancipatory paradigm** extends the naturalistic paradigm by placing human beings and human behavior within the context of their history, culture, gender, and economic, social, and political situations. This paradigm also is referred to as the **critical social theory paradigm**. Research guided by this paradigm emphasizes the influence of oppression and discrimination—in the form of social class and power struggles—on people's behavior. Emphasis is also placed on raising "awareness of social problems and . . . ensur[ing] that the voices and perspectives of marginalized people are heard" (Weaver & Olson, 2006, p. 464). Thus, researchers must be aware of their own and other researchers' biases. The results of research conducted within the context of the critical emancipatory paradigm are directed toward actions that will create changes in society; the goal is emancipation (Weaver & Olson). A general example of research conducted within the context of the critical social theory paradigm is provided by Marcellus' (2003) discussion of the health-related effects of pregnant women's drug and alcohol misuse on their children during infancy and later life. She pointed out,

> Because nursing is a practice profession, it is not enough to critique theories. . . . Criticism that is not connected to action is incapable of affecting change. . . . A key issue [for nurses, expectant and new mothers, children born of women who misused substances during pregnancy, and health-care professionals] then becomes one of working together and developing services that are supportive of women in their drug use and recovery yet responsible enough to identify when a child is at risk. (p. 448)

The **feminist research perspective** can be regarded as a special case of the critical emancipatory paradigm, in that the emphasis is on "gender discrimination and discrimination within patriarchal societies" (Polit & Beck, 2006, p. 225). Im and Chee (2003) used a feminist research perspective to explore issues in the use of e-mail group discussions involving women and men with cancer. Their discussion of the study included comments on the intersubjectivity between the researcher and the research participants. They explained,

> Intersubjectivity between researcher and participant and the mutual creation of data . . . are essential components of research from a feminist perspective. . . . Feminists propose that research should not be conducted on the basis of distant relationships between researchers and research participants, as dictated by traditional scientific research methodology [that is, the postpositivist paradigm]. Rather, in feminist research, "intersubjectivity" is emphasized and findings are usually shared with participants. (p. 291)

The critical social theory paradigm can be an informative lens through which to view nursing education research. For example, Freire (1972) wrote that liberation from oppression occurs through reflection and taking actions directed toward the conditions that encourage or permit oppression. Mooney and Nolan (2006) commented that nursing education research guided by Freire's interpretation of critical social theory "may contribute towards the development of nurses who will be competent to meet the demands of contemporary healthcare practice" (p. 240).

Postpositivist Paradigm

The **postpositivist paradigm**, which is an extension of **logical positivism** and sometimes is referred to as **postmodernism**, **neomodernism**, or **empiricism**, most closely resembles the objective perspective of the physicists, chemists, and other scientists who study the physical world. However, postpositivism allows not only for objectivity but also for subjectivity in that research participants' own words and their perceptions of their health-related experiences are considered as important as objective data from biophysical measures, such as vital signs and laboratory tests. Furthermore, the postpositivist paradigm, which Rawnsley equated with what she called **human science 1**, focuses on "constructing the meaning of experiences" within the context of conceptual models and middle-range theories (Fawcett, 2002, p. 43). Consequently, human science 1 research is **theory laden**.

The emphasis in postpositivist theory-testing research is on falsifying hypotheses, rather than confirming them (Weaver & Olson, 2006). Although research conducted within the postpositivist paradigm is thought to be value free (Lincoln & Guba, 1985), many researchers recognize that what they personally value is an important influence on what they study. For example, Garity's (2006) long-standing interest in the experiences of caregivers of family members with Alzheimer's disease is evident in her study of caregivers' feelings after placing their loved one in a nursing home. In addition, societal values, when translated into policies, influence what researchers study, or at least what can be studied with financial support from federal governments and private foundations. Societal values also influence what is considered ethically acceptable to study. The ultimate goal of postpositivist paradigm research is prediction and control (Weaver & Olson). For example, McCaffrey and Freeman's (2003) interest in helping people control their pain led to their test of a predictive middle-range theory of the effect of a music intervention on pain control.

WHAT ARE THE MAJOR TYPES OF RESEARCH DESIGNS?

Research designs are divided into two major categories—qualitative and quantitative. We have summarized the special features of qualitative and quantitative research designs in Box 7–4 and Box 7–5. A combination qualitative and quantitative research design is also sometimes used. We discuss each category in more detail here.

Qualitative Research Designs

Qualitative research designs, which typically are used to generate descriptive middle-range theories, are most simply characterized by data that are words. The words may be written answers to one or more open-ended questions or they may be spoken answers to one or more open-ended questions asked by the researcher who transcribes them as a written narrative. An example of an open-ended question is: "What does feeling healthy mean to you?"

Most qualitative research designs are associated with the naturalistic paradigm or the critical emancipatory paradigm (see Box 7–3). Accordingly, these research designs are regarded as

BOX 7-4	Characteristics of Qualitative Research Designs

- Associated with the naturalistic paradigm or the critical emancipatory paradigm
- Data are words.
- Reality is viewed from the research participant's perspective.
- Approach is holistic.
- Focuses on understanding the whole of people's health-related experiences
- Small number of participants used
- One or more concepts identified, each of which is made up of several themes or categories
- Research participants are in their natural settings.
- Data collection and analysis may occur simultaneously.

BOX 7-5	Characteristics of Quantitative Research Designs

- Associated primarily with the postpositivist paradigm
- Data are numbers.
- Reality is viewed from the researcher's perspective.
- Focuses on parts rather than wholes
- Targeted to particular aspects of people's health-related experiences
- Large number of participants used
- Few concepts/study variables usually involved
- Research participants may be in natural or contrived settings.
- Data collection typically precedes data analysis.

holistic approaches that focus on understanding the whole of a certain thing—called a **phenomenon**—such as people's health-related experiences.

Qualitative research designs focus on interpretation of the meanings people give to a phenomenon. This type of research design frequently involves collection of data in natural settings—that is, settings where the people whose experiences are of interest are located and where they feel most comfortable. Data collection in the natural setting typically starts with one or more broad, open-ended research questions that are answered in each research participant's own words. If the data are written answers to questions, each person's participation in the study may end once the answers are provided. If, however, the data are spoken answers, each person's participation in the study may continue as the researcher asks additional questions based on the participant's answers to clarify or expand the meaning of the answers to the initial questions. The data, therefore, represent each research participant's subjective response, viewpoint, thoughts, and/or feelings.

Qualitative research typically involves a relatively small number of research participants but a large number of themes or categories making up a concept.

Researchers who use qualitative research designs often are regarded as the research instrument for data collection because they ask questions and analyze answers in an attempt to identify the meaning of the phenomenon being studied to each participant. The researcher may ask questions and analyze answers simultaneously. That is, the researcher may collect data from one person, analyze those data, and then collect more data from another person. As the data are analyzed, the researcher may identify other questions that then are asked of the next person from whom data are collected. Consequently, qualitative research designs tend to be quite flexible.

Quantitative Research Designs

Quantitative research designs, which sometimes are used to generate descriptive middle-range theories but more frequently are used to test descriptive, explanatory, and predictive middle-range theories, are most simply characterized by data that are numbers. Most quantitative research designs are associated with the postpositivist paradigm (Box 7–3), although quantitative designs also can be used within the context of the naturalistic or critical emancipatory paradigm (Ford-Gilboe et al., 1995). Quantitative research designs are regarded as targeted approaches that focus on understanding particular aspects of people's health-related experiences.

These research designs typically involve a relatively large number of research participants who are measured on a small number of concepts, or study variables. Quantitative research designs also typically employ one or more research instruments selected by the researcher prior to the beginning of the study to measure particular concepts. The research instruments usually are biophysiological equipment, such as the equipment used to measure blood pressure, or questionnaires made up of items that are rated by research participants on a numerical scale with word descriptors, such as 0 = none of the time, 1 = some of the time, and 2 = all the time. Additional research instruments rarely are added as the study progresses. Although the data represent each research participant's responses, those responses are limited to readings from technical devices and the scores for questionnaire items. Researchers who use quantitative research designs are not regarded as the research instrument regardless of how involved they may be in the collection and analysis of the data. Typically, most, if not all data are collected before analyses begin. Consequently, quantitative research designs are not flexible.

Combined Qualitative and Quantitative Research Designs

Sometimes, researchers combine qualitative and quantitative research designs concurrently in one study or sequentially in a series of related studies, so that some data are words and other data are numbers (Creswell, 2003). At other times, researchers may attach numbers to word data, such as the number or percentage of research participants whose words reflected a particular theme. Or, words may be converted to numbers by calculating a range of scores from categories of words. For example, within the context of the Roy Adaptation Model, an adaptation score ranging from 0 to 100 can be calculated by dividing the number of responses to an open-ended question classified as positive by the total number of positive plus negative responses and multiplying the result by 100 (Fawcett, 2006).

When qualitative and quantitative research designs are combined, it is likely that more than one philosophical paradigm has guided the research (Weaver & Olson, 2006). For example, the qualitative portion of a study might be guided by the naturalistic paradigm or the critical emancipatory paradigm, and the quantitative portion might be guided by the postpositivist paradigm.

The combination of qualitative and quantitative research designs sometimes is referred to as "**multi-method research**" (Kerlinger & Lee, 2000, p. 592) or a "**mixed method**" design (Polit & Beck, 2006, p. 244). This type of research design is defined as "research in which the investigator collects and analyzes data, integrates the findings, and draws inferences using both qualitative and quantitative approaches or methods in a single study or program of inquiry" (Creswell & Tashakkori, 2006). Sandelowski (2000) pointed out that mixed method designs can involve combinations of "sampling, data collection, and data analysis techniques commonly . . . conceived as qualitative or quantitative" (p. 248).

In mixed method research, a quantitative theory-testing study may include a qualitative component. This approach frequently is accomplished by asking research participants to first respond to research instruments, such as questionnaires, made up of several items that are rated and scored using numbers, followed by one or more open-ended questions that are answered in words. Powel and Clark (2005) referred to the responses to such open-ended questions as "marginalia" (p. 828). Conversely, a qualitative theory-generating study may include a quantitative component. This approach can be accomplished by first asking research participants to respond to one or more open-ended questions that are answered in words followed by one or more questionnaires made up of items that are rated and scored using numbers.

In each approach, the additional data typically are used for one or more of three purposes of mixed method designs: (a) **triangulation**, to achieve or ensure corroboration of data, or convergent validation; (b) **complementarity**, to clarify, explain, or otherwise more fully elaborate the results of analyses; and (c) **development**, to guide the use of additional sampling, and data collection and analysis techniques (Greene, Caracelli, & Graham, cited in Sandelowski, 2000, p. 248).

Polit and Beck (2006) pointed out that the gradual progress that is characteristic of theory development can be facilitated by mixed-method designs, in that the complementary use of qualitative and quantitative data capitalizes on the strengths of both words and numbers, allowing each type of data "to do what it does best, possibly avoiding the limitations of a single approach" (p. 245). In addition, they noted that inconsistencies found in the qualitative and quantitative data of a single mixed method study can advance theory development in previously unexpected ways.

When qualitative and quantitative research designs are combined, one type of design may be dominant and the other type "nested" within the dominant type (Kerlinger & Lee, 2000, p. 593; Padgett, 1998). For example, Lewandowski, Good, and Draucker (2005) explained that they used a "mixed method (QUAN + qual) concurrent nested design (experimental + descriptive)" to study the effects of guided imagery treatments on pain and power as knowing participation in change (p. 60). Their study, which was based on Rogers' Science of Unitary Human Beings, focused primarily on analysis of responses to questionnaires that yielded numerical scores (Lewandowski, 2004) but also included analysis of the words research participants used to respond to the request, "Describe to me your pain right now" (Lewandowski et al., p. 62).

HOW IS THE CRITERION OF OPERATIONAL ADEQUACY APPLIED TO RESEARCH DESIGN?

When applied to the research design element of empirical research methods, the criterion of **operational adequacy** refers to the amount of information about the research design given in a research report and focuses attention on whether the design was appropriate for the theory-generating research or theory-testing research reported.

The operational adequacy criterion, when applied to research design, is met when you can answer "yes" to two questions:

* Is the research design identified in the research report?
* Did the research design allow the research questions to be answered?

Is the Research Design Identified in the Research Report?

The research design may or may not be explicitly identified in a research report. An example of explicit identification of the research design is: "A quasi-experimental, completely randomized design was used" to investigate the effects of guided imagery therapy on ratings of pain and feelings of power for people experiencing chronic pain" (Lewandowski, 2004, p. 235).

If the research design is not identified explicitly, you may be able to identify it by reviewing the purpose of the research. For example, Gigliotti (2004) did not explicitly identify the research design she used to study the etiology of maternal-role stress. However, examination of the main research question—"What is the relationship among maternal role involvement, student role involvement, total network support, and maternal-student role stress in mothers attending college who are and are not in concurrent mid-life developmental transition?" (Gigliotti, p. 160)—suggests that she probably used a correlational research design because the research question referred to the relation between variables. Further examination of Gigliotti's research report revealed that she used correlational statistical techniques, which supports the presumption of a correlational research design.

Did the Research Design Allow the Research Questions to Be Answered?

The most important function of research designs is "to provide answers to research questions" (Kerlinger & Lee, 2000, p. 450). A research design is able to provide answers to research questions when it *fits* those questions. "Fit," Macnee and McCabe (2008) explained, "refers to how well the design matches the question of interest" (p. 195). We prefer to think of "fit" as the extent to which the research design matches the type of middle-range theory that was generated or tested. In other words, we view the research design as the plan for the empirical aspects of the way in which a middle-range theory is generated or tested.

The research question may be written in a research report as one or more actual questions (Box 7–6), or it may be written as a narrative statement of the purpose of the research. For example, the research question for Callaghan's (2005) study, shown in Box 7–6 as an actual question, could be stated as: "The purpose of this correlational study was to examine the relation between adolescents' spiritual growth and their self-care agency."

Alternatively, the research question could be written as one or more specific aims. The research question for Thomas-Hawkins' (2005) study, shown in Box 7–6 as an actual question, could, for example, be stated as: "A specific aim of this instrument development study was to estimate the construct validity of the revised Inventory of Functional Status–Dialysis." Note that in both examples, the research design was identified—a correlational design for Callaghan's study and instrument development (a type of descriptive research design) for Thomas-Hawkins' study.

As we explained in Chapter 5, research questions are also shaped by the conceptual model that guided the study. Two of the studies cited in Box 7–6 serve as examples. DeSanto Madeya (2006b) used Roy's Adaptation Model to guide her theory-generating study and, therefore, focused on how people with a spinal cord injury and their family members adapted to living with the injury. Melancon and Miller (2005) used Levine's Conservation Model to guide their theory-testing study and, therefore, were interested in the extent to which the experimental massage therapy affected patients' perceptions of pain relief from the perspective of Levine's principle of the conservation of structural integrity, which "refers to maintaining or restoring the structure of the body, that is, preventing physical breakdown and promoting healing" (Levine, 1988, p. 227).

BOX 7-6   Examples of Research Questions for Theory-Generating and Theory-Testing Research Designs

Descriptive Theory-Generating Research—Descriptive Research Design

What is the experience of adapting to living with a spinal cord injury for the injured person and family members? (DeSanto Madeya, 2006b)

Descriptive Theory-Testing Research—Descriptive Research Design

What is the construct validity of the revised Inventory of Functional Status-Dialysis? (Thomas-Hawkins, 2005)

Explanatory Theory-Testing Research—Correlational Research Design

What is the relation between adolescents' spiritual growth and their self-care agency? (Callaghan, 2005)

Predictive Theory-Testing Research—Experimental Research Design

What is the difference in perception of relief of low back pain of patients who received massage therapy and patients who received traditional therapy? (Melancon & Miller, 2005)

As explained in Chapters 1 and 2, there are three types of middle-range theories, each generated and tested by a specific type of research. Descriptive middle-range theories are generated and tested by means of descriptive research; the research may be qualitative, quantitative, or a combination of both. Explanatory middle-range theories are tested by means of correlational research, and predictive middle-range theories are tested by means of experimental research. (See Box 7–6 for examples of research questions and research designs for generating descriptive middle-range theories and testing descriptive, explanatory, and predictive middle-range theories.)

Descriptive Research Designs Used to Generate Descriptive Middle-Range Theories

Descriptive research designs are used to generate or to test middle-range theories by providing answers to questions about the characteristics of concepts. A descriptive middle-range theory provides names for things—that is, **phenomena**—or for classifications of the characteristics, also referred to as attributes or properties, of things.

The basic research question answered by all descriptive research designs is:

- What is x?

The letter x is the symbol used for the phenomenon before it has a name. Thus, a phenomenon may be thought of as an unnamed thing. When the phenomenon, x, is named, it is referred to as a concept. Examples of concepts evident in the research questions listed in Box 7–6 include adaptation to spinal cord injury, functional status, spiritual growth, self-care agency, low back pain, and type of therapy (massage or traditional).

Characteristics and Importance of Descriptive Research Designs. Recall from Chapter 2 that **concepts** can be constants or variables and that **variables** can be designated as independent or dependent. Concepts that are **constants** have just one form or score; concepts that are **variables** have more than one form or can take a range of scores. An **independent variable** is a concept that influences another concept; a **dependent variable** is a concept that is influenced by another concept. In descriptive research, the phenomenon, x, may be a constant or a variable, but a concept that is variable is not typically categorized as independent or dependent because the influence of one concept on another is not relevant in descriptive research.

At the start of a descriptive study, participants are not usually placed in groups on the basis of some characteristic for the purpose of comparing them on the phenomenon, x. Comparisons might be made, however, if analysis of the data suggests that differences between groups of research participants may exist. For example, if DeSanto Madeya (2006b) had noticed that people's adaptation seemed to differ on the basis of length of time since the spinal cord injury, she could have described the adaptation of her research participants 5 years and 10 years following the injury (see Box 7–6).

The importance of descriptive research should not be minimized. This type of research is a necessary prerequisite for correlational and experimental research. This is because a phenomenon must be described before any attempt is made to link that phenomenon with another through correlational research or to study the effect of the phenomenon on another phenomenon through experimental research. We must, as Lobo (2005) asserted, "have clear and accurate descriptions of the phenomena as foundational work" (p. 5). This means that descriptive theories must be generated and tested before explanatory theories and then predictive theories are tested. The progression of theory development is illustrated in Figure 7–1.

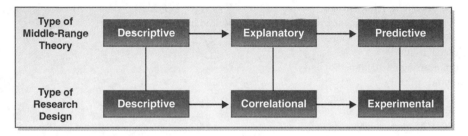

Figure 7-1. Progression of theory development. *Adapted from Fawcett, J. (1999). The relationship of theory and research (3rd ed, p. 20). Philadelphia: F. A. Davis, with permission.*

Types of Descriptive Research Designs.

Descriptive research designs used to generate middle-range theories may be qualitative, quantitative, or a combination of qualitative and quantitative; specific research designs are listed in Box 7–7. In this section and in Table 7–1, which is on the CD that comes with this book, we discuss specific designs in each of the three categories.

Qualitative Descriptive Research Designs

Most descriptive research designs used to generate descriptive middle-range theories are categorized as qualitative. The data, therefore, are words. Each of the many different qualitative research designs offers special instructions for conduct of a study. The highlights and an example of each design are given below; highlights of the various designs also are given in Table 7–1, which is on the CD that comes with this book. These highlights should provide sufficient information for application of the criterion of operational adequacy. (You can read more about each design in the references cited below and in textbooks by Creswell, 1998; Leininger, 1985a; Lincoln & Guba, 1985; and Speziale & Carpenter, 2003 among others. Overviews of the essential features of some qualitative research designs are available in Fitzpatrick and Wallace, 2006.)

Concept analysis, which sometimes is called **concept development**, focuses on enhancing understanding of the meaning of a concept (Rodgers & Knafl, 2000). Different approaches to concept analysis include critical appraisal of the literature (Morse, 2000), a critical paradigm approach (Wuest, 2000), dimensional analysis (Caron & Bowers, 2000), the evolutionary method (Rodgers, 2000), a feminist approach (Wuest, 1994), the hybrid model of concept development (Schwartz-Barcott & Kim, 2000), the Norris method (Lackey, 2000), simultaneous concept analysis (Haase, Leidy, Coward, Britt, & Penn, 2000), and the Wilson method (Avant, 2000; Walker & Avant, 2005), which frequently is referred to as Walker and Avant's approach

BOX 7-7	Types of Research Designs Used to Generate Descriptive Middle-Range Theories

Descriptive Qualitative Research Designs

Concept Analysis
Phenomenology
Hermeneutics
Parse Basic Research Method
Human Becoming Hermeneutic Method of Basic Research
Newman's Research as a Praxis Protocol
Ethnography
Ethnonursing research methodology
Grounded theory
Photo disclosure methodology
Rogerian Process of Inquiry
Unitary Appreciation Inquiry
Unitary Field Pattern Portrait Research Method
Focus group research
Parse's Preproject-Process-Postproject Descriptive Qualitative Method of Applied Research

Descriptive Quantitative Research Designs

Status Survey

Descriptive Qualitative and Quantitative Research Designs

The Delphi Technique
Case study research
Action research

to concept analysis. Each approach involves slightly different steps—from identification of the concept through presentation of findings—that typically are outlined in the method section of the research report. One step of all approaches is a review of theoretical and empirical literature. The literature, then, becomes the data for the study. The hybrid model also includes collection of data from human beings who are thought to have experienced the concept.

A different approach to concept analysis, called **concept inventing**, involves "a multidimensional all-at-once process of analyzing-synthesizing, bring[ing] to life novel unitary concepts" (Parse, 1997, p. 63; Parse, 2006). Although the conceptual or theoretical origins of a concept rarely are taken into account in concept analysis research, Paley (1996) maintained that the meaning of a concept depends on the theory in which it is used.

The specific research question answered by concept analysis is:

• What are the *attributes* of concept *x*?

For example, Holden (2005) used the Wilson method, as interpreted by Walker and Avant, to analyze the concept of complex adaptive systems. The result of the analysis represents a descriptive middle-range theory of complex adaptive systems. Holden discussed the relevance of the concept to nursing within the context of four nursing conceptual models—Johnson's

Behavioral System Model, King's Conceptual System, Rogers' Science of Unitary Human Beings, and Roy's Adaptation Model.

Phenomenology, which was developed within the disciplines of philosophy and psychology, is regarded as a philosophy and a method. Although the origin of phenomenology can be traced to the 19th-century philosopher Brentano, Husserl (1931) is regarded as the father of phenomenonology as a philosophy (Ritzer, 1980). Heidegger (1927/1962) and Merleau-Ponty (1962), among others, extended Husserl's work and made substantial contributions of their own to philosophical phenomenology. As a method, phenomenological research designs emphasize the study of various everyday experiences as lived by human beings. Slightly different approaches to the method of phenomenology have been developed by Colaizzi (1978), Giorgi (1985), van Kaam (1959), and van Manen (1984). In addition, Patterson and Zderad (1976) and Streubert (1991) interpreted the method of phenomenology for the study of lived experiences of particular interest to nurses.

The specific research question answered by all approaches to phenomenology is:

• What is the *lived experience* of *x*?

For example, Bournes and Ferguson-Paré (2005) used van Kaam's phenomenological research design to describe a phenomenon they called "persevering through a difficult time" as experienced by patients, family members of patients, nurses, and allied health professionals during the outbreak of severe acute respiratory syndrome (SARS) in Toronto, Canada. Bournes and Ferguson-Paré interpreted their findings within the context of Parse's Theory of Human Becoming. Their findings can be considered a descriptive middle-range theory of persevering.

Hermeneutics is a type of phenomenological research design that focuses on interpretation of diverse lived experiences that are already available in written form, such as in a book or a journal (Dilthey, 1961). The emphasis in hermeneutics typically is on interpretation of "the social, cultural, political, and historical context in which those [lived] experiences occur" (Polit & Beck, 2006, p. 215). Slightly different approaches to hermeneutics have been developed by Gadamer (1976), Heidegger (1962), and Ricoeur (1976). Furthermore, Alligood (Alligood & Fawcett, 1999) extrapolated Allen's (1995) interpretive hermeneutic method for interpretation of writings about nursing science.

The specific research question answered by hermeneutics is:

• What is the *meaning* of *x*?

For example, Alligood and Fawcett (2004) used a rational hermeneutic research design to interpret the concept of pattern in writings by Martha Rogers, the theorist who developed the Science of Unitary Human Beings. Their interpretation can be considered a descriptive middle-range theory of pattern.

The **Parse basic research method** was developed by Parse (1998) as a way to collect and analyze data from the perspective of her Theory of Human Becoming, which is a nursing grand theory. The Parse method of basic research is a "phenomenological-hermeneutic method in that the universal experiences described by participants who lived them provide the source of information, and participants' descriptions are interpreted in light of the human becoming theory'" (Parse, p. 63).

The specific research question answered by Parse's basic research method is:

• What is the *structure of the universal lived experience* of *x*?

For example, Pilkington (2005) used Parse's basic research method to study the lived experience of grieving a loss from the perspective of elders residing in a long-term care facility. Her findings can be considered a descriptive middle-range theory of grieving a loss.

The **Human Becoming hermeneutic method of basic research** was developed by Cody (1995) as a way to interpret literary texts from the perspective of the Theory of Human Becoming. Cody explained that he drew primarily from Gadamer's (1976, 1989) approach to hermeneutics.

The specific research question answered by the Human Becoming hermeneutic method is:

• What is *the meaning of x as interpreted from a literary text?*

For example, Ortiz (2003) used the Human Becoming hermeneutic method of basic research to describe the meaning of what he called lingering presence, as interpreted in letters from the book *A Promise to Remember: The NAMES Project Book of Letters* (Brown, 1992). The findings can be considered a descriptive middle-range theory of lingering presence.

Research as praxis protocol was developed by Newman (1997) as a way to collect and analyze data from the perspective of her Theory of Health as Expanding Consciousness, which is a nursing grand theory. The protocol is used to generate middle-range theories addressing the process of expanding consciousness as expressed in people's life patterns. The research design is "hermeneutic, to reflect the search for meaning and understanding and interpretations inherent in the researcher's embodiment of the theory; and dialectic because both the process and the content [are] dialectic. The process is the content. The content is the process" (Newman, p. 23).

The specific research question answered by Newman's research as praxis protocol is:

• What are the person's *life patterns* of *x?*

For example, Neill (2005) used Newman's research as praxis protocol to generate a descriptive middle-range theory of new ways of living experienced by women who had multiple sclerosis or rheumatoid arthritis.

Ethnography, which was developed within the discipline of anthropology, is the study of cultures. This descriptive qualitative research design can be traced to ancient Greece (Sanday, 1983). Contemporary ethnography is thought to have originated with Boas' (1948) study of Eskimo culture (Sanday), although Malinowski (1922) and Radcliffe-Brown (1952) contributed substantially to modern ethnographic research design (Atkinson & Hammersley, 1994). The four major approaches to ethnography are the classical, the systematic, the interpretive or hermeneutic, and the critical (Muecke, 1994).

The specific research question answered by ethnography is:

• What are the *behaviors of people of culture* x?

For example, Villarruel (1995) used the systematic approach to ethnography to describe Mexican Americans' meanings and expressions of pain, as well as self-care and dependent-care actions associated with their experiences of pain, within the context of Orem's Self-Care Framework, a conceptual model of nursing. The results of her study can be considered a descriptive middle-range theory of self-care and dependent-care actions to alleviate pain.

The **ethnonursing research methodology**, which Leininger (2006a) adapted for nursing from ethnography, provides a way to study the health-related beliefs, values, and lifeways of people of diverse cultures within the context of her Theory of Culture Care Diversity and Universality, which is a nursing grand theory. The ethnonursing research methodology has been used to study more than 40 Western and non-Western cultures (Leininger 2006b).

The specific research question answered by Leininger's ethnonursing research methodology is:

- What are the *health-related beliefs, values, and lifeways of people of x culture?*

For example, De Oliveira and Hoga (2005) used Leininger's ethnographic research methodology to describe the process by which women residing in a low-income community in Sao Paulo, Brazil, sought and underwent surgical contraception. Their findings can be considered a descriptive middle-range theory of surgical contraception experienced by low-income Brazilian women.

Grounded theory, which was developed by sociologists Glaser and Strauss (1967), can be considered both a conceptual orientation to research and a method. As a conceptual orientation, grounded theory focuses attention on a basic social problem, a basic social process, and the trajectory of the process. The method associated with the conceptual orientation typically is used to generate middle-range theories addressing the trajectory of basic social processes used by people to deal with particular basic social problems, such as a "child's disturbed behavior, which was escalating out of control" (Scharer & Jones, 2004, p. 87) or "nurses striving to provide high quality end-of-life care on an acute medical unit while being pulled in all directions" (Thompson, McClement, & Daeninck, 2006, p. 169). Research conducted within the context of the conceptual orientation of grounded theory contributes primarily to advancement of knowledge within the discipline of sociology. Sometimes, however, the method is used as the research design to generate a middle-range theory within the context of the conceptual orientation of other disciplines (Glaser, 2005). Moreover, as a general method, grounded theory can be used to generate theories from both qualitative and quantitative data (Glaser).

The typical specific research question answered by grounded theory is:

- What theory describes the *trajectory of x social process?*

For example, Radwin (2000; Radwin & Alster, 1999) used the grounded theory method for her study of oncology patients' perceptions of the characteristics and desired outcomes of high-quality nursing care. As Radwin continued her research, she placed her descriptive middle-range theory of oncology patients' perceptions of nursing care and outcomes within the context of the Quality Health Outcomes Model (QHOM) (Radwin & Fawcett, 2002). The QHOM is a relatively new conceptual model of nursing developed by Mitchell and colleagues (1998) to explain how characteristics of health-care systems and of clients influence the link between interventions and outcomes.

The **photo-disclosure methodology** was developed by Bultemeier (1997) as a way to generate descriptions of manifestations of lived experiences within the context of Rogers' Science of Unitary Human Beings, which is a conceptual model of nursing. She explained, "Photo-disclosure emerges from the philosophical base of phenomenology and visual research. Both fields provide avenues for understanding the human condition . . . [and] human experience" (Bultemeier, p. 65). The data used for theory generation include both words and photographs.

The specific research question answered by photo-disclosure methodology is:

- What are the *manifestations of the lived experience* of x?

For example, Bultemeier (1993, 1997) used the photo-disclosure method to generate the descriptive middle-range theory of perceived dissonance as a lived experience manifested in premenstrual syndrome.

The **Rogerian process of inquiry** was developed by Carboni (1995) as an "evolution-centered" way to generate theories focusing on "human and environmental energy field patterns and the nature of human evolution" (p. 36), within the context of Rogers' Science of Unitary Human Beings.

The specific research question answered by the Rogerian process of inquiry is:

• What is the *pattern of evolution of human and environmental energy fields for people in x situation?*

For example, Carboni (1998) used the Rogerian process of inquiry to clarify her descriptive middle-range theory of enfolding health-as-wholeness-and-harmony with residents and staff of a nursing home.

Unitary appreciative inquiry was developed by Cowling (2001) "as a method for uncovering the wholeness, uniqueness, and essence of human existence" (p. 32) within the context of Rogers' Science of Unitary Human Beings. The specific research question answered by unitary appreciative inquiry is:

• What are the *wholeness, uniqueness, and essence of the person's life within the context of x situation?*

For example, Cowling (2004) used unitary appreciative inquiry to develop a descriptive middle-range theory of life pattern profile of despair as reported by women who had experienced despair in the context of depression, addiction, sexual abuse, child abuse, loss of a loved one, terminal illness, infertility, or chronic illness.

The **unitary field pattern portrait research method** was developed in 1994 within the context of Rogers' Science of Unitary Human Beings. Butcher (2006) explained that the purpose of this research design "is to create a unitary understanding of the dynamic kaleidoscope and symphonic pattern manifestations emerging from the pandimensional human/environmental field mutual process as a means to enhance the understanding of a significant phenomenon associated with human betterment and well-being" (p. 180).

The specific research question answered by the unitary field pattern portrait research method is:

• What is the *pattern profile* of *x?*

For example, Butcher (1996) used the unitary field pattern portrait research method to develop a descriptive middle-range theory of dispiritedness in later life.

Focus group research was developed as a way to collect data from groups of people. Although focus groups technically are a strategy for collecting data, the methodology involved can be considered a distinct research design. This method, originally referred to as focused interviews, began in 1941 when Lazarsfeld and Merton collaborated in evaluating studio audiences' responses to radio programs (Stewart & Shamdasani, 1990). Focus group research is "designed to obtain the participants' perceptions of a narrow subject in a setting that is permissive and non-threatening" (Burns & Grove, 2007, p. 379). Research participants typically meet as anywhere between 1 and 50 groups of "8 to 12 individuals who discuss a particular [sensitive] topic under the direction of a moderator [and at least one other researcher] who promotes interaction and assures that the discussion remains on the topic of interest" (Stewart & Shamdasani, p. 10). A hallmark of focus group research design is group, rather than individual, interviews.

The specific research question answered by focus group research is:

- What are the *groups' perceptions* of *x*?

For example, Rujkorakarn and Sukmak (2002) used a focus group research design to generate a descriptive middle-range theory of Thai married women's and men's concepts of health and self-care, within the context of Orem's Self-Care Framework.

The **Parse preproject-process-postproject descriptive qualitative method of applied research** was developed by Parse (1998) as a way to identify and document changes that occur when a project to apply the Theory of Human Becoming in practice is implemented. The specific research question answered by Parse's preproject-process-postproject descriptive qualitative method of applied research is:

- What *changes occur* when Human Becoming theory is applied in practice?

For example, Legault and Ferguson-Paré (1999) used the preproject-process-postproject descriptive qualitative method of applied research to generate a descriptive middle-range theory of changes that occurred when the Theory of Human Becoming was implemented in a 41-bed vascular and general surgery unit at the Vancouver Hospital and Health Services Center in Vancouver, British Columbia, Canada.

A Quantitative Descriptive Research Design

One descriptive research design to generate descriptive middle-range theories—the status survey— is categorized as quantitative. The data, therefore, are numbers.

The status survey, through its essential features, should provide sufficient information for application of the criterion of operational adequacy. (You can read more about survey research in the references provided below and in Babbie, 1990 and Rosenberg, 1968, among others.)

Status surveys can be traced to ancient Egypt, where "rulers conducted censuses to help them administer their domains" (Babbie, 1998, p. 255). In modern times, status surveys have been conducted by researchers since at least the 1830s, and many advances in survey research methodology were made during the 20th century (Kerlinger & Lee, 2000).

The goal of status surveys is "to examine the current status of some . . . characteristic" of a group of people, an organization, a situation, or an event (Kerlinger & Lee, 2000, p. 599). More specifically, the status survey research design focuses on collection of numerical data indicating people's opinions or attitudes about characteristics of themselves, organizations, situations, or events. Status surveys also focus on collection of data that can be considered facts, such as characteristics of people "that are a function of their membership in society [including] gender, income level, political and religious affiliations, ethnicity, occupation, and educational level" (LoBiondo-Wood & Haber, 2006, p. 241). Other facts are the number and type of activities people perform, such as the activities nurses perform when they care for patients or the activities people perform when they are well or ill. Still another fact is the number of times a certain health-related event occurs in a health-care organization, such as the yearly rate of medication errors or wrong-site surgery. Status surveys are conducted by "asking people questions; their answers constitute the [numerical] data" (Fowler, 1993, p. 1).

The specific research question answered by status surveys is:

• What are the *characteristics* of *x*?

For example, Cook, Pierce, Hicks, and Steiner (2006) conducted a status survey of physical and occupational therapists to generate a descriptive middle-range theory of the therapists' beliefs about the self-care information needs of caregivers of persons who had had a stroke, within the context of Orem's Self-Care Framework, a conceptual model of nursing.

Qualitative and/or Quantitative Descriptive Research Designs

Three research designs used to generate descriptive middle-range theories—the Delphi technique, case study research, and action research—involve collection of qualitative and/or quantitative data, or, in other words, involve collection of words and/or numbers. The essential features of these three research designs should provide sufficient information for application of the criterion of operational adequacy.

The **Delphi technique**, which is named for the oracle at Delphi in ancient Greece, is used to identify issues and consensus about those issues in such diverse fields as business, defense, and education, as well as in the discipline of nursing (Keeney, Hasson, & McKenna, 2006). Delphi technique research involves several rounds of data collection from a large group of people who are experts in a particular area, such as nurses who are certified in a particular nursing practice specialty. The first round usually is collection of qualitative data—words—in one-to-one or group interviews focused on issues that each expert thinks are important. The word data are summarized quantitatively, and the numerical results are distributed via questionnaire to the experts. Each expert then is asked to rank-order or prioritize the issues. The rounds continue with updates of the numerical data until consensus is reached.

The specific research question answered by the Delphi technique is:

• What is the *consensus about* x?

For example, McKenna (1994) used the Delphi technique to gain consensus from a group of psychiatric hospital ward managers about a nursing model to guide care of long-stay psychiatric patients. His findings can be considered a descriptive middle-range theory of models preferred by nurses for use with long-stay psychiatric patients.

Case study research, which is thought to have originated within the discipline of sociology (Hammersley, cited in Cohen, 2006), is an in-depth, intensive examination of one or just a few individuals, organizations, or communities. Each case study involves the collection of many details from multiple sources to gain a comprehensive description of the case. Special features of case study research are its "real life context" (Cohen, p. 139) and the "unique stories" that are extracted from the "details and complexities" and "the peculiarities and the commonalities" of a specific case (Liehr & LoBiondo-Wood, 2006, pp. 153, 161). Although much of the data collected for case study research are in the form of words, numerical data also may be collected and sometimes are compared with the word data. Furthermore, the data may be unstructured or structured.

The specific research question answered by case study research, which is adapted from a question formulated by Liehr and LoBiondo-Wood (2006) is:

• What are the *details and complexities* of *x*?

For example, Maldonado, Callahan, and Efinger (2003) conducted a case study of the lived spiritual experiences of participants in a Five Wishes seminar about holistic and end-of-life care decisions guided by Parse's Theory of Human Becoming. Their findings can be considered a descriptive middle-range theory of spiritual experiences.

Action research originated with Lewin's (1938, 1946) studies of how change occurs and the impact of that change when dealing with problems of segregation, discrimination, and assimilation of minority populations. Action research is "a systematic, participatory approach to inquiry that enables people to extend their understanding of problems or issues and to formulate actions directed towards the resolution of those problems or issues" (Stringer & Genat, 2004, p. 4). Action research is participatory because the researcher and the people who are experiencing specific "real world problems" participate together in the research with the goal of empowering those people to "act on their own behalf" to solve the problems (Speziale & Carpenter, 2003, p. 253).

An action research design may be used to evaluate new programs or projects implemented in health-care organizations, schools, or communities. Data may be words or numbers obtained from people's stories, drawings, and paintings or from observation of "plays and skits, and other activities designed to encourage people to find creative ways to explore their lives, tell their stories, and recognize their own strengths" (Polit & Beck, 2006, p. 227). Several variations of action research design exist, including collaborative inquiry, cooperative inquiry, action science or action inquiry, participatory inquiry, participatory action research, and community-based action research (Speziale & Carpenter, 2003).

The specific research question answered by all variations of action research is:

• What *changes are needed to resolve problem* x?

For example, Bent and her colleagues (2005) used participatory action research as the methodological framework to study a project involving the linkage of Watson's Theory of Human Caring, a middle-range nursing theory, with practice and inquiry in health-care services delivery throughout the Veterans Administration Eastern Colorado Health Care System. The study results can be considered a descriptive middle-range theory of the strategies used to link a theory to practice and research.

A Quantitative Descriptive Research Design to Test Descriptive Middle-Range Theories

One descriptive research design that is used to test descriptive middle-range theories is **instrument development** (Box 7–8). It is categorized as quantitative; the data, therefore, are numbers. The essential features of instrument development, given below and in Table 7–2, which is on the CD that comes with this book, should provide sufficient information for application of the criterion of operational adequacy. (You can read more about instrument development in Nunnally and Bernstein, 1994, and Waltz, Strickland, & Lenz, 2005.)

Instrument development refers to the construction of research instruments that measure middle-range theory concepts. We regard instrument development as a theory-testing research design because the concept that is measured by each instrument and the definition of that concept constitute a middle-range theory.

Instrument development begins with identification of a concept—sometimes by means of concept analysis—and proceeds to a theoretical definition of the concept and selection of items

BOX 7-8	Types of Research Designs Used to Test Middle-Range Theories

Quantitative Descriptive Research Design Used to Test Descriptive Theories

Instrument development

Quantitative Correlational Research Designs Used to Test Explanatory Theories—Sample Surveys

Bivariate research design

    Model testing designs

    Regression models

    Canonical correlation models

    Path models

    Structural equation models

Quantitative Experimental Research Designs Used to Test Predictive Theories

True experimental designs

    Pretest-posttest control group design

    Solomon four-group design

    Posttest-only control group design

Quasi-experimental designs

    Single-subject research

    N-of-1 randomized controlled trial

    Crossover design

    Nonequivalent control group design

    Interrupted time-series design

True experiments and/or quasi-experimental designs

    Outcomes research

    Randomized controlled clinical trial

    Factorial designs

Other descriptive, correlational, and experimental research designs

    Evaluation research

    Pilot, or exploratory, research

that address all aspects of the definition. This is followed by administration of the instrument to people to determine whether it consistently measures what it is supposed to measure. The consistency with which the instrument measures the concept is referred to as its **reliability**. The extent to which the instrument measures the concept as it is theoretically defined is referred to as its **validity**. We discuss reliability and validity and the other so-called psychometric properties of instruments in Chapter 9.

The specific research question answered by instrument development is:

• How is x reliably and validly measured?

For example, Lancaster (2004) developed an instrument she called Coping with Breast Cancer Threat to measure the concept of primary prevention coping behaviors used by women who have a family history of breast cancer. Lancaster defined primary prevention coping behaviors as "those actions initiated by an individual before breast cancer develops that serve to assist a woman to effectively cope with her appraised breast cancer threat" (p. 35). The instrument development research was guided by Neuman's Systems Model concept of primary prevention interventions and Lazarus' middle-range theory of coping.

Quantitative Correlational Research Designs Used to Test Explanatory Middle-Range Theories

Correlational research designs are used to test explanatory middle-range theories by providing answers to questions about relations between concepts. Specifically, these research designs are used to test explanatory middle-range theories that include at least two concepts.

Interest in correlational research can be traced to advances in methodology and statistical techniques in the biological and behavioral sciences that began in the late 1800s and early 1900s (Cohen & Cohen, 1975) and continue to the present. Correlational research focuses specifically on testing explanatory theories, which address the extent to which variation in one concept is related to variation in another concept. **Variation** is determined by the range of numerical scores on instruments that measure the concepts. The highlights of correlational designs are given below and in Table 7–2 on the CD. These highlights should provide sufficient information for application of the criterion of operational adequacy. (You can read more about correlational research designs in the references cited below and in a statistics textbook, such as Munro, 2005).

Correlational research designs are quantitative designs. The data, therefore, are numbers. Some textbook authors refer to correlational research designs as ordinary correlational research (Powers & Knapp, 2006), descriptive correlational research (Burns & Grove, 2007; Fain, 2004; LoBiondo-Wood & Haber, 2006; Polit & Beck, 2006), predictive correlational research (Burns & Grove; LoBiondo-Wood & Haber), or causal-comparative correlational research (Powers and Knapp). We prefer the general term **correlational research designs** to avoid confusion with descriptive theory and descriptive research designs and predictive theory and experimental research designs, as well as to avoid the misleading interpretation that correlational research designs are capable of establishing causality.

The basic research question answered by all correlational research designs is:

• What is the relation between x and y?

Characteristics of Correlational Research Designs. In correlational research, concepts must be **variables** because a correlation coefficient cannot be mathematically calculated between concepts that are constants or between constant and variable concepts. Variables and their relation to one another, including the direction of the relation and its symmetry, are essential characteristics of correlational research.

Variables may be independent or dependent. An **independent variable**—that is a concept that influences another concept—is typically indicated by the symbol x and is sometimes called an **explanatory variable** or a **predictor variable**. The letter y is the symbol typically used for a **dependent variable**—that is, a concept that is influenced by another concept.

Correlational research designs may include virtually any number of independent and dependent variables. The number of variables ultimately is determined by the number of concepts making up the explanatory theory that is being tested, as well as by practical limits imposed by the criterion of parsimony for middle-range theories (see Chapter 6) and by available statistical techniques (see Chapter 12).

We believe that correlational research cannot establish causation. Thus, the designation of independent and dependent variables in correlational research should not be interpreted as indicating that change in one variable actually causes a change in another variable. Rather, correlational research can indicate only a relation of some kind between two or more theoretical concepts that are variables.

The **direction of the relation** between each pair of variables can be specified as not known, direct, or inverse (Figure 7–2).

An explanatory theory may simply specify that a relation between x and y exists, but the direction is not known (see Figure 7–2 part A), such that a change in the numerical score for x is related to a change in the numerical score for y. An example of the existence of a relation is: There is a relation between loneliness and cognitive functioning.

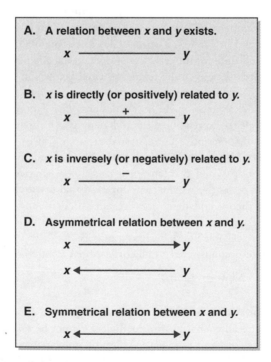

Figure 7-2. Correlational research: Types of relations between x and y.

Alternatively, the explanatory theory may specify that the direction is known, such that *x* is directly related to *y*, or that *x* is inversely related to *y* (see Figure 7–2 parts B and C). A **direct—or positive—relation** means that the change in the numerical score for one variable is in the same direction as the change in the numerical score for another variable; this type of relation is illustrated with a plus sign (+) (see Figure 7–2 part B). An example of a direct relation is: An increase in physical energy is related to an increase in functional status, and conversely, a decrease in physical energy is related to a decrease in functional status.

An **inverse—or negative—relation** means that the change in the numerical score for one variable is in the opposite direction of the change in the numerical score for another variable; this type of relation is illustrated with a minus sign (−) (see Figure 7–2 part C). An example of an inverse relation is: An increase in depression is related to a decrease in functional status, and conversely, a decrease in depression is related to an increase in functional status.

The **symmetry** of the relation between each pair of variables can be specified as not known, asymmetrical, or symmetrical. If an explanatory theory does not specify the symmetry of the relation between *x* and *y*, all that can be proposed is that a relation exists (see Figure 7–2 part A), or if known, that the relation is direct (see Figure 7–2 part B) or inverse (see Figure 7–2 part C).

If an explanatory theory specifies that the relation between *x* and *y* is **asymmetrical**, then the "path" between *x* and *y* can be determined. An asymmetrical relation is not reversible; only one path is evident—from *x* to *y* or from *y* to *x* (see Figure 7–2 part D). An example of an asymmetrical relation is: Maternal age is related to adjustment to motherhood. In this example, the path is from maternal age (*x*) to adjustment (*y*).

An explanatory theory can also specify that the relation between *x* and *y* is **symmetrical**; in this case, the "path" between *x* to *y* is reversible or reciprocal (see Figure 7–2 part E). An example of a symmetrical relation is: There is a reciprocal relation between child health and family health. In this example, the path can be from child health (*x*) to family health (*y*) or from family health (*y*) to child health (*x*).

Comparisons of participants in correlational research are not typically made—that is, participants in correlational research typically are not divided into groups (Burns & Grove, 2007). However, group comparisons are sometimes made as part of a correlational research design (Powers & Knapp, 2006). Such comparisons focus on some aspect of a difference in the relation between *x* and *y* for two or more groups, rather than group differences in *x* or *y* alone (Cohen & Cohen, 1975). An example is: The size of the correlation coefficient between physical energy and functional status is larger for young women than for older women.

Types of Correlational Research Designs

Sample Surveys

Sample surveys, which are studies of some portion of all the people who are of interest to the researcher, can be considered the basic research design for correlational research (Cohen & Cohen, 1975; Kerlinger & Lee, 2000). The goal of sample surveys is to test the relations between concepts that are proposed in explanatory theories.

Different sample survey research designs include different numbers of variables. The simplest design includes two variables and is known as a **bivariate research design**. More complex designs include multiple independent and multiple dependent variables; they are termed **model-testing designs** and are named by the statistical technique used to empirically test the relations between variables. Specific correlational research designs used to test explanatory theories are listed in Box 7–8.

Bivariate Research Design

A **bivariate research design** is a sample survey that focuses on examination of the relation between two concepts that are variables (see Figure 7–2 parts A, B, and C). The basic research question answered by the bivariate research design is:

- What is the relation between x and y?

For example, in a study guided by Orem's Self-Care Framework, Hurst and colleagues (2005) tested an explanatory middle-range theory by examining the bivariate correlations between social support and self-care agency and between social support and self-care practices. The research participants were African American women who had HIV disease.

Model-Testing Designs

Model-testing designs are sample surveys that include several variables (Burns & Grove, 2007). It is important to understand that the word "model," as used in correlational research, does not refer to the C component of C-T-E structures but rather comes from the statistical element of the E component. More specifically, the so-called model of correlational research is typically a diagram of the relations between variables—that is, the concepts of an explanatory theory (see Table 7–2, on the CD that comes with this book, and Figure 7–3). The label for each model is based on the statistical technique used to empirically test the relations between variables (see Chapter 12).

Regression models, which are tested by the statistical technique known as **multiple regression**, include a set of two or more independent variables and one dependent variable (see Figure 7–3 part A). The explanatory theory for a regression model proposes that the scores for each of the two or more concepts that are independent variables explain variation in the score for the concept that is the dependent variable.

The basic research question answered by regression models is:

- What is the relation between a set of independent variables, x_1, x_2, . . . x_n and the dependent variable, y?

(Note that the subscripts 1 and 2 refer to different variables; the subscript n is used to indicate any number of variables.)

For example, in a study guided by the Neuman Systems Model, Gigliotti (2004) tested an explanatory middle-range theory of the relation of three independent variables—maternal role involvement (x_1), student role involvement (x_2), and total network social support (x_3)—to the dependent variable, maternal-student role stress (y). The research participants were two groups of female students enrolled in an associate degree nursing program clinical course. The students in one group were less than 37 years of age; the students in the other group were 37 years of age or older. All students had at least one child less than 19 years of age who lived at home.

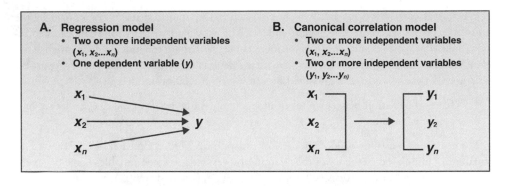

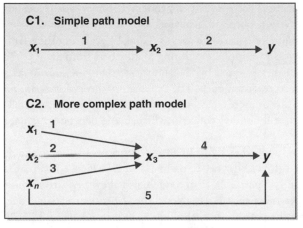

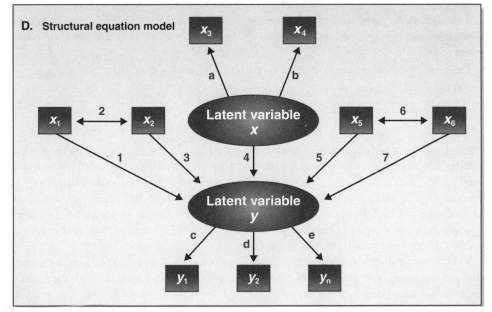

Figure 7-3. Correlational research: Model-testing research designs.

Canonical correlation models, which are tested by the statistical technique known by the same term, are an extension of regression models. The explanatory theory for a canonical correlation model proposes that a set of two or more concepts that are the independent variables are related to a set of two or more concepts that are the dependent variables (see Figure 7–3 part B). The basic research question answered by canonical correlation models is:

- What is the relation between a set of independent variables, x_1, x_2, . . . x_n and a set of dependent variables, y_1, y_2, . . . y_n?

For example, in a study guided by the Roy Adaptation Model, Bournaki (1997) tested an explanatory middle-range theory of the relation of seven independent variables—age (x_1), gender (x_2), past painful experiences (x_3), temperament (x_4), general fears (x_5), medical fears (x_6), and child rearing practices (x_7)—to five dependent variables—pain location (y_1), pain intensity (y_2), pain quality (y_3), observed behaviors (y_4), and heart rate change (y_5). The research participants were children between the ages of 8 and 12 years and their female caregivers. The children were receiving a venipuncture during a visit to an outpatient clinic.

Path models, which are tested by the statistical technique known as **path analysis**, are another extension of regression models. The explanatory theory for a path model proposes that there are paths from one or more concepts to one or more other concepts, all of which are independent variables, to still another concept, which is the dependent variable (see Figure 7–3 parts C1 and C2).

Path models allow paths directly from an independent variable to the dependent variable; these paths are called **direct effects** (see paths 1 and 2 in Figure 7–3 part C1 and paths 1, 2, 3, 4, and 5 in Figure 7–2 part C2). Path models also allow paths from one independent variable through another independent variable to the dependent variable; such paths are called **indirect effects** (see the path from x_1 through x_2 to y in Figure 7–3 part C1, and the paths from x_1, x_2, and x_n through x_3 to y in Figure 7–3 part C2).

Inasmuch as the paths always go the same way, from independent variables to the dependent variable and are asymmetrical (see Figure 7–2 part D), path models are said to be **recursive models**.

The basic research question answered by path models is:

- What are the direct and indirect paths between sets of independent variables x_1, x_2, . . . x_n and the dependent variable y?

For example, in a study guided by the Roy Adaptation Model, Tsai (2005) tested her middle-range theory of chronic pain with data from people 65 years of age and older who had arthritis. The theory proposes paths from chronic pain (x_1), disability (x_2), social support (x_3), financial hardship (x_4), age (x_5), and gender (x_6) to distress (x_7), and from distress (x_7) to depression (y). In this example, the path from chronic pain, disability, social support, financial hardship, age, and gender to distress, and the path from distress to depression are direct; the path from chronic pain, disability, social support, financial hardship, age, and gender to depression is indirect because it goes through distress.

Structural equation models, which are tested by the statistical technique known by the same term, are an extension of path models. The explanatory theory for a structural equation model proposes that some paths between variables may be asymmetrical (see paths 1, 3, 4, 5, and 7 in Figure 7–3 part D; see also Figure 7–2 part D) and that other paths may be symmetrical, or reciprocal (see paths 2 and 6 in Figure 7–3 part D; see also Figure 7–2 part E). Inasmuch as paths can go two ways, structural equation models are said to be **nonrecursive models**.

Furthermore, structural equation models allow one or more concepts to be **latent variables**—that is, unmeasured concepts that are reflected in measured concepts, which may be called **manifest variables** or **indicators** (Norris, 2005). In diagrams, latent variables are usually designated by circles, and indicators are designated by boxes (see Figure 7–3 part D); the lines from the latent variables to the indicators are not paths but rather indicate that the latent variable is indicated by or manifested by the indicators (see lines a, b, c, d, and e in Figure 7–3 part D). For example, severity of illness may be regarded as a latent variable that is reflected in the indicators of stage of disease, number of hospitalizations, and number of complications.

The basic research question answered by structural equation models is:

- What are the asymmetrical and symmetrical relations between sets of independent variables x_1, x_2, . . . x_n and the dependent variable y?

For example, in a study guided by the Roy Adaptation Model, Nuamah and colleagues (1999) tested a middle-range theory of health-related quality of life in people with recently diagnosed cancer. The theory proposes that there are symmetrical relations between four indicators reflecting the latent variable, health-related quality of life (y). The four indicators are physical symptoms (y_1), affective status (y_2), functional status (y_3), and social support (y_4). The theory also proposes that there are asymmetrical relations from age (x_1), gender (x_2), race (x_3), income (x_4), marital status (x_5), type of adjuvant cancer treatment (x_6), and severity of illness (x_7) to the four indicators of health-related quality of life (y_1, y_2, y_3, y_4).

Quantitative Experimental Research Designs Used to Test Predictive Middle-Range Theories

Experimental research designs are used to test predictive middle-range theories by providing answers to questions about the effects of one or more concepts on one or more other concepts. Specifically, experimental research designs are used to test middle-range predictive theories that include at least two concepts. Experimental research designs are quantitative designs; the data, therefore, are numbers.

The basic research question answered by all experimental research designs is:

- What is the effect of x on y?

Experiments are considered to be the most rigorous type of research design. Indeed, the primacy of experimental designs in most disciplines led to classifying all other designs as quasi-experimental or nonexperimental (LoBiondo-Wood & Haber, 2006; Pedhazur, 1982; Polit & Beck, 2006). The inference is that quasi-experimental and nonexperimental designs are not as good as experimental designs. We regard that inference as misleading and prefer the terms descriptive, correlational, and experimental research because of the ease of linkage with descriptive, explanatory, and predictive theories, respectively. Accordingly, what others classify as nonexperimental research designs we consider descriptive or correlational research designs, and we include quasi-experimental research with experimental research designs. In addition, we believe that any research design is as good as any other if it is used appropriately and rigorously.

An **experiment** is defined as "that portion of research in which variables are manipulated and their effects on other variables observed" (Campbell & Stanley, 1963, p. 1). Although experiments have been conducted since ancient times, Fisher (1925, 1935) is credited with major advances in experimental design and related statistical techniques—known as **analysis of variance**—in modern times (Campbell & Stanley; Cook & Campbell, 1979; Kerlinger & Lee, 2000). Campbell and Stanley maintained that Fisher's "most fundamental contribution has been the concept of achieving pre-experimental [equivalence] of groups through randomization" (p. 2). Kerlinger and Lee maintained that Fisher "virtually revolutionized statistical and experimental design thinking and methods," and referred to him as "the father of analysis of variance" (p. 170).

"All experiments," according to Cook and Campbell (1979), "involve at least a treatment, an outcome measure, units of assignment [that is, individuals or existing groups or communities], and some comparison from which change can be inferred and hopefully attributed to the treatment" (p. 5).

Each of the many different experimental research designs offers special instructions for conduct of a study. The highlights of several designs, which should provide sufficient information for application of the criterion of operational adequacy, are given below and in Table 7–2 on the CD. You can read more about each design in the references cited below, especially in Campbell and Stanley's (1963) and Cook and Campbell's (1979) now-classic books, and in many basic and advanced research methods textbooks.

Characteristics of Experimental Research Designs. Experimental research designs have some specific characteristics—manipulation, control, and randomization—as well as constants and variables, which are found in other research designs.

Independent and **dependent variables** in experimental research are, as in other research designs, designated by the symbols x and y, respectively. The letter x is the symbol typically used for the independent variable—that is, a concept that in the case of experimental research is thought to have an effect on another concept, y, which is the dependent variable. More specifically, in experimental research, x refers to a categorical variable made up of the so-called experimental and control treatments. The experimental and control treatments are the categories of one independent variable; they are not different independent variables. Experimental research designs usually involve one independent variable, which encompasses the experimental and control treatments, and one or more dependent variables, the outcome(s).

Complex experimental research designs may include more than one independent variable, in which case the effect of any theoretical relations between the independent variables—called **interaction effects**—can be tested statistically (see Chapter 12). In experimental research, the concepts that are the outcomes must be variables because the relevant statistical tests require variation—a range of scores—for all outcome measures.

The **experimental treatment** is a therapy or intervention that usually is thought to be better than some other therapy or intervention, referred to as the **control treatment**. Research participants who receive the experimental treatment are collectively referred to as the **experimental group**, and those who receive the control treatment are collectively referred to as the **control group**. More than one experimental or control treatment can be included in a study. For example, in women with breast cancer, Samarel and colleagues (2002) compared the effects of an experimental treatment consisting of individual telephone and group support with one control treatment consisting of only individual telephone support and another control treatment consisting of only mailed information.

Ethical standards for experimental research require that each control group receive some intervention. The semantic clarity criterion for middle-range theories requires that a precise description of the experimental treatment and the control treatment(s) be included in the research report. Thus, a statement that the experimental group received a "new treatment" is not sufficient. Similarly, a statement that the control group received "usual care" or "standard care" is not sufficient. Instead, the new treatment and the usual or standard care should be described in detail.

Comparisons in experimental research are of two types. **Between-groups comparisons** involve comparing groups of different people who make up the experimental and control groups. **Within-groups comparisons** involve comparing groups of people with themselves at different times and under different conditions, such as before and after receiving an experimental treatment.

In addition to these characteristics, experimental designs have three other essential characteristics—manipulation, control, and randomization.

Manipulation typically refers to the experimental and control treatment categories of the independent variable. In other words, some therapy or intervention is "manipulated" to form experimental and control treatments. In most experimental research, "the researcher actively initiates, implements, and terminates" the treatments (Abraham & Wasserbauer, 2006, p. 185). For example, a researcher could manipulate a childbirth education intervention so that some people—the experimental group—receive a new curriculum, whereas other people—the control group—receive the standard curriculum.

At times, though, a so-called **natural experiment** that does not involve the researcher's active manipulation of the independent variable occurs as the result of a change in the usual way of doing something. For example, allowing a woman's partner to be in the delivery room during a cesarean birth after many years of excluding partners of cesarean-delivered women from the delivery room is a natural experiment that occurred as a result of a change in maternity unit policy in many hospitals (Rodriguez, 1981).

Control refers to the researcher's ability to rule out threats to valid conclusions about the data and to increase the precision of the research results (Cook & Campbell, 1979). The ways in which researchers can impose control in experimental research are discussed in Chapter 11.

Randomization refers to the selection of research participants, their assignment to groups, and the assignment of groups to experimental and control treatments. Randomization means that each person has an equal chance of being selected for the study, an equal chance of being assigned to a certain group, and an equal chance of receiving the experimental or control treatment (Kerlinger & Lee, 2000). Randomization can be achieved by various methods, including use of a table of random numbers, a coin toss, the so-called sealed opaque envelope technique, or a computer program. Examples of those methods of randomization to experimental and control treatment groups are given in Box 7–9.

Types of Quantitative Experimental Research Designs.
Quantitative experimental research encompasses three true experimental designs and several quasi-experimental designs. A few other research designs may be carried out as either true experiments or

BOX 7-9	Examples of Methods of Randomization to Experimental and Control Treatment Groups

Table of Random Numbers

"Patients were randomly assigned to either the control or experimental group, using a random number table to determine group allocation" (Chair, Taylor-Piliae, Lam, & Chan, 2003, p. 473).

Coin Toss

"[R]andom assignment to the treatment or the compassion group [was accomplished] by use of a computerized coin toss" (McDonald & Nicholson, 2006, p. 53).

Sealed Opaque Envelope Technique

"The process of randomization was accomplished by creating an equal number of slips of paper marked either C for control [group] or E for experimental group. These were placed in envelopes so that 22 control and 22 experimental slips were in one pile for women and 11 control and 11 experimental slips were in another pile for men. Each pile of envelopes [was] sealed and placed in a box and thoroughly mixed. Without unsealing them, the envelopes were stacked. After a potential participant indicated a willingness to be involved in the study, met eligibility criteria and signed the informed consent, he/she picked the top envelope and opened it. Those who opened envelopes with a C slip of paper were in the control group, and those who opened envelopes with an E slip were in the experimental group" (McCaffrey & Freeman, 2003, p. 519).

Computer Program

"Random assignment to the [experimental] treatment ($n = 21$) or control ($n = 21$) group was achieved using a computerized minimization program that controlled for age, antidepressant medication use, anti-anxiety medication use, long-acting opioid medication use, and length of pain" (Lewandowski, Good, & Draucker, 2005, p. 61).

quasi-experimental designs. Specific experimental research designs used to test predictive theories are listed in Box 7–8.

True Experimental Designs

The three major requirements for **true experimental designs** are the manipulation of an independent variable, random assignment of research participants to groups, and random assignment of treatments to groups (Kerlinger & Lee, 2000). Ideally, all three requirements should be met. However, random assignment of treatments to groups frequently is not done. Consequently, some researchers may refer to their use of any of the designs categorized as true experiments as quasi-experimental designs.

Campbell and Stanley (1963) identified three true experimental designs. These are the pretest-posttest control group design, the Solomon four-group design, and the posttest-only control group design.

The pretest-posttest control group design involves randomization to the experimental and control treatments and measurement of the dependent variable before and after the experimental treatment. This design is also referred to as the **true or classic experiment** (Whittemore & Grey, 2006).

For example, Williams and Schreier (2005) used a pretest-posttest control group design to test a predictive middle-range theory of the effects of audiotaped education on self-care behaviors used by women with breast cancer to manage side effects of chemotherapy, including fatigue, anxiety, and sleep disturbances. Women were randomly assigned to the control group or the experimental group. The control group received standard education, which included oral instructions about chemotherapy side effects given by staff nurses and literature from the American Cancer Society (ACS). The experimental group received a 20-minute educational audiotape, which included information about exercise and relaxation, as well as the standard education. Data were collected by telephone before chemotherapy began (pretest) and 1 and 3 months later (posttests). The study was based on Orem's Self-Care Framework.

The Solomon four-group design is an extension of the pretest-posttest control group design. This design involves randomization of research participants to four groups, two of which receive the experimental treatment and two of which receive the control treatment. One experimental group and one control group are measured on the dependent variable both before and after the experimental treatment, and the other experimental group and the other control group are measured on the dependent variable only after the experimental treatment. This design permits examination not only of the effects of the experimental and control treatments but also of the effect of the pretest on the posttest (Sechrist & Pravikoff, 2002). Although this design typically is considered a true experimental design, some researchers categorize their Solomon four-group design studies as quasi-experimental.

For example, McGahee and Tingen (2000) used a Solomon four-group design to test a predictive middle-range theory of the effects of an ACS-developed smoking prevention curriculum, "Do It Yourself—Making Healthy Choices," on fifth-grade children's attitudes toward smoking, their subjective norms about smoking, and their refusal skills. The study was guided by the social-psychology theory of reasoned action. Accordingly, attitude is "considered personal in nature and is based on beliefs about smoking and consequences of smoking" (McGahee & Tingen, p. 7). Subjective norms is the term used to refer to the child's ideas about his or her "significant others' beliefs about smoking and [his or her own] motivation to comply with significant others' beliefs" (McGahee & Tingen, p. 7). Refusal skills refer to "the knowledge and the ability to successfully refuse offers to smoke cigarettes" (McGahee & Tingen, p. 9). One experimental group who received the ACS curriculum provided data 1 day prior to implementation of the curriculum (pretest) and 3 weeks after completion of the curriculum (posttest). A control group who did not receive the ACS curriculum also provided pretest and posttest data. The other experimental group who received the ACS curriculum provided data only at 3 weeks after completion of the curriculum (posttest). The other control group who did not receive the curriculum provided data just once (posttest). Fifth-grade classes from different schools, rather than individual children, were randomly assigned to the experimental and control groups. McGahee and Tingen referred to their study as a "quasi-experimental" design (p. 12) perhaps because the treatments were not randomly assigned to the groups, or individual children were not randomly assigned to treatments.

The posttest-only control group design involves randomization of the experimental and control treatments and measurement of the dependent variable only after the experimental treatment. This design is also called the **after only** design (Whittemore & Grey, 2006).

For example, Chair and colleagues (2003) conducted a posttest-only control group study, based on Orem's Self-Care Framework, designed to test a predictive middle-range theory of the effect of positioning on back pain in Chinese men and women who had undergone coronary angiography in Hong Kong. The men and women were randomly assigned to an experimental group or a control group. The experimental treatment consisted of hourly changes of position while lying in bed, "varying between supine, right side lying and left side lying during the first 7 hours [after coronary angiography]. During side lying, a pillow was placed at the lumbar area for support and the affected leg remained straight. Patients were also instructed to place three fingers over the femoral dressing to apply pressure while turning" (Chair et al., p. 473). The control treatment consisted of "bedrest for 8–24 hours, depending on the protocol of each cardiology team, with the affected leg immobilized during bedrest" (p. 473). Posttests were measures of back pain, vascular complications, and pedal pulses. Back pain was measured at 15 minutes, 2, 4, and 6 hours, and the next morning following angiograpy. Presence of any vascular complications, including femoral bleeding and hematoma at the catheter site, as well as pedal pulses, was assessed at 15, 20, and 45 minutes, every hour for 7 hours, and the next morning following angiography.

Quasi-Experimental Designs

When manipulation and/or randomization are not possible or feasible, true experiments cannot be conducted. **Quasi-experiments**, which Campbell and Stanley (1963) called **pre-experimental designs**, are those for which one or more of the requirements of a true experiment—manipulation of an independent variable, random assignment of research participants to groups, and random assignment of treatments to groups—is not met (Kerlinger & Lee, 2000). In particular, quasi-experiments are research designs "that have treatments, outcome measures, and experimental units, but [may] not use random assignment to create the comparisons from which treatment-caused change is inferred. Instead, the comparisons depend on nonequivalent groups that differ from each other in many ways other than the presence of a treatment whose effects are being tested" (Cook & Campbell, 1979, p. 6).

Quasi-experimental designs are important because some research topics involving human beings as research participants cannot be studied using true experimental designs. For example, an intervention designed to promote comfort only for people who are dying would not be administered to people who are not dying. Similarly, a traumatic event, such as domestic violence, cannot be randomly assigned to experimental and control groups.

Many different quasi-experimental research designs have been identified. One category of quasi-experimental research design involves just one research participant or one group of participants. These are single-subject research designs, N-of-1 randomized clinical trials, and crossover designs. Another category of quasi-experimental research design, nonequivalent control groups, involves just one group of research participants or two groups that are not equivalent because they are not randomly assigned to treatments.

Single-subject research (Backman & Harris, 1999) involves measurement of the dependent variable at least once before administration of the experimental treatment, followed by repeated measurement of a clinically relevant dependent variable. Just one person typically is included in the study, although the study may be repeated with one or more other individuals. Backman and Harris pointed out that single-subject research is "ideally suited to rehabilitation research when individualized goals and treatment plans are important" . . . [and provides] a systematic approach to evaluating clinical change" (p. 173). This design is similar to what Rolfe (2006) called **single-case research**. He explained that single-case research focuses "on the unique individuals the nurse meets in each of her [or his] clinical encounters" (p. 40). Rolfe values this research design as a way to advance what he calls **nursing science of the unique**, which he views as a way to combine practice with experimental research.

For example, Fulk (2004), a physical therapist, used a single-subject design with multiple experimental treatments to test a predictive middle-range theory of the effects of different gait training interventions—which involved walking on a treadmill or on the floor with body weight supported at self-selected or fast speeds—on one woman's ability to walk beginning 5 weeks after she had experienced a stroke. Three dependent variables—gait velocity, gait endurance, and motor control—were measured prior to the beginning of each physical therapy session. Another dependent variable—a walking ability questionnaire—was completed by the woman prior to the beginning of physical therapy and at the end of each treatment phase. The study was guided by a conceptual frame of reference addressing motor control and motor learning, "which advocate for a task oriented approach such as [body weight support] training" (Fulk, p. 21).

The **N-of-1 randomized controlled trial** (Backman & Harris, 1999), which is a type of single-subject research, involves alternating administration of an experimental treatment and a control treatment to just one person. The order of administration of the experimental and control treatments is determined randomly, and the individual serves as his or her own control. McCaffery and Arnstein (2006) explained that "N-of-1 trials evaluate the effectiveness of a procedure or treatment in a single person, rather than a larger [group of people]. In short, N-of-1 trials are thought to evaluate the individual's potential for benefiting from active treatment" (p. 63). This design is most frequently used by physicians to study the effects of drugs that have a rapid effect but then cease to have an effect soon after being discontinued (Backman & Harris, 1999). The experimental treatment typically is a new drug; the control treatment can be another drug with an effect similar to the experimental drug, or a placebo that has no effect.

For example, Jansen and colleagues (2001) conducted five separate N-of-1 trials to test the efficacy of methylphenidate hydrochloride, a central nervous system and respiratory system stimulant marketed as Ritalin™, for three depressed and two chronically apathetic older adults. Each person received 5 mg of methylphenidate (experimental treatment) twice a day for 2 days in random order with a placebo drug (control treatment) twice a day for 2 days, over a total period of 5 weeks. The dependent variables were depression (measured in the three depressed persons), apathy (measured in the two apathetic persons), functional status (measured in all five persons), and adverse effects (measured in all five persons).

A **crossover design** is an extension of the N-of-1 randomized trial to more than one person. This design involves two groups who receive one experimental treatment followed by another experimental treatment (Polit & Beck, 2006). The order of administration of the two treatments to the two groups is determined randomly. The group of research participants serves as its own control.

For example, Schneider and colleagues (2004) used a crossover design to test a predictive middle-range theory of the effects of virtual reality as a distraction intervention on symptom distress, fatigue, and anxiety experienced by women receiving chemotherapy for breast cancer. One-half of the women in the sample received the virtual reality intervention plus standard care during their first chemotherapy treatment, and standard care only during their second chemotherapy treatment, whereas the other half received standard care only during their first chemotherapy treatment and the virtual reality intervention plus standard care during their second chemotherapy treatment. The experimental virtual reality intervention was described as "a computer-simulated technique that allows individuals to hear and feel stimuli that correspond with a visual image by wearing a headset that projects the image with accompanying sounds. . . . Virtual reality is considered a distraction technique because it diverts the focus of attention away from the stressful stimuli" (Schneider et al., pp. 82, 84). The investigators used Lazarus' theory of coping to guide their study.

Nonequivalent control group designs involve just one group of research participants or two groups that are not equivalent because they are not randomly assigned to treatments (Cook and Campbell, 1979). When two groups are involved, one of the groups may not receive any treatment. The group that does not receive any treatment may be called the **comparison group**, rather than the control group (Polit & Beck, 2006). Groups who do not receive any treatment as part of a study may be offered an opportunity to receive the experimental treatment after their participation in the study is concluded. Such groups may be referred to as "delayed treatment" groups (Colling, Owen, McCreedy, & Newman, 2003, p. 118). Colling and colleagues, for example, offered their experimental continence program to control group participants after the program had been received by all experimental group participants (J. Colling, personal communication, June 17, 2006).

Comparison groups may be deliberately formed by the researcher for quasi-experimental research, or they may evolve naturally (Burns & Grove, 2007). For example, Keefe and colleagues' (2005) study included a comparison group that evolved as they tested a predictive middle-range theory of the effects on the behavior of infants with colic of an individualized nursing intervention called REST (Regulation, Entrainment, Structure, and Touch; Reassurance, Empathy, Support, and Time-out). The study was guided by Keefe's (1988) developmental psychobiological theory of infant colic. Infants were randomly assigned to the experimental group, who received the weekly home-based REST routine for 4 weeks, or the control group, who received weekly home visits for 4 weeks from the evaluation team to collect data but did not receive the REST routine. The comparison group evolved when "parents in the control group began to comment on the benefits derived from having the evaluation team members visit their homes. This posttest-only [comparison] group consisted of infants referred to the study [who] where older than the [experimental and control group infants at the beginning of the study], yet comparable in age to those infants completing the intervention program" (pp. 233–234).

The four specific nonequivalent control group designs most frequently used in the social and health sciences are the one-group pretest-posttest design, the one-group posttest only, the nonequivalent control group pretest-posttest design, and the posttest-only with nonequivalent groups design. A summary of the characteristics of these four designs is given in Table 7–2, which is on the CD that comes with this book. Many other less frequently used designs are described in detail by Cook and Campbell (1979).

Interrupted time-series designs involve comparisons of multiple measures of the dependent variable before and after an experimental treatment is administered. This design does not include a comparison group. **Time-series** refers to multiple measures of the same or a similar dependent variable over time; **interrupted time-series** "requires knowing the specific point in the series when a treatment occurred" (Cook & Campbell, 1979, p. 207). Whittemore and

Grey (2006) pointed out that interrupted time-series designs can be used to determine **trends**, or changes over time. The data collected before the treatment is administered are referred to as the **baseline data**; the data collected after the treatment is implemented are referred to as the **outcomes**.

For example, Ravesloot, Seekins, and White (2005) tested a predictive middle-range theory of the effects of the Living Well with a Disability health promotion program on secondary conditions, such as urinary tract infections, pressure sores, and depression; limitations associated with the secondary conditions; number of days that physical or mental symptoms were experienced; and utilization of health-care services in adults with mobility impairments. The Living Well program was given at nine Centers for Independent Living (CILs) throughout the United States; the centers were randomly assigned into two blocks. Baseline data were collected at the beginning of each Living Well program. Outcomes were measured immediately after the end of the program and then at 2, 4, and 12 months. Ravesloot et al. did not identify an explicit conceptual or theoretical frame of reference for the study. However, it can be inferred from the focus of the Living Well program that their work was grounded in a health promotion frame of reference.

True Experiments or Quasi-Experimental Designs

Some theory-testing experimental research may involve a true experiment, a quasi-experimental design, or a combination of the two. Outcomes research, clinical trials, and factorial designs fall into this category of experimental research.

Outcomes research, which may be designed as true experiments or quasi-experimental studies, "is undertaken to document the quality and effectiveness of health care and nursing services" (Polit & Beck, 2006, p. 251). The interrupted time-series study conducted by Ravesloot and colleagues (2005) could be considered outcomes research. Another example, made up of a series of several studies conducted by an oncology nurse, is given here.

For almost 30 years, McCorkle (2006) has been studying the effects of nursing interventions on outcomes experienced by people with cancer and their family caregivers. Her research has focused primarily on the effects of structured nursing interventions provided by advanced-practice nurses in patients' homes. Outcomes studied included patients' physical symptom distress, mood disturbances, functional status, and relationships with family members and friends, as well as family caregivers' psychological distress and burden. As her program of research evolved, McCorkle more explicitly conceptualized her studies within in a health-related quality of life frame of reference. Moreover, one of her correlational studies (Nuamah et al., 1999) was explicitly guided by Roy's Adaptation Model.

The **clinical trial**, which is a term used in the health-care sciences to refer to research designed to test predictive middle-range theories about the effects of interventions, represents a combination of quasi-experimental and true experimental designs over five phases (Whittemore & Grey, 2002). The essential features of each phase of a clinical trial are given in Box 7–10. **Phase III clinical trials**, which frequently are referred to as **randomized clinical trials** or **randomized controlled clinical trials (RCTs)**, are regarded as the "gold standard" of research designs and "the most appropriate research design to answer questions about the effectiveness of an intervention" (Whittemore & Grey, 2006, pp. 222, 226).

An example of a Phase III RCT is given here. McCaffrey and Freeman (2003) conducted an RCT, guided by Rogers' Science of Unitary Human Beings, to test a predictive middle-range theory of the effects of a music intervention on pain in community-dwelling older adults with

BOX 7-10	Phases of Clinical Trials

Phase I—Descriptive or correlational studies to generate and test theories that guide development of the interventions and develop instruments to measure outcomes; quasi-experimental studies to finalize intervention content and dose, such as the length of time the intervention should be administered or its intensity

Phase II—Quasi-experimental studies to obtain preliminary data about intervention effects, including amount of difference in outcomes for experimental and control groups

Phase III—True experiments to determine intervention effects in ideal settings with attention to precise administration of the intervention by research team members

Phase IV—Determination of the extent to which the Phase III experimental intervention is applicable in actual practice settings with people other than the Phase III research participants, monitoring of long-term positive and negative effects of the intervention, and determination of the cost-effectiveness of the intervention

Phase V—Wide-scale studies to determine the effects of the interventions on public health

osteoarthritis. Research participants were randomly assigned to experimental and control groups. The experimental group participants sat in a quiet and comfortable place at home and each day for 14 days listened to a 20-minute audiotape of three relaxing music selections by Mozart. The control group participants also sat in a quiet and comfortable place at home for 20 minutes each day for 14 days but were permitted only to read books or magazines during that time. Pain, the dependent variable, was measured on the 1st, 7th, and 14th days before and after listening to the music (experimental group) or sitting quietly (control group).

Although clinical trials are most frequently conducted to test the safety and effectiveness of drugs and surgical procedures, all phases may be used in any area of health sciences research. For example, McCaffrey and Freeman (2003) did not publish any reports of Phase I, II, IV, or V trials. Suppose, however, that they conducted a Phase I clinical trial to find out how long people were willing to sit quietly and listen to music and how many minutes of music how often were needed to obtain an effect on pain. Suppose also that they conducted a Phase II clinical trial to determine whether people who listened to music experienced less pain than people who did not listen to music. And suppose that when the results of their Phase III clinical trial indicated that listening to music was an effective way to reduce pain experienced by research participants who had osteoarthritis, they decided to conduct a Phase IV clinical trial by administering the music intervention to older adults who experienced pain from osteoarthritis and lived in nursing homes. The Phase IV clinical trial could include measuring not only pain but also mobility and collecting data from research participants for 2, 3, or more months. Finally, suppose they collaborated with many other researchers and clinicians to conduct a Phase V clinical trial by implementing the music intervention in nursing homes throughout an entire country and determining the effects on all nursing home residents who agreed to provide data.

Factorial designs are more complex versions of either true experiments or quasi-experimental designs that involve two or more independent variables, examination of the effects of each independent variable, and the effects of the interaction between the independent variables (Campbell & Stanley, 1963; Polit & Beck, 2006). The name of the design comes from calling the independent variable a **factor**. Each factor—or independent variable—encompasses two or more treatment levels, which usually reflect the dose of the treatment. The effects of the independent variable are called the **main effects**; the effects of the interaction of the independent variables are called the **interaction effects**. The independent variables may be treatments and/or study participant characteristics. The dependent variable may be measured both before and after (pretest and posttest) or only after (posttest only) the treatments have been administered (Campbell & Stanley).

For example, Smith (2001) tested a predictive middle-range theory of the effects of an experimental culture school educational treatment and a control treatment informatics class on cultural self-efficacy, that is, "the degree of confidence . . . nurses have as they provide care to Hispanic, African-American, and Asian clients" (Smith, p. 52), as well as cultural knowledge. The independent variables were the treatment (two levels: experimental culture school and control informatics class), race (two levels: white and nonwhite), and phase of data collection (three levels: pretest prior to administration of the treatment, posttest at the end of the 8.5-hour treatment, and another posttest 3 weeks later). The study was guided by Giger and Davidhizar's (1999) Transcultural Assessment Model and Theory, which focuses attention on culturally unique individuals, culturally sensitive environments, culturally specific health-related behaviors, and culturally competent nursing care involving consideration of space, time, social organization, environmental control, biological variations, and communication.

Other Descriptive, Correlational, and Experimental Research Designs

Some types of research involve descriptive, correlational, and experimental research designs. Among these are evaluation research and pilot, or exploratory, research (see Box 7–8).

Evaluation research, which focuses on determining the effectiveness of programs, policies, or procedures, involves various descriptive, correlational, or experimental research designs. Four types of evaluation research have been identified—process analysis, outcome analysis, impact analysis, and cost-benefit analysis.

Process analysis, which is also called **implementation analysis**, focuses on description of the process used to implement a program, policy, or procedure, and how that program, policy, or procedure actually works in practice (Polit & Beck, 2006). **Outcome analysis** focuses on description of people's health status following implementation of a program, policy, or procedure (Polit & Beck). **Impact analysis** focuses on determining whether implementation of a new program, policy, or procedure resulted in greater effects than those associated with the previously used program, policy, or procedure (Polit & Beck). **Cost-benefit analysis** focuses on comparing the financial costs of the implementation of a program, policy, or procedure with its benefits (Polit & Beck). All four types of analysis are incorporated in the guidelines for policy and program evaluation that are associated with the Conceptual Model of Nursing and Health Policy (Fawcett & Russell, 2001; Russell & Fawcett, 2005). The guidelines are listed in Table 7–3 on the CD that comes with this book.

An example of program evaluation is Dalton, Garvey, and Samia's (2006) evaluation of an experimental diabetes disease management program used by a home health-care agency. The quasi-experimental evaluation project, which involved both outcome analysis and impact analysis, included three groups of diabetic home health-care patients. One group received traditional home health care for diabetes prior to the implementation of the Medicare Prospective Payment System (PPS), another group received traditional home health care for diabetes after the implementation of PPS, and a third group received the experimental diabetes disease management program after the implementation of PPS. The evaluation project was guided by Orem's Self-Care Framework.

An example of policy evaluation is Poirier's 2005 study. Using the Conceptual Model of Nursing and Health Policy (Fawcett & Russell, 2001) and the Piper Integrated Fatigue Model (Piper, Dibble, Dodd, Weiss, Slaughter, & Paul, 1998) as guides for a correlational study, Poirier evaluated the impact of Family and Medical Leave Act benefits and employer sick leave benefits, individual characteristics, and radiation therapy–related fatigue on the employment patterns of men and women with cancer.

Pilot and exploratory studies can be descriptive, correlational, or experimental. An **exploratory study** or a **pilot study** typically is conducted with a small number of research participants to determine the feasibility of conducting the study with a large number of people, including the utility of the selected research design, the adequacy of the approach used to recruit and retain research participants, the adequacy of the instruments used to measure study variables, and the procedures used to collect data, as well as to obtain an estimate of the size of the correlation between study variables or the amount of difference between experimental and control groups (Prescott & Soeken, 1989).

For example, Mock and her colleagues (2001) conducted a pilot study guided by Levine's Conservation Model at five university hospital outpatient cancer units to determine the feasibility of conducting a large-scale study of the effects of an experimental home-based moderate walking exercise intervention on women's experiences of fatigue, as well as their physical functioning, emotional distress, and quality of life while receiving chemotherapy or radiation therapy for breast cancer. The women were randomly assigned to the experimental moderate walking exercise intervention or the control usual care treatment. The investigators found that some women in the usual care control group engaged in active exercise during the study and that some women in the experimental group could not maintain the prescribed amount of exercise. They also found that follow-up was needed to ensure consistent implementation of the experimental intervention. In addition, they realized that some objective measures of outcomes were needed in addition to the women's own reports of outcomes. They used the insights gained from the pilot study to refine the design, instruments, and data collection procedures for a larger study (Mock et al., 2005).

Conclusion

This chapter was not meant to be a comprehensive discussion of research design but rather an overview of the essential features of research designs typically found in the literature of the health sciences, with an emphasis on nursing science. We have included the information needed for evaluation of the research design element of the E component of C-T-E structures for theory-generating research and theory-testing research. If you read a report of a study based on a research design not mentioned in this chapter, you may want to search the literature to find out more about the particular research design or read the references to that design cited in the research report.

It is tempting to get lost in the details of research design and other elements of the E component of C-T-E structures. However, the importance of the C and T components must be emphasized. We agree with Pedhazur (1982), who pointed out, "It is a truism that methods per se mean little unless they are integrated within a theoretical context and applied to data obtained in an appropriately designed study" (p. 3). Accordingly, the researcher's selection of a research design depends partly on what designs are specified in the research methods guidelines associated with the conceptual model (see Table 5–5 on the CD that comes with this book) or grand theory (see Table 5–6, on the CD) that guided the research and partly on the specific research question. The research question, in turn, depends on the research focus guidelines of the conceptual model (see Table 5–3, on the CD) or grand theory (see Table 5–4, on the CD), as well as what already is known about the research topic. If very little is known about the topic, a descriptive research design is appropriate to generate a descriptive theory. If something is known about at least two concepts, a correlational research design is appropriate to test an explanatory theory. If enough is known to test a predictive theory addressing the effect of an intervention on one or more specific outcomes, an experimental research design is appropriate. How much already is known is determined from a critical review of the literature about the topic.

The questions to ask and answer as you evaluate the research design element of empirical research methods are listed in Box 7–11. Application of the criterion of operational adequacy for research designs should help you to better understand the E component of C-T-E structures. The learning activities for this chapter will help you increase your understanding of the operational adequacy criterion and its application to the contents of research reports.

BOX 7-11	Evaluation of Theory-Generating and Theory-Testing Research Designs: *How Good* Is the Information?

Operational Adequacy

* Is the research design identified in the research report?
* Did the research design allow the research questions to be answered?

References

Full citations for all references cited in this chapter are provided in the Reference section at the end of the book.

Learning Activities

Activities to supplement what you have learned in this chapter, along with practice examination questions, are provided on the CD that comes with this book.

Chapter 8

Evaluation of Samples

This chapter continues the focus begun in Chapter 7 on the empirical research methods (E) component of conceptual-theoretical-empirical (C-T-E) structures for research. Recall from Chapter 2 that the E component of a C-T-E structure encompasses five major elements—the research design, the sample, the instruments and any experimental conditions, the procedures used to collect data and protect research participants from harm, and the techniques used to analyze the data. This chapter focuses on the sample, or research participants, element of the E component of C-T-E structures.

KEYWORDS

Attrition	Population
Bias	Power Analysis
Chain Sampling	Probability Sampling
Cluster Sampling	Purposeful Selection
Convenience Sampling	Purposive Sampling
Data Saturation	Quota Sampling
Deviant Case Sampling	Random Sampling
Effect Size	Representative Sample
Exclusion Criteria	Response Rate
External Validity	Sample
Extreme Case Sampling	Selective or Judgmental Sampling
Generalizability	Simple Random Sampling
Inclusion Criteria	Snowball Sampling
Matching	Stratified Random Sampling
Maximum Variation Sampling	Theoretical Sampling
Network Sampling	Transferability
Nonprobability Sampling	Typical Case Sampling

Recall from Chapters 3 and 4 that you began to learn *where* in research reports to look for information about the research participants who made up the sample (Box 8–1) and *what* information you could expect to find (Box 8–2).

BOX 8-1	Evaluation of Samples: *Where* Is the Information?

- Look in the method section of the research report
  - Usually a separate subsection for sample
- Also look in the results section

BOX 8-2	Evaluation of Samples: *What* Is the Information?

- The source of data for theory-generating research and theory-testing research

Recall also that in Chapter 4, where we presented a framework for evaluation of C-T-E structures for research, you began to learn how to determine *how good* the information about the research participants is.

In this chapter, we will help you learn *what* number of research participants is needed for different kinds of theory-generating research and theory-testing research and more about how to determine *how good* the information about the selection and number of research partici- pants is. More specifically, in this chapter we discuss in detail the criterion of operational ade- quacy as it applies to the sample and provide examples that should help you better understand how to apply the criterion as you read research reports. Application of the criterion will facil- itate your evaluation of *how good* the information about the sample provided in the research report is.

WHAT IS A SAMPLE?

Recall from Chapter 2 that the source of data needed to generate or test middle-range theo- ries is referred to as the sample and that the sample can be made up of people, animals, organ- izations, or documents. Samples of people can be individuals as well as members of groups of interest for the research, such as families (Niska, 2001) and communities (Racher & Annis, 2005). Animals, such as rabbits and cats, may be the sample for research (Holtzclaw & Hanneman, 2002) or may be included as companions to people, such as in research designed to investigate the influence of companion animals on the well-being of nursing home residents (Dono, 2005). Organizations, such as hospitals, home health-care agencies, and nursing homes, can be the sample, rather than the people who work in the organization (Almost, 2006). Documents, such as books, book chapters, and journal articles (Almost) or patients' charts (Kelley, Daly, Anthony, Zauszniewski, & Strange, 2002), also can be regarded as the sample.

The people who participate in research may be referred to as **subjects**, **informants**, **respon- dents**, **research participants**, or **study participants**. The particular term used in a research report depends on the philosophical paradigm reflected in the study and the research design used. People who participate in research conducted within the context of the naturalistic paradigm or the critical emancipatory paradigm frequently are referred to as research participants, study participants, or informants, whereas participants in research conducted within the context of the postpositivist paradigm may be referred to as subjects, respondents, research participants, or study participants. Regardless of the term used, the people who participate in theory-generating research or theory-testing research are collectively referred to as the sample.

A **sample** is specifically defined as a portion or a subset of a population. A **population** is defined as "the total number of units from which data can potentially be collected" (Parahoo, 2006, p. 256). In nursing research, the **population units**—also called **elements** (Burns & Grove, 2007; Haber, 2006; Polit & Beck, 2006)—typically are people but also can be animals, organizations, or documents. People's responses to open-ended questions or the recorded observations of people engaged in a certain behavior—rather than the people themselves— also can be considered population units. For example, the responses of caregivers of individuals with Alzheimer's disease to interview questions can be the population units, rather than the caregivers themselves. Or, a researcher's observations of people with Alzheimer's disease can be the population units rather than the people themselves.

The **target population**—also called the **theoretical population** (Parahoo, 2006)—is all units or elements that might be included in a study (Parahoo; Polit & Beck, 2006). An example of a target population is: All individuals with Alzheimer's disease in the state of Massachusetts.

The population units of interest depend, in part, on the conceptual model that guides the theory-generating research or theory-testing research. For example, most conceptual models of nursing include a research methods guideline indicating that research participants should be human beings. Population units of interest also depend on the research question. Suppose, for example, a researcher was interested in conducting a King's Conceptual System–based theory-generating study of individuals' perceptions of caring for a family member recently diagnosed with Alzheimer's disease. The population units would be men and women who were caring for a family member who had recently received the diagnosis of Alzheimer's disease.

Access to the entire target population may not be possible due to inability to identify every population unit. Access to the entire target population also may not be possible if some people are too ill or too disabled to participate. Therefore, a portion or subset of the entire target population—called the **accessible population** (Polit & Beck, 2006) or the **study population** (Parahoo, 2006)—is selected. The sample may be selected from either the target population or the accessible population (Figure 8–1). An example of an accessible population is: All family members of individuals with Alzheimer's disease who are receiving care at adult day care centers in Massachusetts.

How Is a Sample Selected?

The target population or the accessible population can be very precisely identified by specifying criteria for inclusion and exclusion of certain population units. **Inclusion criteria**—also called **sampling criteria** or **eligibility criteria** (Burns & Grove, 2007)—refer to the characteristics the population units must have to be part of the sample. An example of inclusion criteria is: Adult family members of individuals with Alzheimer's disease being cared for at home.

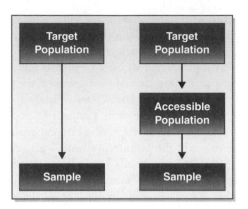

Figure 8-1. Target populations, accessible populations, and samples.

Exclusion criteria are population unit characteristics that exclude those units from being part of the sample. An example of exclusion criteria is: Adult family members of individuals with Alzheimer's disease residing in skilled nursing facilities.

In nursing research, inclusion and exclusion criteria frequently focus on demographic and health-related characteristics but also may specify the setting in which the population units are located. Note that the examples of inclusion and exclusion criteria given here include a demographic characteristic (adults), health condition (Alzheimer's disease), and setting (home or skilled nursing facility).

Why Are Samples Selected?

Samples are selected because it usually is impossible or too expensive to conduct research using the entire target population or accessible population. At times, however, it is possible to include all units of an entire population in a study. For example, a study of the type and frequency of practice activities performed by nurse case managers was conducted using the entire target population of all 20 registered nurses who were, as of fall 2004, working as case managers in the Women's Health Network, a breast and cervical cancer and cardiovascular disease risk screening program for low-income, uninsured, or underinsured women in Massachusetts (Fawcett, Schutt, Gall, Riley-Cruz, & Woodford, 2007).

HOW IS THE CRITERION OF OPERATIONAL ADEQUACY APPLIED TO SAMPLES?

When applied to the sample element of empirical research methods, the criterion of **operational adequacy** refers to the amount of information about the sample given in a research report and focuses attention on whether the sample was selected using an appropriate method and was large enough to provide enough data to generate or test a meaningful middle-range theory.

The operational adequacy criterion, when applied to samples, is met when you can answer yes to three questions:

- Are the population and the sample clearly identified in the research report?
- Is the method of sample selection appropriate?
- Is the size of the sample adequate?

Are the Population and the Sample Identified in the Research Report?

The sample almost always is explicitly identified in a research report, although the target population or accessible population may not be identified. If the population is not explicitly identified, the inclusion and exclusion criteria usually are explained and can be used to describe the population. Examples of identification of the sample are given in Box 8–3.

Just one of the reports cited in Box 8–3 included a statement about the target population, and two reports did not include any information about exclusion criteria. Sufficient information, however, was given in each report for the reader to describe the population. For example, for the study reported by Beanlands and colleagues (2005), the accessible population can be described

BOX 8-3	Examples of Identification of Samples in Research Reports

An example from the report of a descriptive study of the activities of caregivers of adults receiving dialysis (Beanlands et al., 2005)

Sample

- Males and females

Inclusion criteria

- Caregivers of adult patients receiving dialysis
- Over the age of 19 years
- Residents of the Province of Ontario, Canada
- Able to verbally communicate in English
- Willing to participate

Exclusion criteria

- None identified

An example from the report of a correlational study of the relations among maternal role involvement, student role involvement, total network support, and maternal-student role stress (Gigliotti, 2004)

Sample

- Women

Continued

BOX 8-3	Examples of Identification of Samples in Research Reports—cont'd

Inclusion criteria

- Under 37 years of age or 37 years of age and older
- Has at least one child under the age of 19 years presently at home
- Born and raised in the United States
- Married
- Currently taking a clinical nursing course in an associate degree program

Exclusion criteria

- None identified

An example from the report of an experimental study of the effects of exercise on fatigue and quality of life during cancer treatment (Mock et al., 2001)

Sample

- Females

Inclusion criteria

- Receiving treatment for cancer at outpatient clinics
- Recently treated for stage I, II, or IIIa breast cancer
- Scheduled to receive outpatient adjuvant radiation therapy or chemotherapy

Exclusion criterion

- Concurrent major health problem that would contraindicate an exercise program

An example from the report of a correlational study of factors related to exercise participation (Kaewthummanukul, Brown, Weaver, & Thomas, 2006)

Target population

- Female registered nurses

Inclusion criteria

- Employed by a government-operated regional university hospital located in the northern region of Thailand
- Employed full-time
- Between the ages of 18 and 60 years
- Willing to participate in the study

Exclusion criterion

- Nurses currently pregnant

Sample

- 970 female registered nurses who met the inclusion criteria and were not pregnant as English-speaking male and female residents of Ontario, Canada, who were over 19 years of age, were caring for adults receiving dialysis, and were willing to participate in the study.

Is the Method of Sample Selection Appropriate?

Sample selection refers to the way in which people, animals, organizations, or documents are identified for inclusion in a study. In general, the goal of sample selection is to obtain an adequate source of data to generate or test a middle-range theory. Different methods of sample selection are appropriate for use with qualitative and quantitative research designs. Regardless of the research design, however, the research report should include a rationale for the sample selection method.

Sample Selection for Qualitative Research Designs

For qualitative research designs, a specific goal of sample selection is to deliberately select "particular settings, persons, or activities . . . to provide information that can't be gotten as well from other [sources]" (Maxwell, 2005, p. 88). A related goal is to deliberately select a sample that will "maximize the scope and range of information obtained" (Lincoln & Guba, 1985, p. 224). The goals of sample selection for qualitative research designs are met with a method variously called **purposeful selection** (Maxwell), **criterion-based selection** (Maxwell), **purposive sampling** (Burns & Grove, 2007; Polit & Beck, 2006), or **selective or judgmental sampling** (Burns & Grove).

We agree with Maxwell (2005) that the term *purposeful selection* is most descriptive of the way samples are selected for qualitative research designs and that it is the least confusing term, as purposive sampling is also used for quantitative research designs (Kerlinger & Lee, 2000; Polit & Beck, 2006). Parahoo (2006) noted that researchers using qualitative research designs may substitute the term **recruitment** for sampling. In other words, the population units of interest are recruited or deliberately invited to participate in the study.

Purposeful selection can be completed using several different strategies. The results of the research conducted with the sample may or may not be applicable to other sample groups.

Strategies Used for Purposeful Selection. Strategies that can be used for purposeful selection of a sample include typical case sampling, maximum variation sampling, extreme or deviant sampling, and theoretical sampling.

Typical case sampling is a strategy used to obtain people or other sources of data that are known to have typical target population characteristics. Also known as **homogeneous sampling** or **criterion sampling** (Polit & Beck, 2006), this strategy is used to "avoid rejection of information on the grounds that it is known to arise from special or deviant cases" (Lincoln & Guba, 1985, p. 200).

Maximum variation sampling is a strategy used to obtain a sample that has very diverse target population characteristics (Polit & Beck, 2006). Lincoln and Guba (1985) pointed out that maximum variation sampling is used "to document unique variations that have emerged in adapting to different conditions" (p. 200).

Extreme or deviant case sampling is a strategy used to obtain a sample that has extreme target population characteristics (Polit & Beck, 2006). The people making up such samples have unusual characteristics "that may be troublesome or enlightening" (Lincoln & Guba, 1985, p. 200).

Theoretical sampling is used primarily with the grounded theory qualitative research design (Glaser & Strauss, 1967). This strategy differs from the other purposeful selection strategies in that additional sources of data are added to the sample as the categories or themes of a middle-range theory emerge from the data already collected.

Regardless of the purposeful selection strategy used, the research participants should have personal experience of the phenomenon being studied (Brink, 2001). An example of the use of each of these purposeful selection strategies is given in Box 8–4. Other examples of purposeful selection sampling are given in Tables 8–1 and 8–2, which are on the CD that comes with this book.

BOX 8-4	Examples of Types of Purposeful Selection of Samples for Qualitative Descriptive Research Designs

Typical Case Sampling

Mahoney (2001) used typical case sampling as part of purposeful selection of a sample for her ethnographic study of understanding the illness experience in patients with congestive heart failure and their family members.

Maximum Variation Sampling

Heaman, Chalmers, Woodgate, and Brown (2006) used maximum variation sampling to obtain a sample that varied according to "type of participants (public health nurse, home visitors and parents) and location of residence (inner city or suburban)" (p. 293) for their descriptive study of factors that public health nurses, home visitors, and parents considered important for the success of an early childhood home visiting program.

Extreme Case Sampling

Gous and Roos (2005) used extreme case sampling for their case study of a woman suffering from depression who killed her baby.

Theoretical Sampling

Montgomery, Tompkins, Forchuk, and French (2006) used theoretical sampling to obtain a sample for their grounded theory study of the experiences of mothers with serious mental illness.

Transferability of Qualitative Research Findings.   Different samples from the same target population may differ from one another and from the target population in one or more characteristics (Williams, 1978). Consequently, different samples may yield different results. In qualitative research, the extent to which research results can be applied—or transferred—to people other than the particular research participants is referred to as **transferability**, or **fittingness** (Polit & Beck, 2006; Speziale & Carpenter, 2003). More specifically, transferability "refers to the probability that the study findings have meaning to others in similar situations" (Speziale & Carpenter, p. 39). Ford-Gilboe, Campbell, and Berman (1995) explained that when conducting qualitative research, "a rich description of the context and sample participants is sought so that transferability of the study findings to other contexts can be made" (p. 24).

Maxwell (2005) claimed that transferability may be irrelevant because the findings of a qualitative study may be especially "illuminating as an extreme case or 'ideal type'" (p. 115). Although Lincoln and Guba (1985) maintained that transferability is determined primarily by readers of the research report or users of the research findings, rather than by the researcher, the limitations or other section of qualitative research reports may include a discussion of transferability.

For example, Copnell and Bruni (2006) used a sample of 12 critical care nurses who worked in intensive care units of hospitals in Melbourne, Australia, for their descriptive study of nurses' understanding of changes in their practice. In the conclusion section of their research report, they commented, "This paper presents the views of a small group of nurses working in one clinical specialty (critical care) in one country (Australia). No claims of the universality [that is, the transferability] of these views are made" (p. 308).

Sample Selection for Quantitative Research Designs

The specific goal of sample selection for quantitative research designs is to obtain a sample that is representative of the target population (Polit & Beck, 2006). A **representative sample** "means that the sample has approximately the characteristics of the population relevant to the research . . . question (Kerlinger & Lee, 2000, pp. 165–166). The characteristics of the population that are relevant for the research question are specified by the inclusion and exclusion criteria (see Box 8–3).

Sample selection methods used for quantitative research designs are **probability sampling** and **nonprobability sampling**. Probability sampling is thought to yield samples that are more likely to be similar to each other and to the population than those yielded by nonprobability sampling (Williams, 1978). Examples of probability and nonprobability sampling are given in Table 8–3 on the CD that comes with this book.

Probability Sampling. **Probability sampling** is characterized by **random selection** of population units, such that every population unit has an equal chance of being selected for the sample. It is thought that a random sample will be a representative sample, although random selection does not guarantee representativeness.

Strategies used for probability sampling are simple random sampling, stratified sampling, cluster sampling, and systematic sampling.

Simple random sampling is the most commonly used probability sampling strategy. It involves assigning a number to every population unit and randomly selecting the units that will make up the population. Random samples can be selected by drawing the numbers of the population units from a hat or other container (Parahoo, 2006) or by using a table of random numbers, a coin toss, the sealed opaque envelope technique, or a computer program. Simple random sampling is most appropriate when the characteristics of all of the population units are similar, that is, when the population is **homogeneous** (Parahoo).

For example, Roelands, Van Oost, Depoorter, Buysse, and Stevens (2006) conducted a correlational study of the relation of home health-care nurses' intentions, attitudes, subjective norms, and self-efficacy to their introduction of the use of assistive devices for community-dwelling older persons with disabilities. The researchers used simple random sampling to select a sample of home health-care nursing departments from the target population of all local home health-care nursing departments in two provinces in Belgium.

Stratified random sampling is one probability sampling strategy that can be used when the characteristics of the units of the population are quite different—that is, when the population is **heterogeneous** (Parahoo, 2006). Heterogeneous population characteristics could include the age, gender, or health condition of people or animals; various types of organizations, such as small community hospitals, large academic medical centers, nursing homes, or home health-care agencies; or various types of documents, such as books, book chapters, or journal articles. When the population units are heterogeneous, stratified sampling increases the likelihood of obtaining a representative sample. Stratified sampling also can be used to obtain homogeneous groups for experimental research—that is, groups that have the same demographic or other relevant characteristics. This strategy involves separating the units of the population into strata, each one of which—called a **stratum**—is made up of one characteristic. More specifically, population **strata** are nonoverlapping or mutually exclusive "segments of a population based on a specific characteristic" (Polit & Beck, 2006, p. 261). Random sampling of the population units within each stratum is used to obtain the sample. Alternatively, random sampling may take into account the proportion of the population characteristic in each stratum; this approach is called **proportional allocation** (Kerlinger & Lee, 2000).

For example, Nir, Zolotogorsky, and Sugarman (2004) used a "stratified, random-sampling technique, controlling for age, sex, and ethnicity [to generate] two homogeneous groups" (p. 523)—one experimental group and one control group—for their experimental study of the effects of a nursing intervention on stroke patients' functional status, depression, locus of control, self-perceived health, self-esteem, and dietary adherence during rehabilitation. In this example, three strata were considered—age, sex, and ethnicity.

Cluster sampling is another probability sampling strategy that can be used when the population is heterogeneous. This strategy is similar to stratified sampling but differs in that it takes advantage of natural clusters, which are groups of population units having similar characteristics (Parahoo, 2006), such as states, health-care institutions, cardiac rehabilitation programs, or breast cancer support groups. More specifically, a cluster is "a group of things of the same kind. It is a set of sample elements held together by some common characteristic(s)" (Kerlinger & Lee, 2000, p. 180). Proportional allocation can be used with cluster sampling as well as with stratified random sampling. **Two-stage** and **multistage cluster sampling** are types of cluster sampling that occur in successive stages using increasingly narrower clusters. This strategy might start, for example, with sampling of health-care institutions, followed by sampling of cardiac rehabilitation programs offered by the selected health-care institutions.

For example, Ngondi et al. (2005) used two-stage cluster sampling for their status survey that was designed to determine the prevalence and geographic distribution of trachoma, a contagious eye disease that can cause blindness, in Eastern Equatorial and Upper Nile, two states located in southern Sudan, Africa. They explained, "Study sites were selected on the basis of . . . (a) anecdotal reports of blinding trachoma; (b) security and accessibility; and (c) feasibility of initiating trachoma control interventions after the survey. . . . A two-stage random cluster sampling with probability proportional to size was used to select the sample . . . at each site. A cluster was defined as the population within a single village. Using a line listing of all the villages in each study site, villages were grouped into subdistricts. . . . In the first stage, villages were randomly selected with probability proportional to the estimated population of the subdistrict. In the second stage, households were selected from the villages selected in the previous stage. The first household was selected by going to the middle of the village and spinning a pen, after which the household nearest to the ball-tip of the pen was selected. Subsequent households were selected by a random walk around the village" (p. 905).

Systematic sampling is still another probability sampling strategy that can be used when the population is heterogeneous. This strategy frequently involves selecting every *n*th **number**—that is, any randomly selected number—on a numbered list of all units in the population until the desired number of population units is obtained. Selecting every *n*th number ensures that the intervals between the listed numbers remain the same. This strategy requires that the population units be listed randomly, the *n*th number be picked randomly by the researcher before selecting the first population unit for the sample, and the first unit be selected randomly (Parahoo, 2006). Moreover, the *n*th number must be within the limits of the total number of population units. For example, if a list contains 1000 names and a sample of at least 100 units is needed, the *n*th number cannot be larger than 10. Expressing doubt about systematic sampling as a legitimate probability sampling strategy, Kerlinger and Lee (2000) noted, "The representativeness of the sample chosen in this fashion is dependent upon the ordering of the *N* elements of the population" (p. 181).

For example, Liu (2006) used systematic sampling for her correlational study of the relation of physiological, psychological, and situational factors to fatigue in Taiwanese patients receiving hemodialysis. The researcher explained that using a list of names of 513 patients obtained in sequence from a chart review, 100 potential research participants were selected "beginning with the 3rd [name] and at intervals of 6 after that" (p. 43).

Nonprobability Sampling. **Nonprobability sampling** does not involve random sampling, although the representativeness of the sample for the population remains very important. However, every unit in the population does not have an equal chance to be selected for the sample and there is no way to determine the probability of including any particular population unit (Polit & Beck, 2006). Kerlinger and Lee (2000) pointed out that the extent to which a nonprobability sample is representative of a population depends at least in part on the "knowledge, expertise, and care" used by the researcher when selecting the sample (p. 178). Repeating a study, which is called **replication**, with a different nonprobability sample selected from the same population can help researchers to determine whether the results of the research remain the same (Kerlinger & Lee). Strategies used for nonprobability sampling are quota sampling, purposive sampling, and convenience sampling.

Quota sampling is a nonprobability sampling strategy that involves identifying certain strata of a target population and selecting a certain number of units from each stratum to meet a quota for the sample (Polit & Beck, 2006). This strategy is similar to stratified random sampling in that strata of the target population are involved. The quotas are proportions of population units. Kerlinger and Lee (2000) explained, "Quota sampling derives its name from the practice of assigning quotas, or proportions of kinds of people, to interviewers. Such sampling has been used a good deal in public opinion polls" (p. 178).

For example, for her instrument development study designed to estimate the reliability and validity of a modified version of the Hung Postpartum Stress Scale, Hung (2005) used quota sampling to obtain a sample of low-risk postpartum women who had delivered healthy full-term infants at hospitals or clinics with the highest birth rates in Taiwan.

Purposive sampling is a relatively arbitrary nonprobability sampling strategy that relies heavily on the researcher's knowledge about the characteristics of the population that are relevant for the research (Kerlinger & Lee, 2000). Despite the risk of obtaining a sample that is not representative of the population, purposive sampling can be a particularly appropriate strategy for selecting a sample of people who are known to be experts in the research topic (Polit & Beck, 2006). For example, Lancaster (2004) explained that she used "purposive sampling [to obtain a sample of women] known to have a first- and/or second-degree relative with breast cancer" (p. 36) for her instrument development study, which was designed to develop and estimate the reliability and validity of the Coping with Breast Cancer Threat instrument.

Convenience sampling, also called **accidental sampling** (Burns & Grove, 2007; Kerlinger & Lee, 2000), is a widely used nonprobability sampling strategy that involves using readily available sources of data for the sample. It is unlikely, however, that a convenience sample is representative of a population, because readily available sources of data may not have the typical characteristics of that population. Although Kerlinger and Lee pointed out that convenience sampling "is hard to defend," they noted that "with reasonable knowledge and care, it probably does not deserve the bad reputation it has" (p. 179). They advised readers of research based on data from convenience sampling to "use extreme circumspection" (p. 179) when interpreting the research results.

Callaghan (2005), for example, used a "volunteer, convenience sample of adolescents aged 14 to 19 recruited from a Southern New Jersey High School" (p. 92) for her study of the relation between adolescents' spiritual growth and their self-care agency.

Snowball sampling is a variation of nonprobability convenience sampling used with both quantitative and qualitative research designs. Snowball sampling is also referred to as **network sampling** or **chain sampling** (Polit & Beck, 2006). This nonprobability sampling strategy relies on referrals from research participants to other potential research participants who have the same characteristics. Snowball sampling "takes advantage of social networks and the fact that friends tend to have characteristics in common" (Burns & Grove, 2007, p. 346) and typically is used when the target population "consists of people with specific [characteristics] who might be difficult to identify by ordinary means" (Polit & Beck, 2006, p. 262).

For example, Copnell and Bruni (2006) used snowball sampling to recruit a sample of male and female nurses of various ages and with diverse practice experiences for their qualitative study of nurses' understanding of changes in their practice. And, Hasnain, Sinacore, Mensah, and Levy (2005) used "snowball sampling techniques and neighborhood outreach strategies" to recruit a sample of 1,095 active intravenous drug users "living in an impoverished, predominantly African American community in Chicago" (p. 894) for their quantitative research, which was designed to test the relation between religiosity and HIV risk behaviors related to sharing injection paraphernalia.

Comparison of Probability and Nonprobability Sampling. Although probability sampling typically is regarded as better than nonprobability sampling, Kerlinger and Lee (2000) pointed out that each method presents challenges to the researcher. They explained that the weakness of nonprobability sampling, which depends on the extent to which the sample is representative of the population, "can to some extent be mitigated by using knowledge, expertise, and care in selecting samples, and by replicating [that is, repeating] studies with different samples. . . . [Furthermore] probability sampling does not guarantee more representative samples of the [population] under study" (p. 178). They concluded that regardless of the sampling method, "[t]he person doing the sampling must be knowledgeable of the population to be studied and the phenomena under study" (p. 178).

Matching. **Matching** is a particular type of sampling used for research designs that require equivalent groups for comparisons. Each research participant in one group is matched on one or more characteristics, such as age, gender, or severity of health condition, with another research participant in another group (Haber, 2006).

For example, Aschen (1997) used a Solomon four-group design to test a predictive middle-range theory of the effects of assertion training therapy on anxiety and responsiveness—that is, assertiveness, in four groups of male and female psychiatric patients. The study was guided by the model of transactional analysis, popularly known as the "I'm OK, You're OK" model (Harris, 1969). Assertiveness was defined as "the ability to express oneself in a direct and honest manner which is appropriate to the situation and does not infringe on the rights of others" (Aschen, p. 46). One experimental group who received the assertion training therapy provided both pretest and posttest data. A control group who did not receive the assertion training therapy also provided both pretest and posttest data. Another experimental group who received the assertion training therapy provided only posttest data, as did another control group who did not receive the assertion training therapy. Research participants in each group were matched rather than randomly assigned to the groups. Aschen explained, "A total of 37 adult [psychiatric] inpatients were selected, 20 of whom served as experimental subjects and 17 as controls. The majority of patients were diagnosed schizophrenic or depressive. Control subjects were selectively matched on age (plus or minus 2 years), sex, and diagnoses. Experimental subjects represented two groups of 10 subjects each (four men, six women). Control subjects were similarly divided, but the investigator was unable to match three subjects, which left seven subjects in the second control group. Therefore, this group contained three men and four women" (pp. 47–48).

Generalizability of Quantitative Research Results. Representative samples are required to generalize research results to the population. That is, the extent to which the sample characteristics actually represent the population characteristics determines whether and to what extent the research results can be generalized. **Generalizability**—also called **external validity**—means that the research results can be extended from the study sample to all units of the target population. Generalizability is a major issue with quantitative research designs. The limitations section of research reports frequently includes a discussion of generalizability.

For example, Salamonson and Andrew (2006) used a sample of second-year nursing students from a 3-year university-based nursing program in New South Wales, Australia, for their correlational study of the relation of age, ethnicity, and part-time employment to academic performance. When discussing the study limitations, they pointed out that their research "only focused on second year nursing students, which makes it difficult to generalize the results to all nursing students across the 3 years of the nursing programme" (p. 346).

Volunteers as Research Participants and Sampling Bias

Research ethics require that human beings who participate in research do so voluntarily and not be coerced. Thus, all samples made up of human beings are **volunteer samples**. Parahoo (2006) mentioned that convenience samples sometimes are made up of people who respond to newspaper advertisements or other public notices about the research. In that situation, the researcher has little or no control over who volunteers for the research are and does not know whether the motivation to volunteer stems from the offer of a financial or other inducement. Similarly, the researcher may have little or no control over who volunteers to participate in research when the population is made up of "captive" population units, such as hospitalized patients, students, prisoners, or even members of various types of support groups, such as those for breast cancer or weight management. It may not be clear whether individuals have volunteered willingly or from a sense of moral obligation, gratitude, fear of reprisal, fear of being considered uncooperative, or a need to conform (Parahoo).

Using volunteers for samples is thought to introduce bias into a research design. **Bias** means that a systematic distortion of an expected result has occurred (Oxford English Dictionary, 2007). When applied to sampling, bias refers to selection of research participants whose characteristics specifically differ from those of the population (Burns & Grove, 2007). Williams (1978) explained that bias is introduced when the sampling strategy is not carried out as planned, and therefore "population units are actually selected into the sample with chances other than those specified in the sampling [strategy]" (p. 68). Bias also can result if people selected for a study decline to participate and are found to differ on one or more characteristics from those people who agreed to participate.

For example, Croteau, Marcoux, and Brisson (2006) used random sampling to obtain a sample for their correlational study of risk factors associated with birth of a small-for-gestational-age infant. They denied any selection bias, explaining, "A selection bias seems improbable, since 95% of all births were reported to us, 93.8% of the women reported were contacted, and only 1.7% refused to participate" (p. 852). Mock et al. (2001) used convenience sampling with random assignment to experimental and control groups for their pilot study of the effects of walking exercise on fatigue, physical functioning, emotional distress, and quality of life among women receiving chemotherapy or radiation therapy for breast cancer. Acknowledging selection bias, they noted, "Selection bias may be represented in this study in the following manner. Women who lived more active lifestyles or had higher levels of physical fitness may have elected to exercise regularly, while women who lived more sedentary lifestyles or had lower levels of physical fitness may have had more difficulty exercising regularly during the study period" (p. 123).

Is the Size of the Sample Adequate?

Sample size refers to the number of population units used as sources of data for a study. The adequacy of the size of a sample depends primarily on the type of research design used. Relatively small samples obtained by purposeful selection typically are used for qualitative theory-generating research designs, whereas relatively large samples obtained by probability or nonprobability sampling are used for quantitative theory-testing research designs.

The actual size of the sample sometimes is based on such practical considerations as the amount of data the researcher can deal with and, in the case of qualitative research, the amount of time the researcher has for "intensive and prolonged contact" with research participants (Haber, 2006, p. 278). The sample size also may depend on the financial resources available to the researcher. The cost of a study includes "the amount of labor in data collection and data analysis" (Kerlinger & Lee, 2000, p. 179). In general, the larger the sample, the greater the cost of data collection and analysis.

The size of a sample also should be based on ethical considerations. King (2001) declared that researchers have an ethical responsibility to recruit an adequate-size sample. Elaborating, Lenth (2001) and Parahoo (2006) pointed out that it is unethical to include more research participants than are needed to obtain accurate data, or so few participants that knowledge cannot be advanced. In both cases, the time and effort of the participants may be wasted. Lenth added that in the case of experimental research, especially when conducted in a health-care setting, if the sample is too small, participants are exposed "to potentially harmful treatments without advancing knowledge," whereas if the sample is a too large, "an unnecessary number of subjects are exposed to a potentially harmful treatment, or are denied a potentially beneficial one" (p. 187).

Factors Affecting Sample Size

In addition to type of research design being used, ethical considerations, and costs, the sample size is also affected by response rate and attrition.

Response Rate. The research participants who actually provide data for a study may be referred to simply as the sample or as the **data-generating sample**. When human beings are the population units, the actual sample size may depend on the number of people who volunteer to participate in a study. Some people selected for a study may refuse to participate. The **response rate**—also referred to as the **refusal rate** (Burns & Grove, 2007)—is the percentage of people who decline an invitation to participate in a study or who accepted the invitation to participate but then did not provide any data. The response rate is calculated as the number of people who declined participation divided by the number of people selected for participation (Polit & Beck, 2006).

For example, Callaghan (2005) reported that she distributed 550 forms containing an explanation of the study along with parental consent and adolescent assent forms. Questionnaires were distributed to the 265 students who returned the consent and assent forms. She explained that 262 of the questionnaires were returned but that "6 were unusable because of missing data, resulting in a response rate of 47%" (p. 92) for her correlation study of the relation between adolescents' spiritual growth and their self-care agency. Thus, the data-generating sample was 256 adolescents.

Sometimes, the research report includes reasons for refusal. Liu (2006) reported that 4 of 36 potential research participants for the pilot phase of her correlational study of the relation of physiological, psychological, and situational factors to fatigue in Taiwanese patients receiving hemodialysis "refused due to physical discomfort," and one person "refused to participate without giving a reason" (p. 43).

Attrition. In addition, the size of the sample depends on the number of people who remain in a study when data are collected more than once. **Attrition**, also called **sample mortality**, refers to the number or percentage of people who withdraw from or drop out of a study after they began to provide data. For example, Smith (2001) collected data in three phases—a pre-intervention pretest, a posttest immediately after the intervention, and another posttest 3 weeks later—for her quasi-experimental study of the effects of an experimental culture school educational treatment and a control treatment informatics class on cultural self-efficacy and cultural knowledge. With regard to attrition, Smith reported, "Four experimental subjects and five control subjects were excluded from the study due to non-completion of follow-up evaluation activities" (p. 55).

Sample Size for Qualitative Research Designs

The ultimate criterion for adequacy of the sample size for qualitative theory-generating research designs is **data saturation** or **saturation of the categories**, which means that no new information would be obtained from additional sources of data, and therefore no new categories or themes would be identified in the words of the research participants (Speziale & Carpenter, 2003). Data saturation may, however, be a myth because it is always possible that other research participants, sampled at another time, might provide data that differ from those provided by the original participants. Consequently, Speziale and Carpenter recommend repeated study—**replication**—of the same research topic with participants having diverse characteristics. This approach is rarely used by nurse researchers. Exceptions were three studies of the universal lived experience of feeling very tired, which was guided by the Theory of Human Becoming and the Parse Method of Basic Research. Baumann (2003) collected data from a sample of 10 girls who attended suburban public schools in the Northeast region of the United States; Huch and Bournes (2003) collected data from a sample of 10 community-dwelling individuals, ranging from college juniors to retired professionals, who had no expressed health concerns and who lived in the southern United States; and Parse (2003) collected data from a sample of 10 women, all over 65 years of age, who were volunteers in community projects in a large metropolitan setting in North America. Bunkers (2003) discussed the similarities and differences in the findings from each study, pointing out that although the findings of each study were expressed in a different way, all three studies contributed to understanding the universal lived experience of feeling very tired.

Many researchers who conduct qualitative theory-generating research claim that data saturation is achieved with a small sample. For example, phenomenological research may be conducted with 10 or fewer participants, whereas grounded theory research designs frequently include 20 to 30 participants, and ethnographic research may involve 25 to 50 informants (Polit & Beck, 2006). Sandelowski (1995) argued that the small samples used for many qualitative studies may not support claims of no new themes or categories emerging from the data, whereas the larger samples typically used for theory-testing research may make in-depth analysis of the data from each research participant very difficult or impossible. She concluded that the size of a sample for qualitative theory-generating research depends on the type of theory-generating research design, the purpose of the research, and the strategy used for obtaining the sample.

Sample Size Justification for Qualitative Designs. Regardless of the sample size, the researcher should provide a justification or rationale for the size of the sample that highlights data obtained from an adequate number of participants "to ensure a rich and complete set of data" (Currie, 2005, p. 11) that permits "the deep, case-oriented analysis that is a hallmark of all qualitative inquiry and that results in . . . a new and richly textured understanding of experience" (Sandelowski, 1995, p. 183). All too often when qualitative research designs are used, the research report ends with a recommendation for additional research about the phenomenon with a larger sample (Cohen, Kahn, & Steeves, 2002). Use of an adequate-size sample for the initial research would, of course, be preferable to recommending additional research just because the sample was not large enough. Examples of sample sizes actually used with different types of qualitative theory-generating research designs are given in Table 8–1. Examples of sample sizes actually used with different types of qualitative or quantitative theory-generating research designs are given in Table 8–2. Both tables are on the CD that comes with this book.

Sample Size for Quantitative Research Designs

The ultimate criterion for adequacy of the sample size for quantitative theory-testing research designs is accurate results from a sample that is representative of the population (Haber, 2006; Polit & Beck, 2006). In general, the larger the sample, the more representative the sample and the more accurate the results. However, few researchers have resources that allow them to collect data from hundreds or thousands of participants. And very large samples yield findings that are statistically significant but practically meaningless (Kerlinger & Lee, 2000; Munro, 2005). Suppose, for example, a researcher conducted a sample survey of 5000 young adults and found a correlation of 0.10 between scores for a measure of performance of activities of daily living and scores for a measure of feelings of well-being. Although such a small correlation coefficient would be statistically significant with such a large sample size, when considering that correlation coefficients range from 0.00 to 1.00, we probably would conclude that the finding has minimal practical value. Conversely, suppose a researcher conducted a survey of 10 older adults and found a correlation of 0.60 between scores for a measure of health status and a measure of quality of life. Although the relatively large correlation coefficient would not be statistically significant with such a small sample, we probably would conclude that the finding has some practical value. Use of small samples for pilot studies, however, is not considered a waste of time, because the researcher is attempting to determine whether a study with a larger sample is feasible and might yield meaningful results. Examples of sample sizes for different types of quantitative theory-testing research designs are given in Table 8–3 on the CD that comes with this book.

Sample Size Justification for Quantitative Designs. Sample size for quantitative research designs can be justified using general rules or power analysis.

General rules are used by some researchers to identify and justify the size of a sample. A **general rule** is a relatively arbitrary formula for calculating the number of research participants needed for a particular research design. General rules for the multiple regression model-testing design, for example, require between 10 and 30 participants for each independent variable

(Kline, 2005; Osborne & Costello, 2004). A more specific general rule for the multiple regression model-testing research design is: The total sample (N) should be equal to or greater than ($\geqslant$) 50 + 8m participants, where m is the number of independent variables (Tabachnick & Fidell, 2001). Suppose, for example, a researcher included four independent variables in a multiple regression model; the required sample size would be: $N \geqslant 50 + (8 \times 4) = 50 + 32 = 82$ participants.

General rules for the structural equation modeling research design require from 100 to at least 500 participants (Kline, 2005; Norris, 2005). General rules for instrument development research designs range from a requirement of at least 10 participants per instrument item (Osborne & Costello, 2004) to at least 300 participants regardless of the number of instrument items (Tabachnick & Fidell, 2001). A more definitive general rule for instrument development research designs was given by Comfrey and Lee (1992), who maintained that "the adequacy of sample size might be evaluated very roughly on the following scale: 50 = very poor; 100 = poor; 200 = fair; 300 = good; 500 = very good; 1000 or more = excellent" (p. 217).

Power analysis is now being used by many researchers as an objective way to identify and justify the smallest sample size needed for accurate and practically meaningful results of quantitative theory-testing research. Power analysis can be done using printed tables available in Cohen's book (1988) and journal article (1992) or using a computer program, such as G*Power 3 (www.psycho.uni-duesseldorf.de/aap/projects/gpower/).

The description of the power analysis in a research report should include the name of the statistical test, the level of one-tailed or two-tailed statistical significance, the level of power, and the effect size used, along with a rationale for the effect size selected. For correlational research designs, the number of independent variables also should be given. For experimental research designs and other designs involving groups, the sample size for each group should be given (see Table 8–3 on the CD).

Power analysis can be applied with almost every **statistical test** used with correlational and experimental research designs. Examples of statistical tests are the Pearson correlation coefficient and multiple regression, both of which are used with correlational research designs; and analysis of variance, which is used with experimental research designs.

Statistics are used to test the so-called **null hypothesis**, which asserts that there is no relation between two or more variables or no difference in scores between two or more groups. The **level of statistical significance**, called **alpha**, refers to the probability of rejecting a null hypothesis. The typical alpha level used for power analysis is 0.05, which means there is a 5% probability of obtaining an inaccurate result—or a 95% probability of obtaining an accurate result. The level of statistical significance is specified for one-tailed and two-tailed tests. A *one-tailed test* of statistical significance is used when the hypothesis asserts that there is a positive or negative relation between variables or that one group will have higher scores than another group. A *two-tailed test* of statistical significance is used when the hypothesis simply asserts that there is a relation between variables or a difference between groups.

Power refers to "the probability of getting a statistically significant result, given that the null hypothesis is false" (Thomas & Juanes, 1996, p. 856). In other words, power refers to obtaining an accurate result from a statistical test. The level of power typically is set at 0.80, which means there is an 80% probability of obtaining an accurate result.

Effect size is a standardized numerical index of the magnitude—or size—of a research finding, including the magnitude of a correlation between variables or the magnitude of the difference between groups. Different numerical indices are associated with different statistical tests. For example, the numerical index for the effect size associated with a Pearson correlation coefficient (r) is the actual Pearson correlation coefficient, whereas the numerical index for the effect size associated with a t-test is d. Cohen (1988, 1992) identified the values for small, medium, and large effect sizes for various statistical tests. For example, for a Pearson correlation coefficient, a small effect size is $r = 0.10$, a medium effect size is $r = 0.30$, and a large effect size is $r = 0.50$. In contrast, for a t-test, a small effect size is $d = 0.20$, a medium effect size is $d = 0.50$, and a large effect size is $d = 0.80$.

Examples of power analysis found in research reports are given in Box 8–5. Note that some examples do not include the numerical index used for effect size (Chan et al., 2006; Kaewthummanukul, Brown, Weaver, & Thomas, 2006; Tsai, Tak, Moore, & Palencia, 2003), and some examples do not include justification for the effect size selected (Callaghan, 2005; Tsai et al., 2003). Note also that Callaghan substituted p for the alpha level; p is the symbol used for probability. In addition, note that none of the examples of correlational research (Tsai et al.; Kaewthummanukul et al.; Callaghan) included the number of independent variables.

BOX 8-5   Examples of Power Analysis in Published Research Reports

- Tsai, Tak, Moore, and Palencia (2003) reported a power analysis for their correlational study of relations between physical disability, social support, daily stress, depression, and pain. They explained, "The sample size of 71 was chosen to achieve enough statistical power for further path model analysis. . . . The recommended sample size according to the power analysis was 65 when a power of 0.80, effect size of 0.20, and alpha level of 0.05 were set for regression and correlational procedures" (p. 161).

- Kaewthummanukul, Brown, Weaver, and Thomas (2006) conducted a power analysis to determine the sample size for their correlational study of variables associated with participation in exercise. They stated, "The required sample size, based on a power analysis for partial correlation and regression analyses, was 329. . . . For this study, the statistically significant level was set at 0.05 and the level for power at 0.80. Because the effect size in a new area of research inquiry is likely to be small, and previous estimates of the effect sizes are unavailable . . . , the effect size of 0.20 as generally applied in nursing research was used" (p. 666).

- Callaghan (2005) conducted a power analysis to determine the size of the sample needed for her correlational study of the relation of between adolescents' spiritual growth and their self-care agency. She reported, "A power analysis revealed that at least 235 subjects were needed to attain a power $= .99$, medium effect size ($f^2 = .15$) and $p = .05$" (p. 92) to test a canonical correlation model. Her actual sample size was 256 adolescents.

- Chan et al. (2006) conducted an experimental study of the effects of an experimental music therapy treatment and control no-music treatment on pain and various physiological measures, including heart rate. They stated, "The power of the study was estimated based on the primary outcome measure, [heart rate] scores. A two-tailed independent t-test was used to test for differences between the two groups, and moderate effect size (0.845) was chosen based on an earlier local study. The required sample for each group was 23 (total $= 26$), and this number should have achieved 80% power at a 5% level of significance. . . . However, three participants in the study group refused to continue during the 15-minute intervention because they did not like the choice of music. Thus, 43 participants were recruited (20 music and 23 controls) and it was possible to reach a 5% alpha, and with a power of 76%" (p. 672).

Conclusion

In this chapter, you learned how to determine how good the information about the sample given in a research report is. Specifically, you continued to learn more about how to evaluate the E component of C-T-E structures using the criterion of operational adequacy. This chapter is not meant to be a comprehensive discussion of sampling and sample size. Rather, we presented an overview of the basic information needed to understand how the sample was obtained. If you read a report of a study in which a sampling strategy not mentioned in this chapter was used, you may want to search the literature to find out more about the particular sampling strategy or read any references to that strategy cited in the research report. We also presented basic information needed to understand whether the size of the sample was adequate, as well as how the size of the sample was justified. We agree with Osborne and Costello (2004) that larger samples usually are more adequate than smaller samples. Larger samples are more adequate because they have greater potential than smaller samples to increase the transferability of results obtained with qualitative research designs and the generalizability of results obtained with quantitative research designs.

The questions to ask and answer as you evaluate the sample element of empirical research methods are listed in Box 8–6. Application of the criterion of operational adequacy for samples should help you continue to better understand the E component of C-T-E structures. The learning activities for this chapter will help you increase your understanding of the operational adequacy criterion and its application to the contents of research reports.

BOX 8-6	Evaluation of Samples: *How Good Is the Information?*

Operational Adequacy

• Are the population and the sample clearly identified in the research report?

• Is the method of sample selection appropriate?

• Is the size of the sample adequate?

References

Full citations for all references cited in this chapter are provided in the Reference section at the end of the book.

Learning Activities

Activities to supplement what you have learned in this chapter, along with practice examination questions, are provided on the CD that comes with this book.

Chapter 9

Evaluation of Research Instruments and Experimental Conditions

This chapter continues the focus on the empirical research methods (E) component of conceptual-theoretical-empirical (C-T-E) structures for research and the criterion of operational adequacy. Recall from Chapter 2 that the E component of a C-T-E structure encompasses five major elements—the research design, the sample, the instruments and any experimental conditions, the procedures used to collect data and protect research participants from harm, and the techniques used to analyze the data. This chapter focuses on the instruments used to collect the data and on the experimental conditions—the experimental treatments and the control treatments—that are used with experimental research designs. Research instruments and experimental conditions are considered empirical indicators.

KEYWORDS

Biophysiological Equipment	Open-Ended Question
Checklists	Participant Observation
Clinimetrics	Psychometric Properties
Coding Sheets	Questionnaire
Credibility	Rating Scales
Cultural Equivalence	Reliability
Dependability	Research Instruments
Empirical Indicator	Sensitivity
Experimental Conditions	Specificity
Fixed-Choice Items	Trustworthiness
Interview Guide	Validity

In Chapter 3, you began to learn *where* to look for information about instruments and any experimental conditions in research reports (Box 9–1) and *what* information you could expect to find (Box 9–2). In Chapter 4, you began to learn how to determine *how good* the instruments and any experimental conditions are by using our framework for evaluating C-T-E structures for research.

In this chapter, you will learn *what* instruments are used to collect data for theory-generating research and theory-testing research and more about how to determine *how good* they are. You will also learn more about *what* experimental conditions are and how to determine *how good* they are. We discuss the criterion of operational adequacy as it applies to the research instruments and experimental conditions in detail and provide examples that should help you to

BOX 9-1	Evaluation of Instruments and Experimental Conditions: *Where* Is the Information?

- Look in the method section of the research report.
  - There are usually separate subsections of the method section for instruments and experimental conditions.
  - Experimental conditions may be part of the procedures subsection of the Method section

BOX 9-2	Evaluation of Instruments and Experimental Conditions: *What* Is the Information?

Instruments = Empirical Indicators

- Very concrete and specific real-world proxies—or substitutes—for middle-range theory concepts

Experimental Conditions = Empirical Indicators

- Protocols or "scripts" that direct actions in a precise manner
- Experimental treatments and control treatments

better understand how to apply the criterion as you read research reports. Application of the operational adequacy criterion will facilitate your evaluation of *how good* the information about the empirical indicators provided in the research report is.

WHAT IS AN EMPIRICAL INDICATOR?

An **empirical indicator** is a very concrete and specific real-world proxy—or substitute—for a middle-range theory concept that is used to measure the concept (DeVellis, 2003). The information obtained from empirical indicators typically is called **data**. The data may be words, which are associated with qualitative research designs, or numbers, which are associated with quantitative research designs.

Research Instruments as Empirical Indicators

Research instruments—also referred to simply as **instruments**—are one type of empirical indicator. The selection of a research instrument is one of the most important decisions made by a researcher. Regardless of how good a research instrument may be, if it does not measure the middle-range theory concept as that concept is constitutively defined by the researcher, it is not appropriate for use in the researcher's study.

Inasmuch as development of a new instrument can take several years, many researchers select existing instruments for their studies. Information about existing instruments can be found in several books and an online database that are listed in the Directories of Instruments on the CD that comes with this book.

Research instruments are used to collect qualitative (word) data or quantitative (number) data for all types of theory-generating and theory-testing research designs. The function of a research instrument is to provide the means by which concepts are measured so that theories can be generated or tested. More specifically, instruments provide word data that can be sorted into qualitative categories or themes, or numeric data that can be calculated to yield quantitative scores.

Research Instruments Used to Collect Qualitative Data

Data that are words are frequently obtained from research participants' responses to an **interview guide** made up of **declarative requests** ("Please tell me about your experience of . . .") or **open-ended questions** ("What has been your experience of . . . ?"). The word data then are analyzed to yield categories or themes. An example of an interview guide is given in Box 9–3.

BOX 9-3 **Example of an Interview Guide Used for Collection of Word Data**

DeSanto-Madeya (2006a) used an interview guide to collect the data for her theory-generating study of the meaning of living with spinal cord injury. She explained, "An interview guide was used to help the spinal cord injured person and family member describe the experience of living with spinal cord injury without leading the discussion. . . . The initial statement asked was 'Please describe your experience, including circumstances, situations, thoughts, and feelings that you think reflect your experience of living with spinal cord injury'" (p. 269).

The initial statement is considered a **declarative request**. That statement also could have been asked as an **open-ended question**, such as "What circumstances, situations, thoughts, and feelings reflect your experience of living with spinal cord injury?"

Research Instruments Used to Collect Quantitative Data

Data that are numbers typically are obtained from research participants' responses to **questionnaires** made up of fixed-choice items. **Fixed-choice items**, also called **closed-ended questions** or **fixed alternative questions** (Polit & Beck, 2006), that make up research instruments are similar to multiple-choice items found on examinations, such as a test given in a nursing research course. Specifically, the response categories for fixed-choice items are selected by the researcher before the research begins, and a number is attached to each response category. The research participants then answer each item by indicating which category or number best represents their feelings, perceptions, attitudes, or whatever aspect of a concept the questionnaire was designed to measure. The number data then are subjected to mathematical calculations that yield a score. An example of a questionnaire with fixed-choice items is given in Box 9–4.

Experimental Conditions as Empirical Indicators

Experimental conditions, which are another type of empirical indicator, are protocols or "scripts" that direct actions in a precise manner. Experimental conditions encompass the

BOX 9-4	Example of a Questionnaire Used for Collection of Number Data

Thomas-Hawkins (2000) used a questionnaire to measure functional status, defined as performance of usual activities, in her theory-testing study of correlates of change in functional status reported by patients receiving hemodialysis. The questionnaire, called the Inventory of Functional Status–Dialysis (IFS-Dialysis®), contains 23 items, arranged in three subscales—Personal Care Activities (5 items), Household Activities (9 items), and Social and Community Activities (9 items). Research participants are asked to indicate whether they did or did not perform the activity within the past 24 hours. A response of "No" is scored as 1, and a response of "Yes" is scored as 2. A "Never Did" option is available if the person responding to the IFS-Dialysis® had never performed the activity. The score for the IFS-Dialysis® is calculated by adding up all the "Yes" responses to items in each of the three subscales and in the total 23-item instrument and then dividing the sums by the number of items answered "Yes" or "No" for each subscale and the total instrument. Thus, the range of possible scores for each subscale, as well as the total instrument, is 1.00–2.00.

Thomas-Hawkins (2005) revised the response options to include four levels of performance for each activity during the past week, with "1 = did not perform, 2 = performed with a lot of help, 3 = performed with a small amount of help, and 4 = performed all by myself" (p. 690). The revised IFS-Dialysis® is scored by calculating a mean score for each subscale and the total IFS-Dialysis® for each respondent. The range of possible scores is 1.00–4.00, with higher scores indicating greater independence in activity performance.

experimental treatments and control treatments that are the focus of experimental theory-testing research. An example of experimental conditions is given in Box 9–5.

BOX 9-5	An Example of Experimental Conditions

Headley, Ownby, and John (2004) conducted an experimental study designed to determine the effects of an experimental seated exercise treatment and a control usual physical activity treatment on fatigue and quality of life in women with metastatic breast cancer.

The **experimental treatment** consisted of "a 30-minute seated exercise program three times a week with at least a one-day break between sessions. The [treatment] involved using a commercially available video called *Armchair Fitness: Gentle Exercise* (Bernstein, 1994). The program includes a five-minute warm-up, 20 minutes of moderate-intensity repetitive motion exercises, and a five-minute cool down. Participants sit in a straight-backed chair while performing stretching and repeated flexion and extension of the arms, head, upper torso, and legs" (p. 979).

The **control treatment** consisted of any usual physical activity engaged in by the control group participants; they did not do the seated exercise program.

WHAT APPROACHES ARE USED TO COLLECT DATA?

Three approaches are used to collect either qualitative (word) data or quantitative (number) data—observing people, examining documents, and listening to or questioning people (Ford-Gilboe, Campbell, & Berman, 1995). Each approach is associated with particular types of research instruments and research designs. Examples of research designs and associated research instruments used with the various approaches to collecting data are given in Tables 9–1, 9–2, and 9–3 on the CD that comes with this book.

Observing People

Observing people can be accomplished while the researcher is engaging in activities with the research participants, such as performing nursing care activities for hospitalized patients. This approach to observing people, which is called **participant observation**, is used more often with ethnography or ethnonursing research methodology than with other research designs (Speziale & Carpenter, 2003).

Observing people also can be accomplished while the researcher is not engaged in any activities or interacting with the research participants. This approach to observing people, which is called **nonparticipant observation**, can be used with any type of descriptive, correlational, or experimental research design.

Instruments used to observe people—to record what was seen by the researcher—include checklists, cameras, and biophysiological equipment. **Checklists** typically are made up of a list of items, such as people's behaviors, as well as categories used to rate whether or to what the extent each item is observed or the way in which the behavior was performed by the research participant (Polit & Beck, 2006). For example, Tyberg and Chlan (2006) used the Checklist of Nonverbal Pain Indicators to record observations of pain-related behaviors exhibited by surgical intensive care unit patients who were intubated and sedated (Figure 9–1).

Observing people also can be done by using a **camera** to take still photographs or motion pictures, including movies and video recordings. For example, the women who participated in Bultemeier's (1997) study used a Polaroid camera to photograph themselves as they experienced premenstrual syndrome.

In addition, observing people can be done using **biophysiological equipment**, which also may be called **biomedical instruments** (Waltz, Strickland, & Lenz, 2005). These research instruments are used to observe people's physiological responses. For example, blood pressure may be measured by equipment such as a sphygmomanometer and stethoscope or by computer readings from a catheter placed in a major blood vessel of the body. In addition, physiological responses, such as an infection or cholesterol level, can be observed in blood or other body fluids by use of microscopes and centrifuges. Bournaki (1997), for example, used a Nellcor electronic pulse oximeter to measure heart rate in her study of correlates of children's pain-related responses to venipuncture.

Examining Documents

Data obtained from examining documents are frequently recorded on a coding sheet. **Coding sheets** typically contain a list of items or elements the researcher considers important. For example, Skalski, DiGerolamo, and Gigliotti (2006) used a coding sheet to record the information they extracted from Neuman Systems Model–based studies of client system stressors, including "purpose statement, client population, sample size, data collection method . . . assessment

Checklist of Nonverbal Pain Indicators (CNPI)

Directions: Use a checkmark (✔) to indicate whether each behavior is present or absent when the patient is at rest and when the patient is active.

When observed, the patient was: At rest _____ Active_____

Nonverbal Pain Behaviors	No	Yes
Verbal complaints **(e.g., "ouch," "stop," "that hurts,"** **"that's enough")**		
Nonverbal vocalization **(e.g., cries, sighs, groans, gasps,** **moans)**		
Bracing **(e.g., clutching or holding onto** **furniture or equipment or the affected area** **of the body during movement)**		
Restlessness **(e.g., constant or periodic shifting of** **position, rocking, hand motions, inability to** **remain still)**		
Facial grimacing or wincing **(e.g., clenched teeth, tightened lips,** **dropped jaw, distorted expression,** **narrowed eyes, furrowed brow)**		
Rubbing **(e.g., massaging the affected area of the body)**		

Figure 9-1. Example of a checklist with a yes/no rating scale. *(Constructed from information given in Feldt [2000], p.17; and Tyberg and Chlan [2006], p. 326.)*

instrument, stressor terminology . . . and evidence of categorization of intra-, inter- and extra-personal stressors" (p. 71). If the documents were reports of research based on different conceptual models or were studies designed to test different middle-range theories, the coding sheet could also be used to record the name of each conceptual model or theory. An example of a coding sheet is displayed in Figure 9–2.

Listening to or Questioning People

Instruments used to listen to or question people include the researcher(s), as well as interview guides and questionnaires (see Boxes 9–3 and 9–4), which are frequently considered self-report instruments because the research participants themselves provide the answers (Polit & Beck, 2006).

Citation	Conceptual Model or Theory	Research Design	Sample Size and Characteristics	Research Instruments Experimental Conditions	Research Findings	Quality of the Research*

*1 = Poor   2 = Adequate   3 = Very good

Figure 9-2. Example of a coding sheet for review of documents.

The Researcher as the Research Instrument

In theory-generating qualitative research designs, the **researcher may be considered the research instrument**. Creswell (1998) explained that the "researcher is an instrument of data collection who gathers words or pictures, analyzes them inductively, focuses on the meaning of [participants' experience], and describes a process that is expressive and persuasive in language" (p. 14). This means that researchers do not try to separate themselves from the research but rather recognize the role they play in the collection of the data by observing participants or recording their answers to interview questions (Speziale & Carpenter, 2003). Butcher (1996) explained that the researcher acts as a human instrument "by obtaining descriptions of the phenomenon . . . through an in-depth interview conducted in a person-to-person encounter between researcher and participant" (p. 46). Carboni (1998), who derived a research design known as the Rogerian process of inquiry from Rogers' Science of Unitary Human Beings, added, "The Rogerian researcher elects to use him- or herself as well as the co-participants in the research as the primary data-gathering instruments" (p. 113).

Interview Guides

Interview guides—also called **interview schedules**—can be unstructured, semi-structured, or structured. Sometimes, the interview guide used with an ethnographic research design is referred to as the **ethnographic interview**.

Most interview guides are made up of open-ended questions or declarative requests, although some may contain fixed-choice questions or a combination of open-ended and fixed-choice questions. Researchers frequently use unstructured or semi-structured interview guides to provide some organization for collection of qualitative data. The data may be recorded as written or oral answers to open-ended questions or declarative requests. The answers may be written by the research participant or by the researcher. Oral answers may be audiotaped or videotaped. Researchers may use structured interview guides to provide some organization for collection of quantitative data.

Unstructured interview guides, which are typically used with phenomenological and ethnographic research designs, start with a broad initial open-ended question or declarative request. For example, an unstructured interview guide used with a phenomenological research design might start with a request such as "Please tell me about your experience of." An interview guide used with an ethnographic research design might start with a question such as "What is the value placed on health in your culture?"

Semi-structured interview guides may be used with various types of research designs, especially qualitative ones. Semi-structured interview guides usually include several open-ended questions or a list of topics that are relevant to the study. An example of a semi-structured interview guide used to collect data from caregivers of family members who had Alzheimer's disease following the family members' placement in a nursing home is given in Box 9–6.

Structured interview guides are used with various types of qualitative and quantitative research designs. Structured interviews typically include a list of specific fixed-choice questions that are relevant to the study. For example, a study designed to examine the correlation between readiness for hospital discharge following childbirth and adaptation to motherhood 10 days after hospital discharge includes a structured interview guide to measure adaptation to motherhood by asking the new mothers the fixed-choice questions listed here:

On a scale of 0 to 10, with 0 indicating "Very sick" and 10 indicating "Very well," how do you feel physically?
On a scale of 0 to 10, with 0 indicating "Very sad" and 10 indicating "Very excited," how do you feel emotionally?
On a scale of 0 to 10, with 0 indicating "Not at all" and 10 indicating "Totally," to what extent have you resumed your usual daily activities?
On a scale of 0 to 10, with 0 indicating "None" and 10 indicating "A lot," to what extent are you receiving help from your family and friends? (Weiss, Aber, & Fawcett, 2006–2009)

Questionnaires

Questionnaires are used with many different types of research designs, especially quantitative ones. Questionnaires may be referred to as **paper and pencil questionnaires** because they are usually printed on paper and are answered using a pencil or pen. Questionnaires do not, however, have to be printed; instead, the items making up the questionnaire can be administered via a computer or telephone.

Questionnaires may be used as the basis for structured interviews or they may be given to the research participants to complete. Questionnaires—which may also be called **surveys, survey instruments**, or **scales**—are made up of one or many items.

BOX 9-6	Example of a Semi-Structured Interview Schedule

I realize you are no longer the primary caregiver for [name of family member with Alzheimer's disease] now that he/she is in a nursing home but I imagine you still have some caretaking responsibilities. Could you tell me what they are?

How do you feel about them?

What's it like to fit this into your schedule?

How is caregiving similar or different now that [name of family member] is in the nursing home rather than at home?

Some people express concerns about their family member being placed in a nursing home. Please describe any concerns you have about [name of family member] being in the nursing home.

Please describe the thoughts or feelings you experience when visiting [name of family member] in the nursing home.

What do you do to cope with [name of family member] being in the nursing home?

Please describe the people who help you to cope with [name of family member] being in the nursing home.

Please describe the things that help you to keep a sense of self or balance as a caregiver.

Please describe the people who help you to keep a sense of self or balance as a caregiver.

Please describe the things that help you to bounce back as a caregiver.

Please describe the people who help you to bounce back as a caregiver.

Please describe the things that help you to persevere or have stick-to-it-ness as a caregiver.

Please describe the people who help you to persevere or have stick-to-it-ness as a caregiver.

(Constructed from information in Garity, 2006, p. 42)

A questionnaire made up of just one item sometimes is referred to as a **single-item indicator**. The one item that Ravesloot, Seekins, and White (2005) used to measure life satisfaction is displayed in Figure 9–3. The five items Tsai (2005) used to measure physical disability are displayed in Figure 9–4.

Life Satisfaction Questionnaire
In general, how satisfied are you with your life?
1 = Very dissatisfied
2 = Dissatisfied
3 = Satisfied
4 = Very satisfied

Figure 9-3. Example of a single-item indicator with a Likert-type scale. *(Constructed from information given in Ravesloot, Seekins, and White [2005], p. 240.)*

Physical Disability Questionnaire

Use a checkmark (✔) to indicate the degree of difficulty you have for each activity, using the ratings listed here:

1 = No difficulty   2 = Some difficulty   3 = A great deal of difficulty

Activity	1	2	3	Never Did the Activity
Going up and down stairs				
Kneeling or stooping				
Lifting or carrying objects weighing less than 10 pounds				
Doing household tasks				
Shopping or getting around town				

Figure 9-4. Example of a multiple-item questionnaire with a Likert-type scale. *(Constructed from information given in Ravesloot, Seekins, and White [2005], p. 240.)*

Rating Scales for Questionnaires

The one or more items making up a questionnaire may be rated on a scale. A **rating scale** "is a device designed to assign a numeric score to people to place them on a continuum with respect to [the concept] being measured" (Polit & Beck, 2006, p. 297).

Scales can have two or more rating points. A two-point rating scale typically is in the form of "Yes" and "No," "True" and "False," or "Correct" and "Incorrect." For example, the items making up the original version of the Inventory of Functional Status–Dialysis (Thomas-Hawkins, 2000) are rated as "Yes" and "No" (see Box 9–4). The items on the Checklist of Nonverbal Pain Indicators are also rated as "Yes" or "No" (see Figure 9–1).

Multiple-point rating scales may be as simple as a numeric scale made up of one or more items. For example, Chair, Taylor-Piliae, Lam, and Chan (2003) used a one-item rating scale to measure the severity of back pain (Figure 9–5). Their instrument is another example of a single-item indicator (see Figure 9–3).

Other commonly used multiple-point rating scales used by nurse researchers include the Likert scale, the semantic differential scale, and the visual analog scale. These rating scales are sometimes referred to as **summated rating scales** because the total score is usually calculated by adding—or summing—the number score for each item (Polit & Beck, 2006).

The **Likert scale**—sometimes referred to as a **Likert-type scale**—is made up of one or more items rated by research participants with regard to how much they agree or disagree with the item. For example, a Likert scale may be made up of several items that are rated on a scale of 1 to 4, with 1 = strongly disagree, 2 = disagree, 3 = agree, and 4 = strongly agree or other rating categories (see Figures 9–3 and 9–4).

Numeric Pain Intensity Scale

On a scale of 0 to 10, where 0 = no pain and 10 = severe pain, circle the number that indicates how much pain are you experiencing right now.

0   1   2   3   4   5   6   7   8   9   10

Figure 9-5. Example of a single-item numeric rating scale. *(Constructed from information in Chair, Taylor-Piliae, Lam, & Chan [2003], p. 474).*

The **semantic differential scale** is made up of one or more items that are rated on a series of bipolar adjective scales. Semantic differential scales are used to measure the meaning of each item to the respondent. Each item may be considered a separate concept or may be a component of a concept. Questionnaires may include one or more of the three dimensions of semantic differential scales. The three dimensions, with examples of bipolar adjectives used to rate them, are:

- Evaluative: good—bad, kind—cruel, beautiful—ugly
- Potency: hard—soft, heavy—light, strong—weak
- Activity: active—passive, fast—slow, hot—cold (Osgood, Suci, & Tannenbaum, 1957)

Semantic differential scales frequently include seven rating points, although other numbers of rating points sometimes are used. Cohen et al. (2005), for example, used a five-point rating scale to measure the meaning of nursing (Figure 9–6). In this example, each bipolar adjective pair was regarded as a characteristic of nursing.

Please place a mark (**X**) on the space that indicates what nursing means to you

Nursing is:

Risky	____ : ____ : ____ : ____ : ____	**Not Risky**
Respected	____ : ____ : ____ : ____ : ____	**Not Respected**
Good	____ : ____ : ____ : ____ : ____	**Bad**
Satisfactory	____ : ____ : ____ : ____ : ____	**Not Satisfactory**
Hard Work	____ : ____ : ____ : ____ : ____	**Easy Work**
Important	____ : ____ : ____ : ____ : ____	**Not Important**
Busy	____ : ____ : ____ : ____ : ____	**Not Busy**
Interesting	____ : ____ : ____ : ____ : ____	**Not Interesting**
Female Oriented	____ : ____ : ____ : ____ : ____	**Male Oriented**
Doing	____ : ____ : ____ : ____ : ____	**Not Doing**
Thinking	____ : ____ : ____ : ____ : ____	**Not Thinking**
Awful	____ : ____ : ____ : ____ : ____	**Pleasant**
Powerful	____ : ____ : ____ : ____ : ____	**Powerless**
Independent	____ : ____ : ____ : ____ : ____	**Dependent**

Figure 9-6. Example of a semantic differential scale. *(Constructed from information given in Cohen et al. [2005], pp. 92, 93.)*

The **visual analog scale** (VAS) is made up of one or more items that are rated by placing a mark at the point on a vertical or horizontal 100-mm line that best indicates the experience of the concept that is measured by the VAS. Each end of the 100-mm line is labeled as one extreme of the experience. For example, McCaffrey and Freeman (2003) used a VAS to rate the experience of pain from the extremes of "no pain" to "worst pain possible" (Figure 9–7).

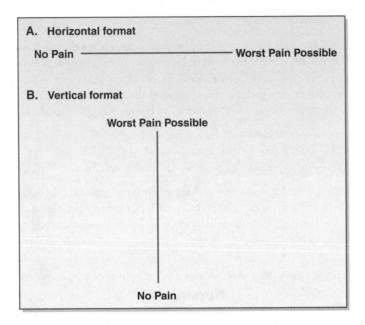

A. Horizontal format

No Pain ————————————— Worst Pain Possible

B. Vertical format

Worst Pain Possible
|
|
|
|
No Pain

Figure 9-7. Examples of a visual analog scale. *(Constructed from information given in McCaffrey and Freeman [2003], p. 520.)*

Standardized and Unstandardized Questionnaires

Sometimes, an instrument may be referred to as a **standardized questionnaire**. The four essential characteristics of a standardized questionnaire are:

1. A fixed set of items . . . designed to measure a clearly defined concept . . . based on a theoretical framework
2. Explicit rules and procedures for administration and scoring
3. Provision of norms to assist in interpretation [**Norms** are typical scores associated with a particular population.]
4. An ongoing development process that involves careful testing, analysis, and revision in order to ensure high technical quality (Waltz et al., 2005, pp. 190–191).

The Scholastic Aptitude Test (SAT®; 2007) is a well-known example of a standardized questionnaire.

Many instruments used by researchers are **nonstandardized questionnaires**. Although such questionnaires "may have incorporated one or more of the four essential characteristics of standardized [questionnaires]" (Waltz et al., 2005, p. 191), they do not reflect all four characteristics, especially norms for the scores with one or more populations. An example of a nonstandarized questionnaire is the Inventory of Functional Status–Dialysis (Thomas-Hawkins, 2000, 2005; see Box 9–4).

HOW IS THE CRITERION OF OPERATIONAL ADEQUACY APPLIED TO RESEARCH INSTRUMENTS?

When applied to the research instruments of empirical research methods, the criterion of operational adequacy refers to the amount of information about the instruments given in a research report and focuses attention on whether the instruments were good enough to provide consistent and appropriate data to generate or test a middle-range theory. The operational adequacy criterion, when applied to research instruments, is met when you can answer yes to two questions:

- Are all research instruments clearly identified and fully described in the research report?
- Are the research instruments consistent and appropriate measures of the middle-range theory concepts?

Are All Research Instruments Clearly Identified and Fully Described in the Research Report?

Every research instrument used in any theory-generating or theory-testing study should be explicitly identified in the research report. Some researchers, however, may not explicitly identify some of the instruments used—for example, to collect background information, such as age, gender, race, ethnicity, and education, about the people who are the research participants.

The research instruments should be not only identified but described (Box 9–7). The description of each instrument should include:

- The name of the middle-range theory concept measured by that instrument
- The number and type of items or questions making up each instrument

For research instruments used to collect quantitative data, the description should also include:

- The scale used to rate the items
- An explanation of the range of possible scores and how the scores are interpreted

Are the Research Instruments Used Consistent and Appropriate Measures of the Middle-Range Theory Concepts?

Each research instrument should provide a consistent and appropriate measure of a middle-range theory concept. The terms used to describe consistency and appropriateness differ for research

BOX 9-7	Example of Description of a Research Instrument

The Self-Esteem Scale (RSES) (Rosenberg, 1965) was used to measure self-esteem [name of the middle-range theory concept measured]. The RSES consists of 10 items that generally deal with favorable and unfavorable attitudes toward oneself [number and type of items]. Caregivers were asked to rate each item on a 4-point scale of *strongly agree, agree, disagree,* or *strongly disagree* [rating scale]. "Positive" and "negative" items are presented alternatively to reduce the effect of response set [additional information about items]. "Negative" items are recoded for consistency in scoring [additional scoring information]. The range of possible scores is 10 to 40 [range of possible scores]; the higher the score, the higher the self-reported self-esteem [interpretation of scores]. (Newman, 2005, p. 418)

   Note: **Response set** is a bias that refers to the tendency, when completing questionnaire items, to "use certain types of responses: extreme responses, neutral responses, agree responses, disagree responses" (Kerlinger & Lee, 2000, p. 713).

instruments used to collect qualitative (word) data and research instruments used to collect quantitative (number) data. The terms typically used for research instruments that provide qualitative data are **dependability and credibility**, which are aspects of **trustworthiness**. The terms typically used for research instruments that provide quantitative data are **reliability** and **validity**, which are referred to as **psychometric properties** of instruments. Other terms, which are associated with the psychometric property of reliability, include efficiency, feasibility, comprehensibility, linearity, simplicity, speededness, and responsiveness. Still other terms, which refer to special psychometric properties of assessment and diagnostic tools, are sensitivity and specificity. The term calibration refers to a special psychometric property of biophysiological equipment. And the term cultural equivalence refers to the psychometric properties of questionnaires that were developed for use with people of one culture and then are used with people of another culture. Psychometric properties may be referred to as **clinimetrics** when the instrument is used as a practice tool to assess "symptoms, physical signs, and other distinctly clinical phenomena" (Feinstein, 1987, p. 5).

   Regardless of the terms used, the language used to report results of tests of the consistency and appropriateness of an instrument should be tentative rather than definite. Specifically, the description of the consistency and appropriateness of a research instrument should be written as "evidence of, estimates of, or support for" rather than "established" or "proven" (Froman, 2000, p. 421).

   Sometimes the reader cannot determine whether the instruments provided consistent data and were appropriate measures of the middle-range theory concepts because the research report contains no relevant information. At other times, however, the researcher may refer the reader to another source for that information. For example, Bournes and Ferguson-Paré (2005) did not list the specific criteria they used to evaluate the trustworthiness of the data they collected, although they stated, "The criteria for the critical appraisal of qualitative research developed by Parse (2001) were used to ensure the overall rigor and credibility of this study" (p. 326).

   If the information about consistency and appropriateness is not given and another source for that information is not cited, the reader may attempt to locate the information by reading the report of another study in which the instruments were used. For example, Tsai (2005) used data originally collected by Mirowsky and Ross (2001) for her theory-testing study of the relation of chronic pain, disability, social support, financial hardship, age, gender, and distress to depression experienced by people 65 years of age and older who had arthritis. Review of Mirowsky and Ross' research report revealed some information about reliability reported for the instrument used to measure depression. Alternatively, the reader may attempt to locate information about the consistency and appropriateness of the instruments from a book or electronic database containing descriptions of many instruments (see the Directories of Instruments on the CD that comes with this book).

Evaluation of the Consistency and Appropriateness of Research Instruments That Provide Qualitative Data

The consistency and appropriateness of research instruments used to collect qualitative data—or the word data themselves—are evaluated in terms of trustworthiness (Ford-Gilboe et al., 1995). **Trustworthiness** refers to the rigor or goodness of the data (Speziale & Carpenter, 2003)—that is, the extent to which the researcher can "persuade his or her audiences (including self) that the findings of an inquiry are worthy of paying attention to, worth taking account of" (Lincoln & Guba, 1985, p. 290).

Two criteria used to evaluate the trustworthiness of research instruments used to collect qualitative (word) data are **dependability** and **credibility**. The two criteria are related: If the data are not dependable, they cannot be credible. Examples of research reports that include information about dependability and credibility are given in Tables 9–1 and 9–2 on the CD that comes with this book.

Dependability. **Dependability** refers to the extent to which the data are dependable—that is, the extent to which they are consistent (Lincoln & Guba, 1985). Activities used by researchers to estimate dependability are inquiry audit and replication.

Inquiry audit—also called **audit ability**—is typically used to estimate dependability. This activity requires a person other than the researcher to review the data and the processes used for analysis and to indicate the extent to which the same conclusions are reached (Polit & Beck, 2006; Speziale & Carpenter, 2003). The example of an inquiry audit given in Box 9–8 is from DeSanto-Madeya's (2006a) phenomenological study of the meaning of living with spinal cord injury.

Replication of research, also referred to as **stepwise replication**, requires two teams of researchers to independently conduct the same study and then compare results. Given the flexibility of qualitative research designs, Lincoln and Guba (1985) pointed out that the two teams must be in constant communication regarding any changes in design. Replication is a very cumbersome approach to estimation of dependability and, therefore, is seldom used. Indeed, Lincoln and Guba stated that they do not recommend use of this approach to estimating dependability because of the difficulties involved. Furthermore, given the focus of qualitative research on individuals' experiences, it may be impossible for the data from the two studies to reveal the same themes or categories. Sandelowski (1993) explained, "Even when confronted with the same qualitative task, no two researchers will

BOX 9-8	Example of an Inquiry Audit Used to Estimate Dependability

Auditability was ensured by providing a written decision trail of the abstraction process from raw data to significant statements, formulated meanings, supportive data, themes, and thematic categories. An expert in phenomenological research audited the study process and confirmed that the data and findings were internally consistent (DeSanto-Madeya, 2006a, p. 271).

produce the same result . . . [because] repeatability is not an essential (or necessary or sufficient) property of things themselves (whether the thing is qualitative research or the qualitative interview)" (p. 3).

Polit and Beck (2008) interpreted stepwise replication to be independent analyses of the same data by two or more researchers. They cited a study of coping with results from predictive gene testing by Williams, Schutte, Evers, and Holkup (2000) as an example. Williams et al. explained:

Three investigators read through the first set of interviews and made marginal notes to code meaningful responses. The investigators compared and revised these codes until there was agreement among the investigators regarding the descriptive codes and their definitions. All data from subsequent interviews were coded independently by the three investigators. The investigators met regularly to compare application of codes and to resolve any differences. As coding of the . . . dataset continued, descriptive categories were developed to reflect the experiences and coping processes used by participants. (Williams et al., pp. 262–263)

Polit and Beck's (2008) interpretation of stepwise replication does not, however, seem consistent with Lincoln and Guba's (1985) explanation of replication.

Credibility. **Credibility** refers to "activities that increase the probability that credible findings will be produced" (Speziale & Carpenter, 2003, p. 38). When research findings are credible, researchers and readers of research reports have confidence in the appropriateness of those findings.

Activities used by researchers to estimate credibility of qualitative data include prolonged engagement, persistent observation, triangulation, peer debriefing, member checks, and negative case analysis. The credibility of the researcher must also be established.

Prolonged engagement with or **immersion in literature about** the phenomenon studied and the data collected involves "the investment of sufficient time in data collection activities to have an in-depth understanding of the [phenomenon studied] . . . and to test for misinformation" (Polit & Beck, 2006, p. 332).

Persistent observation means that the "researcher's focus [is] on the aspects of a situation that are relevant to the phenomenon being studied" (Polit & Beck, 2006, p. 333). Together, prolonged engagement and persistent observation provide scope and depth in data collection. The example of prolonged engagement and persistent observation given in Box 9–9 is from Carboni's (1998) study of enfolding health-as-wholeness-and-harmony. Carboni used the Rogerian process of inquiry research design.

BOX 9-9

Example of Prolonged Engagement and Persistent Observation Used to Estimate Credibility

"A nurse researcher spent four to six hours a day, two to three days a week during a thirty-six week period fieldwork" (Carboni, 1998, p. 146). "The nurse-researcher's immersion in the field entailed becoming deeply involved with all co-participants of the study as well as becoming involved in the day-to-day activities of the unit. Emphasis was placed on dialog and other forms of communication such as touch, rather than observation. There were instances that the researcher, as a nurse, participated in appropriate nursing activities relevant to traditional nursing practice with the elderly institutionalized person. . . . Any and all of these experiences were viewed as opportunities to develop shared understanding. . . .

"Prolonged engagement in the field assisted the nurse-researcher to be open to the multiple and changing potentialities of energy field patterns. The immersion in the field of eight months allowed the nurse-researcher time to become thoroughly familiar with the site and thus be sensitive to all the complexities as they emerged, as well as provided the nurse-researcher with sufficient time to establish trust with the co-participants. Prolonged engagement provided the scope necessary to establish credible knowledge. . . . Persistent observation assisted the nurse-researcher in identifying manifestations of field patterning most relevant to the questions being pursued. This was accomplished through the nurse-researcher's commitment to focusing on these significant manifestations and providing a complete and thorough description and understanding of them. Persistent observation provided the depth necessary to establish credible knowledge" (Carboni, p. 161).

Triangulation involves using multiple methods to collect the data, such as interviews and observations; multiple sources of data, such as nurses, patients, and patients' family members; multiple researchers, to collect, analyze, and interpret the data; or multiple theoretical perspectives to interpret the data (Speziale & Carpenter, 2003). The use of triangulation can help the researcher and reader distinguish accurate data from data that have errors (Polit & Beck, 2006). The example of triangulation given in Box 9–10 is from Maldonado, Callahan, and Efinger's (2003) study of lived spiritual experiences of several women and a man who worked with older adults in end-of-life care units. The researchers used a case study research design.

Peer debriefing is accomplished when the researcher and one or more colleagues who can provide an objective perspective together review and discuss the data that were collected (Speziale & Carpenter, 2003). An example of peer debriefing—also from Maldonado and colleagues' (2003) study—is given in Box 9–11.

BOX 9-10

Example of Triangulation Used to Estimate Credibility

This study employed triangulation to enhance trustworthiness. The use of the software [Atlas.ti], separate analyses by the three researchers, member checks, and post analysis literature reviews provided a triangulated analysis (Maldonado et al., 2003, p. 17).

BOX 9-11	Example of Peer Debriefing Used to Estimate Credibility

Peer review provided feedback regarding methodology, coding procedures, and reliability procedures and verified that the sub-categories, core categories, and themes accurately reflected the
meanings of the participants' experiences. Transcripts of two randomly selected cases were read and
analyzed by two [end-of-life] care experts, who checked for undisclosed biases of the researchers,
confirmation of emerging findings, and rigor of the analysis (Maldonado et al. 2003, p. 17).

Member checks are accomplished when the researcher shares the results of analysis of the
data with the research participants to determine whether the results are consistent with the
participants' understanding of their experiences of the phenomenon (Lincoln & Guba, 1985).
An example of member checks, from DeSanto-Madeya's (2006a) phenomenological study of
the meaning of living with spinal cord injury, is given in Box 9–12.

BOX 9-12	Example of Member Checks Used to Estimate Credibility

Credibility was demonstrated when the study participants recognized the transcribed data as their
own experiences. . . . Of the 20 family dyads, 18 were contacted by phone to assure that the
interpretation was truly reflective of their experience of living with spinal cord injury. The spinal
cord injured persons and family members reflected and concluded that the essence of the phenomenon of living with spinal cord injury was captured. Not every family member and injured
person experienced every theme but all the themes were recognized as accurate representations of
the meaning of living with spinal cord injury (DeSanto-Madeya, 2006a, p. 271).

Negative case analysis—also referred to as **searching for disconfirming evidence**—
involves the researcher's review of all data for any instances that do not support the theory
that is being generated (Lincoln & Guba, 1985; Polit & Beck, 2006). This activity may
be accomplished by means of the purposeful selection strategies of maximum variation
sampling and extreme or deviant case sampling of research participants that we discussed
in Chapter 8. The example of negative case analysis used to estimate credibility given in
Box 9–13 is from a study of older women's perspectives of the care they received during
treatment for breast or gynecological cancer. The investigators used a grounded theory
research design.

BOX 9-13	Example of Negative Case Analysis Used to Estimate Credibility

In keeping with the [research] team's commitment to avoid stereotyping older women and adhere
to principles of qualitative analysis . . . the investigators deliberately read for and discussed negative cases (i.e., instances where participants' experiences or commentary departed from or challenged an emerging theme) (Sinding, Wiernikowski, & Aronson 2005, p. 1171).

The credibility of the researcher also must be established because researchers are sometimes considered the research instrument in qualitative research designs. **Researcher credibility** refers to "the faith that can be put in the researcher" (Polit & Beck, 2006, p. 334). The credibility of the researcher is estimated by review of the researcher's credentials, such as training in and experience with the particular qualitative research design used, as well as any personal experience with the phenomenon studied. The extent to which the reader regards the researcher as credible influences confidence in the analysis and interpretation of the data. For example, Gagliardi provided information that can be used to establish her credibility as a researcher in a prologue to the description of a Roy Adaptation Model–based qualitative study of living with multiple sclerosis (Gagliardi, Frederickson, & Shanley, 2002). She explained:

> I am a nurse researcher. The Roy adaptation model is the lens through which I view nursing, and I have used that model to guide my previous research. . . . I also am one of the approximately 250,000 to 350,000 people who have multiple sclerosis (MS). My experiences with MS led me to this study. As my condition became increasingly debilitating, I wanted to learn more than I already knew about MS, both from the literature and from other people who have MS. As the study progressed, I sought assistance from two other researchers (K.F. and D.S.) [the research report co-authors, K. Frederickson and D. Shanley]. I collected and did the initial analysis of the data. D.S. served as the auditor for the data analysis. K.F. contributed valuable insights into the data analysis and interpretation of the findings within the context of the Roy adaptation model. Their contributions helped me to bracket [that is, set aside] my personal experience of living with MS as I reviewed the study data. In turn, K.F. and D.S. learned a great deal about living with MS. (p. 230)

In addition, all three researchers' academic and professional credentials are included under the title of the journal article.

Evaluation of the Consistency and Appropriateness of Research Instruments That Provide Quantitative Data

The consistency and appropriateness of research instruments used to collect quantitative data are evaluated in terms of their psychometric properties, especially **reliability** and **validity** (Ford-Gilboe et al., 1995). The two criteria are related: If a research instrument is not reliable, it cannot be valid. An instrument can, however, be reliable but not valid. Examples of research reports that include information about reliability and validity are given in Tables 9–2 and 9–3 on the CD that comes with this book. The instruments used to collect quantitative data also must be calibrated to ensure accuracy and must be used in a culturally sensitive manner in order to ensure their usefulness and value.

Reliability. **Reliability** refers to "the extent to which [an instrument] provide[s] consistent results" (Carmines & Zeller, 1979, p. 12)—that is, the extent to which an instrument provides a consistent measure of a middle-range theory concept. Each instrument used to collect quantitative (number) data should be a reliable measure of a middle-range theory concept for the population of interest and for the specific sample.

Types of Reliability

Three major types of validity have been identified—internal consistency reliability; equivalence reliability; and stability, or test-retest, reliability (Carmines & Zeller, 1979; DeVon et al., 2007; Higgins & Straub, 2006; Nunnally & Bernstein, 1994).

Internal consistency reliability refers to the extent to which the items making up a questionnaire measure the same concept. In other words, an estimate of internal consistency reliability indicates the extent to which the instrument items are highly interrelated (DeVellis, 2003). The two approaches to estimating internal consistency reliability are split-half reliability and coefficient alpha reliability.

Split-half reliability involves dividing the items making up one questionnaire into two groups, such as the even-numbered items and the odd-numbered items (**odd–even reliability**) or the first and last halves of the items (**first-half last-half split**); the two groups may also be made up of randomly selected items (**random halves**) (DeVellis, 2003). The scores for the two groups of items are then compared by means of a correlation coefficient, sometimes referred to as the **Guttman split-half coefficient**. The example of split-half reliability given in Box 9–14 is from Tsai and Chai's (2005) study of the development and psychometric testing of an instrument to evaluate nursing Web sites.

BOX 9-14	Example of Internal Consistency Reliability: Split-Half

Tsai and Chai (2005) reported split-half internal consistency reliability for the Nursing Web site Evaluation Questionnaire, which they developed as a way to evaluate nursing Web sites: Part I of the Nursing Web site Evaluation Questionnaire is made up of 17 items addressing the overall impression (3 items), download and switch speed (2 items), accessibility and convenience (8 items), and web page content (4 items) aspects of nursing websites. Each item was rated on a scale of 1 to 5. Tsai and Chai reported, "With respect to the internal consistency of Part I of the questionnaire, the Guttman split-half value was 0.85" (p. 409).

Coefficient alpha, usually called **Cronbach's alpha**, is a "sophisticated and accurate method" of estimating internal consistency reliability (Polit & Beck, 2006, p. 326). The coefficient alpha approach to estimating internal consistency reliability is a statistical procedure that provides an estimate of the split-half reliability for all possible ways of dividing the questionnaire into two halves. A special feature of some computer software programs used to calculate Cronbach's alpha is a display of coefficient alpha if each item were to be removed from the questionnaire. That information allows researchers to refine questionnaires by removing items that decrease the coefficient and then recalculating the questionnaire scores with the most internally consistent set of items. Cronbach's alpha is used when questionnaire items can be rated on more than two points, such as a 5- or 10-point rating scale. A statistic called **Kuder-Richardson 20** is used to estimate internal consistency reliability when instrument items are scored as categories, such as 0 = wrong and 1 = right, 0 = no and 1 = yes, or 1 = false and 2 = true, or other categories (Knapp, 1991). Examples of internal consistency reliability estimates are given in Boxes 9–15 and 9–16.

Equivalence reliability refers to the extent of consistency of scores or codes obtained from the data collected by use of questionnaires. The three approaches to estimating

BOX 9-15	Example of Internal Consistency Reliability: Cronbach's Alpha

Ravesloot, Seekens, and White (2005) reported an internal consistency reliability estimate for the Secondary Conditions Surveillance Instrument (SCSI), which they used to measure the amount of time people are limited due to such secondary conditions as urinary tract infection, pressure sores, and depression in their study of the effects of the Living Well With a Disability health promotion program: "Cronbach's alpha for the SCSI in this study was .89" (Ravesloot et al., p. 240).

Ravesloot et al. (2005) also reported an internal consistency reliability estimate for the Health-Promoting Lifestyle Profile II (HPLP), which they used to measure lifestyle: "The [HPLP] measures six dimensions of lifestyle: health responsibility, physical activity, nutrition, spiritual growth, interpersonal relations, and stress management. . . . [C]oefficient alphas ranged from .68 to .89 for the subscales and [it was] .93 for the total score" (Ravesloot et al., p. 240).

BOX 9-16	Example of Internal Consistency Reliability: Kuder-Richardson 20

Li and Wang (2006) reported a Kuder-Richardson 20 estimate of internal consistency reliability for the Knowledge of ETS Scale, which they used in their study of correlates of adolescents' behavior to avoid environmental tobacco smoke (ETS): "The 14-item [Knowledge of ETS Scale] . . . was used to assess the participants' knowledge regarding ETS, side effects of exposure to ETS, and ways to avoid ETS. The items were given the response choices 'true,' 'false' or 'do not know.' A total score was obtained by summing up the correct responses (1 point each) across the 14 items. The possible scores ranged from 0 to 14, with higher scores indicating better knowledge. In this study, the Kuder-Richardson 20 reliability of this scale was .67" (Li & Wang, pp. 105–106).

equivalence reliability are alternate forms reliability, intrarater reliability, and interrater reliability.

Alternate forms reliability—also called **parallel forms reliability**—refers to the extent to which two different versions of the same questionnaire yield the same score when administered to the same people. The two versions of the instrument may be administered sequentially in one testing session or at different times. This type of reliability is usually estimated by calculating a correlation coefficient or by some other way of comparing the scores from the two versions of the questionnaire. A major issue associated with alternate forms reliability is construction of two versions of a questionnaire measuring the same concept. As Carmines and Zeller (1979) pointed out, "It is often difficult to construct one form of a [questionnaire], much less two forms, that display the properties of parallel measurements" (p. 41). Consequently, alternate forms reliability is not often estimated. An example of alternate forms reliability is given in Box 9–17.

Intrarater reliability refers to the extent to which one researcher codes or scores the same data in the same way two or more times. This type of reliability can be estimated by calculating the **percentage of agreement** between the codes or scores obtained each time. Intrarater reliability also can be calculated using a statistic known as the **intraclass correlation coefficient**, which, in the case of intrarater reliability, is an estimate of the consistency or agreement

BOX 9-17	Example of Equivalence Reliability: Alternate Forms

Beyer, Turner, Jones, Young, Onikul, and Bobaty (2005) developed alternate forms of the Oucher Pain Scale for use by 3- to 12-year-old children of three ethnic origins—Caucasian, Hispanic, and African American: "The three ethnic versions of the Oucher each has two scales, a photographic scale on the right side of the poster and a numeric scale labeled 0 to 100, by tens, on the left side of the poster. On the numeric scale, 0 means 'no hurt,' 10 to 30 means 'little hurts,' 30 to 60 means 'middle hurts' 60 to 90 means 'big hurts' and 100 means the 'biggest hurt you could ever have.' On the photographic scale, six color photographs of one preschool child in varying levels of discomfort are displayed. . . . The alternate form of the Oucher is actually a mirror image of the original large form, just smaller in size. . . . Children who could count to 100, by ones or tens, and could identify which of two numbers [was] larger used the numeric scale. Children who could not perform both these tasks but could successfully complete a Piagetian seriation task . . . used the photographic Oucher scale" (Beyer et al., pp. 12–13).

The researchers reported reliability coefficients for the alternate forms of the photographic scale of 0.875 for the Caucasian children, 0.909 for the African American children, and 0.912 for the Hispanic children. The reliability coefficients for the alternate forms of the numeric scale were 0.906 for the African American children, 0.984 for the Hispanic children, and 0.998 for the Caucasian children (Beyer et al.).

of scores assigned by the rater at two different times. In addition, intrarater reliability can be calculated using a statistic known as **Cohen's kappa**, which, in the case of intrarater reliability, is an estimate of the agreement between the scores assigned by the rater at two different times. An example of intrarater reliability is given in Box 9–18.

BOX 9-18	Example of Equivalence Reliability: Intrarater Reliability

Howe, Innes, Venturini, Williams, and Verrier (2006) reported intrarater reliability for the 19–item Community Balance and Mobility Scale, which they developed to measure balance in ambulatory individuals who had experienced a traumatic brain injury and who were participating in a neurorehabilitation program: "Four teams, each comprised of two physical therapists, assessed a total of 32 patients. . . . The initial assessment was videotaped and scored independently by the same physical therapist three weeks later to evaluate intra-rater reliability. . . . [F]or intra-rater reliability, weighted [Cohen's] kappa values were above 0.80 for six of the 19 items and between 0.61 and 0.80 for ten of the 19 items (Howe et al., pp. 889–892). The intraclass correlation coefficient for all 19 items was 0.977" (Howe et al.).

Interrater reliability refers to the extent to which two or more researchers independently code or score the same data in the same way. This type of reliability can be estimated by calculating the **percentage of agreement** between the codes or scores obtained from each researcher or by calculation of an **intraclass correlation coefficient**, which, in the case of interrater reliability, is an estimate of consistency or agreement of scores assigned by two or more independent raters. **Cohen's kappa** also can be used to estimate interrater reliability; in this case, the statistic indicates the extent of agreement of scores assigned by two or more independent raters to the same behaviors at the same time. Examples of interrater reliability are given in Box 9–19.

Intrarater reliability and interrater reliability can be used to estimate the reliability of codes or scores assigned to direct observations of research participants or to estimate the reliability of codes or scores assigned to participants' responses to questions. The data may be words or numbers. The examples in Boxes 9–18 and 9–19 refer to number data. An example for word data is Bultemeier's (1997) calculation of interrater reliability for the results of coding participants' word data by three independent coders.

Stability reliability, also referred to as **test-retest reliability** or **temporal reliability**, involves administration of a questionnaire to the same research participants two different times. The scores obtained from the two administrations then are compared, typically by means of calculating a correlation coefficient. A major issue associated with test-retest reliability is the amount of time between the two administrations of the questionnaire. Nunnally and Bernstein (1994) indicate that there is no satisfactory resolution of that issue and, therefore, do not recommend obtaining estimates of test-retest reliability. However, some researchers continue to estimate test-retest reliability; an example is given in Box 9–20.

BOX 9-19	Examples of Equivalence Reliability: Interrater Reliability

Example Using Percentage of Agreement

Tyberg and Chlan (2006) reported interrater reliability of the Checklist of Nonverbal Pain Indicators (CNPI), which they used to measure pain experienced by patients who were intubated and sedated: "A total of 22 paired nurse observations were collected. . . . Overall inter-rater agreement of nurses' observations of patients' pain behaviors using the CNPI [was] high (mean = 97.2%, range 90.91–100% overall)" (Tyberg & Chlan, p. 326).

Example Using Intraclass Correlation Coefficient

Chair, Taylor-Piliae, Lam, and Chan (2003) reported interrater reliability for an instrument used to assess the presence of hematoma and bleeding in their study of the effect of positioning on back pain following coronary angiography. "Since six research assistants were used for data collection, 10 patients were examined by all research assistants to establish the level of agreement on hematoma and bleeding assessment. None of the 10 patients developed hematoma but bleeding amount estimation was done. Inter-rater reliability by Intraclass Correlation Coefficient was established at 0.91 for the bleeding assessment" (Chair et al., p. 474).

Reliability Across Samples

An instrument that has demonstrated an adequate estimate of reliability for one sample may not be reliable with another sample even when selected from the same population. That is because errors in measurement, variability of instrument scores, and other factors affecting the reliability of an instrument can vary from sample to sample. For example, to measure the frequency and severity of nausea and vomiting during pregnancy, Steele, French, Gatherer-Boyles, Newman, and Leclaire (2001) used a daily log questionnaire that they modified and

BOX 9-20	Example of Stability Reliability: Test-Retest Reliability

Hill, Aldag, Hekel, Riner, and Bloomfield (2006) reported an estimate of test-retest reliability for the Maternal Postpartum Quality of Life questionnaire (MAPP-QOL), which they used to measure quality of life for women following childbirth. The 41 items on the MAPP-QOL include five sub-scales: Psychological/Baby, Socioeconomic, Relational/Spouse-Partner, Relational/Family-Friends, and Health & Functioning.

For the total scale, support for temporal (test-retest) reliability was provided by test-retest correlations of 0.74 with a 2-week interval. Temporal reliability also was supported by test-retest correlations with a 2-week interval for all five subscales: Psychological/Baby ($r = 0.76$), Socioeconomic ($r = 0.76$), Relational/Spouse-Partner ($r = 0.72$), Relational/Family-Friends ($r = 0.69$), and Health & Functioning ($r = 0.66$).

adapted from a questionnaire that had been adapted from yet another questionnaire. They explained:

> The daily log was a modified and abbreviated version of the Rhodes Index of Nausea and Vomiting (Rhodes, Watson, & Johnson, 1984), which had been adapted by Brown, North, Marvel, and Fons (1992) for their study of acupressure wristbands to relieve nausea and vomiting in hospice patients. The Rhodes Index of Nausea and Vomiting has been used extensively in research and . . . has an estimated reliability of at least 0.83. The version of the instrument used in the current study was that used in the Brown et al. (1992) study, with two changes. In the Brown et al. version, the third question asked participants how long they were nauseated. The version used in this study asked women how many times they were nauseated. In this study, a fifth question about wear-ing of [sea] bands also was added. (p. 65)

Although Steele et al. reported a reliability coefficient for the original version of the ques-tionnaire, they did not report a reliability estimate for the version they used. The reader can-not assume that the instrument is reliable, especially because it was a twice-modified version of the original instrument for which a reliability estimate was reported.

In contrast, Tsai (2005) reported internal consistency reliability estimates for both the financial hardship instrument used in an earlier study and in her own study of the relation of chronic pain, disability, social support, financial hardship, age, and gender to distress, and the relation of distress to depression. She explained, "Financial hardship was measured by three items. . . . Internal consistency reliability was 0.82 in a study by Mirowsky and Ross (2001) and 0.79 for this study" (p. 160).

Interpretation of Reliability Coefficients

In general, the higher the reliability coefficient, the more acceptable the estimate of reliability. Reliability coefficients can range from 0.00 to 1.00 or 0% to 100%. Coefficients of at least 0.70 or 70% are typically considered acceptable reliability estimates. Knapp (1991) pointed out that Cronbach's alpha "can actually take on any value between minus infinity and +1" (p. 459). He went on to point out that negative alphas "are reflective of very bad measuring instruments, as far as internal consistency is concerned" (p. 460).

Other Psychometric Properties Related to Reliability

Psychometric properties related to reliability include efficiency, feasibility, comprehensiveness, linearity, simplicity, speededness, and responsiveness.

Efficiency refers to the number of items that need to be included on a questionnaire to obtain or retain adequate reliability, as well as the amount of time required to complete the questionnaire (Polit & Beck, 2008). In general, the fewer the items, the lower the reliability, but the quicker the questionnaire can be completed. Too many items may impose too great a burden on research participants, who may refuse to respond to all items or give responses that do not reflect their actual experiences, perceptions, attitudes, or beliefs. Consequently, researchers can use a mathematical formula—the **Spearman-Brown prophecy formula**—to calculate the number of items needed to obtain an acceptable estimate of reliability. An example of application of the Spearman-Brown prophecy formula is given in Box 9–21.

BOX 9-21 Example of Application of the Spearman-Brown Prophecy Formula

The Spearman-Brown prophecy formula is:

$r' = kr/(1 + [(k - 1)r])$,

where k = the factor or percentage by which the instrument items are being increased or decreased;
r = the original reliability coefficient; and
r' = the reliability coefficient after deleting or adding items.

Suppose that a researcher has developed an instrument with 50 items, which had an estimated reliability of 0.90. Suppose also that the researcher would like to estimate the reliability of a short form of the instrument, made up of 25 items, so that 50% of the original number of items will remain. Applying the Spearman-Brown prophecy formula, the researcher found out that the estimated reliability of a 25-item form of the instrument would be a still acceptable 0.82:

$r' = 0.50(0.90) /(1 + [0.50 - 1.0)0.90]) = 0.45/(1.0 + (-0.50)0.90]) = 0.45/0.55 = 0.82.$

Suppose that a researcher has developed an instrument with 20 items, which had an estimated reliability of 0.65. Suppose also that the researcher would like to estimate the reliability of the instrument if 10 items were added, so that 150% of the original number of items would make up the longer questionnaire. Applying the Spearman-Brown prophecy formula, the researcher found out that the estimated reliability of a 30-item form of the instrument would be a more acceptable 0.74.

$r' = 1.50(0.65)/(1.0 + [1.50 - 1.0)0.65]) = 0.975/(1.0 = (0.50)0.65]) = 0.975/1.325 = 0.74$

Feasibility, which refers to the suitability of an instrument for its intended use, is related to reliability especially if the instrument is to be used as an assessment tool in practice. As part of their critical review of instruments used to measure burden experienced by caregivers of persons with a stroke, Visser-Meily, Post, Riphagan, and Lindeman (2004) identified five aspects of instrument feasibility—time needed for administration, scoring ease or difficulty, number of items to be answered, percentage of missing data for each item, and response rate. They found that the feasibility of instruments is not always reported. Indeed, reports about the development of just five of the nine caregiver burden scales they reviewed included data for some aspect of feasibility, and none of the reports included data for all aspects of feasibility.

Feasibility overlaps, in part, with efficiency in that both properties consider the time needed for administration of the instrument. Scoring ease and response rate are somewhat dependent on **comprehensibility**, which refers to the extent to which the research participant and researcher are able to comprehend the behaviors needed to obtain an accurate measure of the concept (Polit & Beck, 2008). Scoring ease and response rate are also dependent on **precision**, which refers to the extent to which the instrument differentiates between respondents with differing amounts of the concept (Polit & Beck), as well as on **range**, which refers to the extent to which the obtained scores encompass the full range of possible scores for the concept measured by the instrument (Polit & Beck).

Linearity, another psychometric property, refers to the extent to which the instrument is an accurate measure of the full range of possible scores (Polit & Beck, 2008). Linearity is related to **simplicity**, which refers to the extent to which the instrument is a simple measure of the concept. Polit and Hungler (1999) pointed out that more complex measurement leads to more errors than does simple measurement. It is likely, then, that a simple instrument will display greater linearity than a more complex one.

Speededness, which refers to the extent to which adequate time is given to obtain complete data without rushing (Polit & Beck, 2008), also may be related to linearity and simplicity. It is likely that when adequate time is given to obtain complete data, those data will be more accurately recorded. It is also likely that it is easier to estimate the amount of time needed to obtain data if the instrument is simple than if it is complex.

Responsiveness, which is defined as "the ability of an instrument to accurately detect change when it has occurred" (Faber, Bosscher, & van Wieringen, 2006, p. 945), is an especially important psychometric property related to reliability when instruments are used as assessment tools in practice situations or for repeated measurements of a concept over time in the same study. The example of responsiveness given in Box 9–22 is from Faber et al.'s study of the clinimetric properties of the Performance-Oriented Mobility Assessment (POMA) scale.

BOX 9-22	**Example of Responsiveness of an Instrument Used for Assessment in Practice Situations**

Faber et al. (2006) estimated the responsiveness of the Performance-Oriented Mobility Assessment (POMA) scale for individuals and for a group. Their results are reported as the minimal detectable change (MDC) in the measurement units of the POMA. Each POMA item is rated on a two- or three-point scale, with a maximum possible score of 28.

The POMA responsiveness findings indicated that "changes in scores at the individual level should be at least 5 points and that changes in mean group scores should exceed 0.8 to be deemed reliable with a confidence interval of 95%" (Faber et al., p. 949).

Validity. **Validity** refers to the extent to which a questionnaire "measures what it purports to measure" (Carmines & Zeller, 1979, p. 12). Estimates of validity, therefore, provide an answer to the question "Are we measuring what we think we are measuring?" (Kerlinger & Lee, 2000, p. 666). When applied to research instruments, validity focuses on the appropriateness of those instruments as measures of middle-range theory concepts (Macnee &

McCabe, 2008). Each questionnaire should be a valid measure of a concept as the concept is constitutively defined in the middle-range theory. This point cannot be overemphasized because many concepts have different constitutive definitions. For example, some questionnaires that are designed to measure functional status may measure the concept defined as the actual performance of usual daily activities, whereas other questionnaires may be designed to measure functional status defined as the capacity to perform usual daily activities (Richmond, Tang, Tulman, Fawcett, & McCorkle, 2004). Thus, the constitutive definition of each concept must be considered when evaluating the validity of any questionnaire.

Types of Validity

Three types of validity have been identified—content validity, construct validity, and criterion-related validity (DeVon et al., 2007; Higgins & Straub, 2006; Nunnally & Bernstein, 1994). Examples of various types of validity are given in Tables 9–2 and 9–3, which are on the CD that comes with this book

Content validity refers to the adequacy of coverage of the items that make up a questionnaire with regard to the constitutive definition of the concept the instrument was designed to measure. Content validity estimates answer the question."Is the substance or content of this [instrument] representative of the content or the universe of content of the [concept] being measured?" (Kerlinger & Lee, 2000, p. 667).

Content validity is typically estimated for questionnaires and other research instruments, such as checklists and structured interview guides, that are used to collect quantitative data. This type of validity may, however, also be estimated for unstructured or semi-structured interview guides and other research instruments used to collect qualitative data.

Adequacy or representativeness of coverage takes two qualities of instruments into account— unidimensionality and balance (Polit & Hungler, 1999). **Unidimensionality** refers to the extent to which the instrument measures just one concept. **Balance** refers to the extent to which the instrument contains items that reflect balanced coverage of the concept. It is noteworthy that a balanced instrument tends to minimize **response-set bias**—that is, the tendency to respond to questionnaire items in a particular way. Various types of response-set bias are listed in Box 9–23.

Content validity may be estimated in several ways, including face validity, a systematic examination of the literature, and judgment by experts.

Face validity, which is regarded as a very weak approach to estimating content validity (Carmines & Zeller, 1979), is determined by examination of the instrument items to determine whether the items look like they are measuring the concept of interest. DeVellis (2003) pointed out that one issue related to face validity is that the assumption that an instrument measures what it looks like it measures "can be wrong" (p. 57). Another issue is that sometimes the concept being measured should not be obvious, such as when an instrument is measuring whether a person is telling the truth (DeVellis). Still another issue is to whom what the instrument measures should be obvious—the researcher, the researcher's peers, or the person responding to the instrument (DeVellis).

Systematic examination of the literature is a more rigorous approach to estimating content validity about the concept the instrument was designed to measure. The researcher may use a checklist to document whether the definition of the concept or the components of the concepts are reflected in the instrument items and then calculate a **percentage of agreement** for the questionnaire items.

BOX 9-23	Types of Response-Set Bias

Social Desirability

Research participants tend to give responses that are consistent with current social views or societal values.

Extreme Responses

Research participants tend to rate items at the extreme of a rating scale, such as *strongly agree* or *strongly disagree,* regardless of item content.

Neutral Responses

Research participants tend to select the midpoint on a rating scale or indicate no opinion to many items regardless of item content.

Agree Responses: Yea-sayers

Research participants tend to agree with many items regardless of the item content; also referred to as acquiescence response-set bias.

Disagree Responses: Nay-sayers

Research participants tend to disagree with many items regardless of the item content.
(Kerlinger & Lee, 2000; Polit & Beck, 2006)

Judgments of experts is an even more rigorous approach to estimating content validity. The experts typically are asked to rate each item on a scale, as, for instance, *not relevant, undecided,* or *relevant.* The content validity of the instrument may be reported as a **percentage of agreement** among the experts or as a **Content Validity Index** (CVI). The CVI "is derived from the rating of the content relevance of the items on an instrument using a 4-point ordinal rating scale, where 1 connotes an irrelevant item and 4 an extremely relevant item. The actual CVI is the proportion of items that received a rating of 3 or 4 by the experts" (Lynn, 1986, p. 384). Examples of content validity are given in Box 9–24 and in Tables 9–2 and 9–3 on the CD.

BOX 9-24	Examples of Content Validity

McKenna (1994) reported three approaches to estimating content validity for instruments he used in a study of identification of a nursing model to guide care of long-stay psychiatric patients.

Face Validity

Since the research tools appear to focus on the topic of investigation, namely nursing models, "face validity" can be claimed. (McKenna, 1994, p. 46)

Review-of-Literature Approach

If research instruments are constructed from relevant literature, content validity can be claimed. . . . This was the case with the instruments in the present study. (McKenna, 1994, p. 46)

BOX 9-24	Examples of Content Validity—*cont'd*

Judgments-of-Experts Approach

[I]n a further attempt to establish content validity, the instruments were sent to a panel of 13 selected nurse academics who were affiliated with institutions of higher learning throughout Great Britain. The criteria for inclusion were:

1. The academic [is lecturing] on psychiatric nursing in tertiary educational establishments.

2. The academic has been the author of articles/books on the utilization and implementation of nursing models. (McKenna, 1994, pp. 46–47)

Judgments-of-Experts Approach With Content Validity Index

Lancaster (2004) included a Content Validity Index in her report of content validity of the Coping with Breast Cancer Threat (CBCT) instrument: "Content validity of the CBCT items was assessed by four clinical nurse specialists, three of whom had oncology certification. The fourth was doctorally prepared. The content validity index . . . for this measure was .81 and all four content experts indicated that the 11 items on the instrument appropriately represented the domain of available content and that none were repetitive in nature" (p. 35).

Popham's average congruency procedure is a special case of the approach using percentage of agreement among experts to estimate content validity (Popham, 1978). This approach is a measure of the average percentage of agreement for all questionnaire items across all content validity experts. The example of Popham's average congruency approach to estimating content validity given in Box 9–25 is from Newman's (2005) study of the relation of personal health and self-esteem to functional status in caregivers of children in body casts.

BOX 9-25	Example of Content Validity: Popham's Average Congruency Approach

Two versions of the IFSCCBC [Inventory of Functional Status–Caregiver of a Child in a Body Cast] were developed by the investigator to ensure content validity of items for caregivers of young and older children. Content validity for both versions was estimated to be 90% using Popham's (1978) average congruency procedure. (Newman, 2005, p. 419)

Construct validity answers the question "What middle-range theory concept does the questionnaire actually measure?" Various approaches are used to estimate construct validity—the known-groups technique, the test of a theoretical proposition, factor analysis, and convergent and discriminant validity.

The known-groups technique for estimating construct validity, which is also called the **contrasted groups approach** (Waltz et al. 2005), involves administering the questionnaire to two or more groups that theoretically should have different scores on the questionnaire and then comparing the scores. The example of the known-groups technique given in Box 9–26 is from Fulk's single-subject study of the effects of different gait training interventions on a woman's ability to walk after experiencing a stroke.

BOX	Example of Construct Validity: Known-Groups
9-26	Approach

[T]o assess the client's reported functional walking ability, she completed a walking ability questionnaire . . . during the initial examination and at the end of every phase [of the study]. In community dwelling individuals with stroke, the questionnaire was found to be able to distinguish between the functional walking categories of physiological ambulator, limited household ambulator, unlimited household ambulator, most limited community ambulator, least limited community ambulator, and community ambulator. (Fulk, 2004, p. 22)

The **test of a theoretical proposition** approach to estimating construct validity, also referred to as the **hypothesis testing approach** or the **experimental manipulation approach** (Waltz et al., 2005), involves use of "the theory or conceptual framework underlying the [instrument's] design to state hypotheses regarding the behavior of individuals with varying scores on the [instrument]. . . . [The researcher then] gathers data to test the hypotheses, and makes inferences on the basis of the findings regarding whether . . . the rationale underlying the instrument's construction is adequate to explain the data collected" (Waltz et al., p. 157). The example of the test of a theoretical proposition given in Box 9–27 is from Bournaki's (1997) study of the relation of age, gender, past painful experiences, temperament, general fears, medical fears, and child-rearing practices to pain location, pain intensity, pain quality, observed behaviors, and heart rate change in school-age children who had a venipuncture.

BOX	Example of Construct Validity: Test
9-27	of a Theoretical Proposition Approach

The Adolescent Pediatric Pain Tool (APPT) . . . is a self-report measure of location, intensity, and quality of pain in children aged 8 to 17 years. Pain location is measured using a body outline figure on which children are instructed to mark the location(s) of their current pain. The number of locations is summed, with scores ranging from 0 to 43. . . . A postoperative decrease in pediatric surgical patients' pain sites was found, thus supporting construct validity. (Bournaki, 1997, p. 150)

(In this example, the proposition tested focused on the number of pain sites that would be identified by patients before and after surgery. It was hypothesized that fewer sites would be identified following surgery.)

The **factor analysis** approach to estimating construct validity involves administering the questionnaire to a large number of research participants—at least 5 to 10 times the number of items—and then analyzing the scores using the statistical procedure of factor analysis. This statistical procedure is used to identify clusters of related items, which are called factors. If the concept measured by the questionnaire is thought to have just one dimension—or component—the factor analysis is expected to yield just one factor. If, however, the concept is thought to have two or more dimensions, the factor analysis is expected to yield the same number of factors as the concept has dimensions. The example of the factor analysis approach to estimating construct

BOX 9-28	Example of Construct Validity: Factor Analysis Approach

The Perceived Multiple Role Stress Scale . . . is an eight-item scale that measures role stress resulting exclusively from the maternal and student roles. . . . [C]onstruct validity was supported by confirmatory factor analysis showing three correlated (.75, .69, .71) factors (emotional role ambiguity, person-role, and inter-role conflict). (Gigliotti, 2004, p. 160)

validity given in Box 9–28 is from Gigliotti's study of stress experienced by nursing students who were mothers of children under the age of 19.

The **convergent validity** and **discriminant validity** approaches to estimating construct validity—also referred to as the **multitrait-multimethod matrix method** (Campbell & Fiske, 1959)—involve administration of two or more different types of questionnaires, such as a Likert scale and a visual analog scale, that are thought to measure the same concept, as well as another questionnaire thought to measure a different yet theoretically related concept. **Convergent validity** is supported if correlations of the scores for the questionnaires measuring the concept of interest and the scores for other questionnaires measuring the same concept are relatively high. In other words, the different ways of measuring the concept "converge" on the concept (Kerlinger & Lee, 2000, p. 671). **Discriminant validity**, which sometimes is called **divergent validity**, is supported if the correlations of the scores for the questionnaires measuring the concept of interest and the scores for the questionnaire measuring the related concept are relatively low. In other words, the scores for the two questionnaires diverge. An example of the convergent and discriminant validity approaches to estimating construct validity is given in Box 9–29.

The discriminant validity approach is sometimes confused with the known-groups approach to estimating validity. For example, Schneider, Prince-Paul, Allen, Silverman, and Talaba (2004) incorrectly claimed that discriminant validity for the Symptom Distress Scale (SDS) was supported by differences in SDS scores between "survivors of myocardial infarction and patients with cancer . . . as well as between patients in home care and healthy controls" (p. 84).

BOX 9-29	Example of Construct Validity: Convergent Validity and Discriminant Validity Approaches

Hill et al. (2006) reported estimates of convergent and discriminant validity for the Maternal Postpartum Quality of Life questionnaire (MAPP-QOL): "Convergent validity of the MAPP-QOL was supported by a strong correlation between the MAPP-QOL and . . . [a] measure of life satisfaction ($r = .69$). Further construct validity was supported by discriminability. The MAPP-QOL was negatively correlated with the overall poor sleep score ($r = -.27, p = .0001$), and the four negative mood scales of the MAACL-R [Multiple Affect Adjective Checklist–Revised, which measures moods]: anxiety ($r = -.41, p < .001$), depression ($r = -.53, p < .001$), hostility ($r = -.36, p < .001$), and dysphoria ($r = -.50, p < .001$). The MAPP-QOL was positively correlated with the three positive mood subscales of the MAACL-R: positive affect ($r = .51, p < .001$), sensation seeking ($r = .35, p < .001$), and the PASS [sum of positive affect and sensation seeking scores] ($r = .54, p < .001$)" (Hill et al., p. 212).

Criterion-related validity involves comparison of the scores obtained from a questionnaire for which validity is being tested with the scores obtained from another questionnaire (the criterion) that measures the same concept. The criterion sometimes is regarded as the best—or "gold standard"—instrument available to measure the concept. Knapp (1985) pointed out that the criterion must be another measure of the concept rather than a measure of a related concept, and that the validity test must be distinct from a study of the relation between two variables. Criterion-related validity is estimated by administering the two questionnaires to research participants and then calculating the correlation between the scores for the two questionnaires. If the correlation is relatively high, criterion-related validity is supported. The two types of criterion-related validity are concurrent validity and predictive validity.

Concurrent validity refers to the ability of a questionnaire to differentiate between individuals on current performance or behavior. The questionnaire for which concurrent validity is to be estimated is administered, and the criterion questionnaire is administered at the same time or a short time later. Waltz et al. (2005) explained, "For concurrent validity, the measure being tested for validity and the related criterion measure are given within a short period of time and their results compared to make statements regarding present standing in regard to the criterion" (p. 168). The example of concurrent validity given in Box 9–30 is from Fulk's (2004) single-subject study of the effects of different gait training interventions on a woman's ability to walk after experiencing a stroke.

BOX 9-30	**Examples of Criterion-Related Validity**

Concurrent Validity

The concurrent validity of the 3-minute walk test as a measure of gait endurance was estimated with the criterion of the 6-minute walk test: "Gait endurance was measured as the distance the client could walk at her comfortable pace over 3 minutes. Leerar and Miller [2002] recently demonstrated that the results of a 3-minute walk test were concurrently valid to the results of a 6-minute walk test" (Fulk, 2004, p. 22).

Predictive Validity

Each of the 43 items on the Breastfeeding Self-Efficacy Scale (BSES) is preceded by the phrase "I can always." Respondents are asked to indicate on a scale from 1 to 5 the degree of confidence they felt, with 1 = not at all confident and 5 = always confident (Dennis & Faux, 1999, p. 402). Self-efficacy is defined as "a dynamic cognitive process in which an individual evaluates his or her capability to perform a given behavior" (p. 400). The BSES was administered while the women were in the hospital following childbirth. They were telephoned at 6 weeks postpartum to determine the criterion behavior of infant feeding method. "The predictive validity of the BSES was assessed by determining the relationship between breastfeeding mothers' self-efficacy and their infant feeding patterns at 6 weeks postpartum. Study participants were classified into three feeding patterns: bottle-feeding, combination feeding, or exclusive breastfeeding. . . . [A] significant difference at the .05 level was found between the exclusive bottlefeeding and exclusive breastfeeding groups' mean scores. The higher the BSES score the more likely the mother was exclusively breastfeeding at 6 weeks postpartum" (p. 406).

Predictive validity refers to the ability of a questionnaire to differentiate between individuals on future performance or behavior. Waltz et al. (2005) explained, "With predictive validity the criterion measure is administered much later than the measure being tested for validity, and the results are compared to assess the ability of the measure being tested to predict future standing in regard to the criterion" (pp. 168–169). The example of predictive validity given in Box 9–30 is from an instrument development study of the psychometric properties of the Breastfeeding Self-Efficacy Scale (Dennis & Faux, 1999).

Interpretation of Validity Coefficients

In general, the higher the validity coefficient, the more acceptable the estimate of validity. Validity coefficients can range from 0.00 to 1.00 or 0% to 100%. Coefficients of at least 0.70 or 70% are typically considered acceptable estimates. However, in the case of some approaches to estimating validity, such as discriminant validity, a very low coefficient may indicate a more acceptable estimate of validity.

Other Psychometric Properties Used to Evaluate Assessment and Diagnostic Tools. Two other psychometric properties are used to evaluate screening or assessment tools and diagnostic aids—sensitivity and specificity.

Sensitivity refers to "the ability of an instrument to identify a 'case' correctly, that is, to screen in or diagnose a condition correctly" (Polit & Beck, 2008, p. 464). **Specificity** refers to "the instrument's ability to identify non-cases correctly, that is, to screen out those without the condition correctly" (Polit & Beck, p. 464). An example of sensitivity and specificity is given in Box 9–31.

Some researchers use sensitivity and specificity data to estimate predictive validity. Faber et al. (2006), for example, used this approach to estimate the predictive validity of the POMA scale, which is "a widely used tool for assessing mobility and fall risk in older people" (p. 945). The investigators explained, "Predictive validity was expressed in terms of sensitivity and specificity. Sensitivity, in this context, is defined as the probability that a future faller is indeed predicted to be a faller, whereas specificity is defined as the probability that a future non-faller

BOX 9-31	Example of Sensitivity and Specificity of a Research Instrument

Vanderwee, Grypdonck, De Bacquer, and Defloor (2006) reported the sensitivity and specificity of two methods—finger and transparent disk—of measuring nonblanchable erythema (NBE), which is defined as "discoloration of the skin" (p. 156) associated with Grade 1 pressure ulcers. In the finger method of measuring NBE, "a finger is used to press on the erythema. If the erythema does not blanch when the finger is removed, it is considered NBE" (p. 156). In the transparent disk method, "a transparent plastic disk is used to press on the erythema. If the skin under the transparent disk does not blanch, it is regarded as NBE" (p. 156).

With the researcher's observations as standard, the sensitivity (the percentage of NBE that was correctly classified as NBE) was 73.1% for the finger method and 74.5% for the transparent disk method. . . . The specificity (the percentage of absence of NBE that was correctly classified) was 95.5% for the finger method and 95.6% for the transparent disk method. (Vanderwee et al., p. 160) is indeed predicted to be a non-faller" (p. 949). They reported the sensitivity of the POMA as 64% and the specificity as 66.1%, and concluded that the "predictive validity with regard to falling was not satisfactory" (p. 952).

Calibration of Biophysiological Equipment

To determine if the research instruments used are consistent and appropriate measures of middle-range theory concepts, the consistency and precision of the instruments themselves—the biophysiological equipment used to measure physiological responses—must be determined. This is usually done by calibrating the equipment against a standard.

Another approach, which is similar to alternate forms reliability, is to **compare the scores** obtained from two versions of the same piece of equipment used to collect the same data from the same research participant at the same time. **Signal-to-noise ratio** sometimes is considered when evaluating biophysiological equipment. This psychometric property addresses the extent to which the equipment maximizes the signal reading (the true differences in participants' scores) and minimizes interference noise (differences in scores caused by anything and everything but true differences) (DeVellis, 2003; Polit & Hungler, 1999).

The example of calibration of biophysiological equipment given in Box 9–32 is from Stepans, Wilhelm, and Dolance's (2006) experimental study of the effects of a smoking hygiene intervention on infants of breastfeeding mothers who smoked cigarettes.

BOX 9-32	Example of Calibration of Biophysiological Equipment

Stepans, Wilhelm, and Dolance (2006) measured breast milk and infant urinary levels of nicotine and cotinine to examine the effects of a smoking hygiene intervention.

Breast milk and [infant] urine samples were analyzed for nicotine and cotinine using a capillary gas-liquid chromatographic assay. A Model 6890 Agilent gas chromatograph equipped with a nitrogen phosphorus detector and a 10 m $\times$ 0.53 mm cross-linked fused-silica capillary column inlet system were used. Statistical analysis of the calibration curve revealed an adjusted r^2 of 0.93 for urinary nicotine levels between 25 and 200 ng/mL and 0.98 for levels from 250 to 2000 ng/mL. The adjusted r^2 was 0.94 for urinary cotinine levels between 25 and 200 ng/mL and 0.95 for levels between 250 and 2000 ng/mL. For breast milk, the adjusted r^2 for nicotine was 0.93 for levels between 25 and 200 ng/mL and 0.99 for levels between 250 and 2000 ng/mL. The r^2 for breast milk cotinine levels was 0.93 for levels between 25 and 200 ng/mL and 0.96 for levels between 250 and 2000 ng/mL. (Stepans et al., 2006, p. 110)

Cultural Equivalence of an Instrument

As more nurses and other health professionals from many parts of the world conduct research and as electronic technology increases ease of communication among researchers, the list of research instruments that have been translated into various languages grows. "A central concern of any translation process," according to Beck, Bernal, and Froman (2003), "is to yield a linguistic and cultural equivalent of the original" (p. 64). Beck et al. went on to point out that the translation should not be literal because the connotative—or implied—meaning of terms may be overlooked. Thus, "a culturally equivalent translation of an instrument is one that has a connotative meaning that is equivalent with the original" (Beck et al., p. 64). A culturally equivalent translation means that the instrument may be appropriately used with members of the culture for which the translation was done (Garity, 2000).

Back-translation is a frequently used procedure to translate instruments from one language to another (Varricchio, 2004). This procedure involves translation of the instrument from the language in which it was originally written to another language and then translation from the other language back to the original language. For example, Ip, Chan, and Chien (2005) used the back-translation procedure to translate the Childbirth Self-Efficacy Inventory (CBSEI) from English into Chinese. They explained, "[The] translation and back-translation procedure . . . was used to develop a culturally equivalent CBSEI. Two bilingual experienced midwives translated the CBSEI into Chinese and another two bilingual midwives back-translated it independently. The researchers and the four translators discussed the clarity of the translation work and examined discrepancies between the two versions; and finally amended a few items to ensure the appropriateness of the translation" (p. 627). Ip et al. also explained that they tested and found acceptable estimates for the content validity, construct validity, and internal consistency reliability of the Chinese version of the CBSEI.

Determining the cultural equivalence of an instrument requires a great deal of effort to maintain the original meaning of the concept being measured and the words used for each item of the instrument (Cha, Kim, & Erlen, 2007). Flaherty et al. (1988) identified five separate types of cross-cultural equivalence for instruments:

- **Content equivalence** refers to the relevance of each item to the culture of interest.
- **Semantic equivalence** refers to the extent to which the connotative meaning of each item is the same in the original culture and the culture for which the instrument is being translated.
- **Technical equivalence** refers to the extent to which the way the data were collected—such as interviews or survey questionnaires—is similar in each culture.
- **Criterion equivalence** refers to the extent to which the interpretation of the data is similar across the cultures.
- **Conceptual equivalence** refers to the extent to which the researcher is able to measure the same middle-range theory concept in each culture.

Beck et al. (2003) pointed out that few instruments used for cross-cultural research achieve the goal of equivalence in all five areas. They, for example, focused on determining the semantic equivalence of the Postpartum Depression Screening Scale for English- and Spanish-speaking cultures. Ip et al. (2005) also focused on the semantic equivalence of the CBSEI. Lin, Kao, Tzeng, and Lin (2007) focused on the content, semantic, and technical equivalences of the Cohen-Mansfield Agitation Inventory, which they translated from English to Chinese.

HOW IS THE CRITERION OF OPERATIONAL ADEQUACY APPLIED TO EXPERIMENTAL CONDITIONS?

When applied to the experimental conditions element of empirical research methods, the criterion of operational adequacy refers to the amount of information about the experimental conditions given in a report of experimental research and focuses attention on whether the experimental conditions were good enough to use when testing a middle-range predictive theory by means of experimental research. The operational adequacy criterion, when applied to experimental conditions, is met when you can answer yes to two questions:

- Are the experimental conditions clearly identified and fully described in the research report?
- Are the experimental conditions an appropriate measure of a concept of a middle-range predictive theory?

Are the Experimental Conditions Clearly Identified and Fully Described in the Research Report?

When evaluating the operational adequacy of experimental conditions, it is important to understand that the experimental and control treatments are the dimensions—or components—of one concept, which is typically called the independent variable. The concept, however, usually does not have an explicit label. If no label is given for the concept, we recommend using a term such as "type of treatment" as a generic label. Sometimes, researchers mistakenly regard the experimental and control treatments as separate concepts, which they refer to as variables. For example, Melancon and Miller (2005) referred to the experimental conditions as "each independent variable (massage and traditional therapies) was measured 3 times" (p. 118), rather than as one independent variable that might be called "type of therapy," made up of an experimental massage therapy treatment and a control traditional therapy treatment.

The experimental conditions used in experimental studies should be clearly identified in the research report. That means that the experimental and control treatments should be clearly and concisely explained. Although the experimental treatment usually is explained in some detail, the control treatment may not be. Sometimes, no information about the control treatment is given other than the number of research participants who received that treatment. At other times, the experimental treatment is explained in detail but the control treatment is very briefly described. For example, as can be seen in Box 9–3, Headley et al. (2004) did not provide the same level of detail for the control treatment as they did for the experimental treatment. In contrast, McCaffrey and Freeman (2003) provided detailed descriptions for both the experimental treatment and the control treatment for their study of the effect of listening to music on chronic pain from osteoarthritis (Box 9–33). Other examples of experimental conditions and associated experimental research designs are given in Table 9–4 on the CD that comes with this book.

Are the Experimental Conditions an Appropriate Measure of a Concept of a Middle-Range Predictive Theory?

The appropriateness of experimental conditions refers to the validity of experimental and control treatments. The research report should provide enough information to determine the validity of the experimental conditions. The validity of experimental conditions depends on the linkage of experimental and control treatments to the middle-range theory concept that is operationalized by the experimental conditions (Carmines & Zeller, 1979). For example, McCaffrey and Freeman (2003) used Rogers' Science of Unitary Human Beings, a conceptual model of nursing, to guide

BOX 9-33	**Example of Detailed Description of Experimental and Control Treatments**

The experimental group was given a cassette tape player and a cassette prepared by the primary investigator on which 20 minutes of relaxation music was recorded. The tape consisted of three musical selections by Mozart: (1) Andantino from *Concerto for Flute, Harp, and Orchestra in C,* K.299; (2) Overture to *La nozze di Figaro,* K.492; and (3) the Sonata Symphonie No. 40, first movement. Participants in the experimental group were asked to listen to the entire tape each day for 14 days at approximately 1 hour after completing their morning toilet. Participants were instructed to sit in the same comfortable chair each day and to avoid other distractions such as reading, speaking on the telephone, listening to the radio, or watching television. The control group sat in a quiet comfortable place for 20 minutes each day approximately 1 hour after completing their morning toilet for 14 days. They were asked to sit in a relaxed manner in a comfortable chair and avoid distractions such as speaking on the telephone, listening to the radio, or watching television during the 20 minutes sitting period. Reading newspapers, books, or magazines [was] permitted in the control group. (McCaffrey & Freeman, 2003, p. 520)

their study of the effect of listening to music on chronic pain from osteoarthritis. As can be seen in Figure 9–8, they clearly linked Rogers' concept of environmental field pattern to the middle-range theory concept of music listening, which they brought to life—or operationalized— as the experimental conditions (see Box 9–33) consisting of the experimental listening to music treatment protocol and the control sitting quietly treatment protocol.

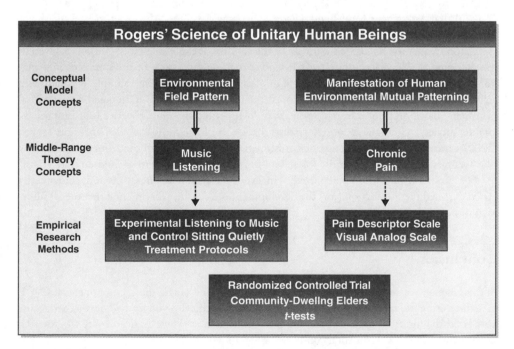

Figure 9-8. Conceptual-theoretical-empirical structure for McCaffrey and Freeman's (2003) experimental study.

To determine if the experimental conditions are an appropriate measure of a concept of a middle-range theory, the outcomes of the experimental conditions must be evaluated.

Outcomes are the effects that experimental conditions have on one or more middle-range concepts. The middle-range theory concepts that are outcomes also are linked to conceptual model concepts and then are operationalized by research instruments. As can be seen in Figure 9–8, McCaffrey and Freeman (2003) linked Rogers' concept of manifestations of human environmental mutual patterning to the middle-range theory concept of chronic pain, which they regarded as the outcome of music listening. They used two sections of the Short Form McGill Pain Questionnaire to operationalize chronic pain—the Pain Descriptor Scale and the Visual Analogue Scale.

Estimation of the validity of experimental conditions usually is limited to **content validity**. When applied to experimental conditions, content validity refers to the appropriateness of the content of the experimental and control treatments. An estimate of the content validity of experimental conditions may be documented by a description of the results of judgments from people who are regarded as experts in the middle-range theory concept that is operationalized by the experimental and control treatments. Statistics such as percentage of agreement or the CVI might be given. Or a claim of content validity for the experimental conditions may be based on a description of how the experimental and control treatments reflect the constitutive definition of the middle-range theory concept that is operationalized by the experimental conditions. For example, Smith (2001) explained that the experimental treatment culture school "is based on the [concepts of Giger and Davidhizar Transcultural Assessment Model and Theory] and includes clear guidelines and intervention strategies for care of culturally diverse clients" (p 52). In this example, the researcher operationalized several concepts of the Transcultural Assessment Model and Theory when she developed the experimental treatment culture school curriculum.

All too frequently, no explicit estimate of the validity of experimental conditions is given in research reports. However, some research reports include discussion of the source of information for the experimental treatment, which implies content validity. For example, Williams and Schreier (2005) reported that they developed the transcript for their audiotaped experimental treatment "based on prior research studies that documented the most effective [self-care behaviors] for anxiety . . . fatigue . . . and sleep disturbance" (p. 139). Similarly, McGahee and Tingen (2000) explained that the experimental treatment "is consistent with guidelines published by [the Centers for Disease Control] for school-based programs targeting children and youth" (p. 11). And, Fathima (2004) reported, "An extensive review of literature and guidance by experts formed the foundation [for] the development of . . . [the experimental treatment] information booklet" (p. 81).

Conclusion

In this chapter, you continued to learn more about how to evaluate the E component of C-T-E structures using the criterion of operational adequacy. Specifically, you learned how to determine how good the information about the empirical indicators is. These indicators are the research instruments and the experimental conditions given in a research report.

It is tempting to focus on the dependability and credibility of qualitative data or the reliability and validity of quantitative data without paying sufficient attention to the middle-range theory concept that was measured by the instrument used to collect the qualitative or quantitative data. It is crucial, instead, to also consider the C and T components of C-T-E structures when evaluating the research instruments and experimental conditions element of the E component.

The questions to ask and answer as you evaluate the research instruments and experimental conditions element of empirical research methods are listed in Box 9–34. Application of the criterion of operational adequacy for research instruments and experimental conditions should help you continue to better understand the E component of C-T-E structures. The learning activities for this chapter will help you continue to increase your understanding of the operational adequacy criterion and its application to the contents of research reports.

BOX 9-34	Evaluation of Research Instruments and Experimental Conditions: *How Good Is the Information?*

Operational Adequacy

Research Instruments

• Are all research instruments clearly identified and fully described in the research report?

• Are the research instruments consistent and appropriate measures of the middle-range theory concepts?

Experimental Conditions

• Are the experimental conditions clearly identified and fully described in the research report?

• Are the experimental conditions an appropriate measure of a concept of a middle-range predictive theory?

References

Full citations for all references cited in this chapter are provided in the Reference section at the end of the book.

Learning Activities

Activities to supplement what you have learned in this chapter, along with practice examination questions, are provided on the CD that comes with this book.

Chapter 10

Evaluation of Procedures for Data Collection

This chapter continues the focus on the empirical research methods (E) component of conceptual-theoretical-empirical (C-T-E) structures for research and the criterion of operational adequacy. Specifically, we focus on the procedures used for data collection, which is the E element concerned with *where, when*, and *by whom* the data were obtained.

KEYWORDS

Concurrent Data Collection

Cross-Sectional Data Collection

Existing Data

External Validity

Internal Validity

Laboratory Setting

Longitudinal Data Collection

Measurement Validity

Naturalistic Setting

New Data

Prospective Data Collection

Researcher Credibility

Retrospective Data Collection

Rigor

Secondary Data Analysis

Threats to Internal Validity or Rigor

Threats to Transferability or Generalizability

Recall from Chapter 2 that the E component of a C-T-E structure encompasses five major elements—the research design, the research participants, the instruments and any experimental conditions, the procedures used to collect data and protect research participants from harm, and the techniques used to analyze the data. In Chapter 3, you began to learn *where* to look for the data collection procedure in research reports (Box 10–1) and *what* information you could expect to find (Box 10–2). In Chapter 4, you began to learn how to determine *how good* the data collection procedures were by using our framework for evaluating C-T-E structures for research.

In this chapter we discuss in detail the criterion of operational adequacy as it applies to data collection procedures and provide examples that should help you better understand how to apply the criterion as you read research reports. Application of the operational adequacy criterion will facilitate your evaluation of *how good* the information about the data collection procedures provided in the research report is.

BOX	Evaluation of Procedures for Data Collection:
10-1	*Where* Is the Information?

Look in the design and procedure subsections of the method section of the research report.

BOX	Evaluation of Procedures for Data Collection:
10-2	*What* Is the Information?

- Where the data were collected
- When the data were collected
- Who collected the data

WHAT ARE PROCEDURES FOR DATA COLLECTION?

Data are collected in various settings at various times and by various people. Evaluation of procedures for data collection, therefore, takes into account where the data were collected, when the data were collected, and who collected the data.

Where Were the Data Collected?

There are several settings in which data can be collected, including a laboratory, a naturalistic setting, a library, or the Internet.

Laboratory

One setting in which data can be collected is a **laboratory** or **testing room**. The environment and testing conditions in a laboratory setting or testing room can be highly controlled. Environmental controls include light, heat, sound, and the color of walls and floor, as well as colors and types of furnishings. Testing conditions can be controlled by administering questionnaires and using biophysiological equipment without interruptions or distractions. In laboratory settings, questionnaire data are usually collected via face-to-face interviews by a member of the research team or are completed by the participants themselves.

Data are collected in laboratories for descriptive, correlational, and experimental research designs. An example of a laboratory setting where data were collected for an experimental study is given in Box 10–3.

Naturalistic Setting

Another setting in which data can be collected is referred to as a **naturalistic setting**. The environment and testing conditions in a naturalistic, or **real-world**, setting cannot be closely

BOX 10-3	Example of a Laboratory Setting Where Data Were Collected

Ludomirski-Kalmanson (1984) collected data in a laboratory setting for her Rogers' Science of Unitary Human Beings–based study of the relation between light waves and human field motion, defined as a holistic sense of movement, in adults who had intact visual sensory perception or total blindness. The surfaces of the laboratory, referred to as an experimental room, were "covered with off-white reflective material and room temperature was maintained at 72 to 74 degrees Fahrenheit. Equal intensity of relative energy in adjusted foot candles was provided by a six-to-one ratio of red to blue florescent bulbs placed in ceiling fixtures equidistant above the [participants]. . . . Each participant was provided with a robe to wear of black absorbent material and [was] requested to be seated" (p. 2094B).

controlled because data are collected in places such as hospital waiting rooms, patients' rooms, and nurses' stations; clinics; and people's homes. Interruptions and distractions in these settings are common, since real-world activities continue in the midst of data collection. In naturalistic settings, questionnaire data may be collected via face-to-face or telephone interviews by a member of the research team. The questionnaires can also be completed by participants themselves while a research team member and each participant are together, or the participants may both receive questionnaires and submit them completed via postal service mail.

Data are collected in naturalistic settings for descriptive, correlational, and experimental research designs. An example of a naturalistic setting where data were collected for a descriptive study is given in Box 10–4. Several other examples are given in Tables 10–1, 10–2, and 10–3, which are on the CD that comes with this book.

BOX 10-4	An Example of a Naturalistic Setting Where Data Were Collected

Garity's (2006) sample was made up of "post–nursing home placement caregivers for their family members with AD [Alzheimer's disease]" (p. 42). She recruited the caregivers from "several AD support groups offered in three nursing homes located in a southern New England state. . . . The researcher telephoned everyone who expressed an interest in study participation to answer any additional questions about the study and to arrange a convenient time for conducting individual interviews. . . . Interviews were conducted in a private area at the nursing homes and at times convenient for the study participants and staff" (p. 42).

Library

Still another setting in which data can be collected is a **library**. This setting is used most frequently when the data are obtained from documents, such as journal articles, books, and other documents available in an actual or electronic library. Libraries are the setting for data collection primarily with descriptive research designs. An example of a library setting where data were collected is given in Box 10–5. Other examples are given in Table 10–1 on the CD that comes with this book.

BOX 10-5	An Example of a Library Setting Where Data Were Collected

Skalski, DiGerolamo, and Gigliotti (2006) reviewed Neuman Systems Model–based literature addressing stressors experienced by diverse client populations. They reported that "a total of 87 studies published as journal articles or book chapters between 1983 and 2005 were reviewed" (p. 71). All of the journal articles and book chapters were retrieved from library holdings.

The Internet

The **Internet** can be used as the setting for data collection for descriptive, correlational, and experimental research designs. An example of an early descriptive nursing study for which the Internet was used for data collection is given in Box 10–6; another example is given in Table 10–1 on the CD.

BOX 10-6	An Example of a Library Setting Where Data Were Collected

Fawcett and Buhle (1995) used the Internet to collect data for a descriptive study of cancer survivors' needs and coping mechanisms. They explained that the Cancer Survivors Survey Questionnaire "was composed and printed out by the first author using the word processing program Word Perfect 5.1 and then reformatted by the second author into plain text for dissemination on Compuserve's Cancer Forum, the Internet newsgroup, and the gopher server side of OncoLink. The plain text was formatted into HyperText Markup Language for placement on the World Wide Web (WWW) portion of OncoLink" (p. 274).

When Were the Data Collected?

Data may be collected prospectively, concurrently, or retrospectively. Data also may be collected once or repeatedly over time and as new data or existing data.

Prospective, Concurrent, and Retrospective Data Collection

Prospective, concurrent, and retrospective data collection may be used for descriptive, correlational, and experimental research designs. Examples are given here and in Tables 10–1, 10–2, and 10–3 on the CD that comes with this book.

Prospective data collection refers to collecting data about the effects of an experience, such as a health condition, that has already occurred. Williams and Schreier (2005), for example, collected data from women who had a diagnosis of breast cancer about four dependent variables—the women's self-care behaviors, and their levels of fatigue, anxiety, and sleep disturbances—three times: before their first cancer treatment (pretest) and 1 and 3 months later (posttests).

Concurrent data collection refers to collecting data as an experience is occurring. Radwin (2000), for example, collected data from patients with cancer about their perceptions of the characteristics of high-quality oncology nursing care during the time they were receiving care from oncology nurses.

Retrospective data collection refers to collecting data about recall of an experience. Pilkington (2005), for example, asked nine men and one woman, ranging in age from 70 to 92 years of age and living in a long-term care facility, to recall their experiences of grieving a loss. Examples of the losses were a man's divorce from his second wife after 10 years of marriage, deaths of a man's close friends, and the death of a man's wife shortly after the deaths of his brother and sister-in-law one year prior to data collection.

Cross-Sectional and Longitudinal Data Collection

Evaluation of when the data were collected also requires consideration of how often the data were collected. Data may be collected cross-sectionally or longitudinally. Cross-sectional or longitudinal data collection may be used for descriptive, correlational, or experimental research designs. Examples are given here and in Tables 10–1, 10–2, and 10–3 on the CD.

Cross-sectional data collection refers to collecting data just one time. Cross-sectional may be thought of as a sample that is a cross section of the target population. Cross-sectional studies frequently take into account differences in research participant characteristics, such as gender, age, education, health condition, or severity of a health condition, when selecting the sample and analyzing the data. Radwin (2000), for example, collected data from a cross section of patients with cancer to identify their perceptions of the characteristics of high-quality oncology nursing care.

Longitudinal data collection, also called **repeated measures** data collection, refers to collecting data more than one time. Williams and Schreier (2005) collected longitudinal data for their pretest-posttest experimental study of the effects of audiotaped education on the self-care behaviors, fatigue, anxiety, and sleep disturbances of women with breast cancer.

Collection of New or Existing Data

Another aspect of when data were collected is whether the data were new or already existed. New data or existing data may be collected for descriptive, correlational, or experimental research designs, although existing data are used more frequently with descriptive and correlational research designs than with experimental designs. Examples are given here and in Tables 10–1, 10–2, and 10–3 on the CD.

New data are specifically collected for a study. Pilkington (2005) collected new data from the men and women who participated in her descriptive study of grieving a loss, and Williams and Schreier (2005) collected new data from the women with breast cancer who participated in their experimental study of the effects of audiotaped education on self-care behaviors, fatigue, anxiety, and sleep disturbances.

Existing data already exist but were collected and/or analyzed for a new study. Existing data are used when the focus of the research is examination of documents, such as books, book chapters, journal articles, or other published or unpublished reports. Holden (2005) collected existing data from published journal articles and books for her analysis of the concept of complex adaptive systems. Existing data are also used for **secondary data analysis** studies, which involve a new or different approach to the analysis of data that already were collected for a study. Tsai (2005) used existing data from a completed study for her secondary analysis of the relation of chronic pain, disability, social support, financial hardship, age, and gender to distress, and the relation of distress to depression.

Who Collected the Data?

Data are typically collected by researchers and research assistants. Polit and Beck (2008) pointed out that researchers usually collect their own data when the research design calls for a relatively small number of participants, as is often the case with descriptive qualitative research and exploratory research designs. Research assistants may be employed to help the researchers when the number of research participants is relatively large, when the research design involves collection of data several times, or when an experimental research design requires complex experimental and control treatments. Chair, Taylor-Piliae, Lam, and Chan (2003), for example, stated that six research assistants collected the data for their experimental study of the effect of positioning after coronary angiography on back pain. Tables 10–1, 10–2, and 10–3 on the CD include information about who collected data for each study.

Researcher credibility, which is evaluated for qualitative research designs, is also relevant for quantitative research designs. Research assistants should be carefully trained so that consistency of the data collection procedures is maintained. Some researchers mention only that research assistants collected data, and others mention only that research assistants were trained. Still other researchers provide a detailed description of research assistant training (Box 10–7).

BOX 10-7	Example of Description of Research Assistant Training

Coleman et al. (2005) provided detailed information about how research assistants, who were oncology nurses, were trained to conduct an experimental study of the most effective way to provide social support for women with breast cancer. The experimental conditions were an experimental treatment of telephone social support and a mailed resource kit, containing an information manual, audiotapes, videotapes, and pamphlets, and a control treatment of the mailed resource kit only. Coleman et al. stated, "For consistency and standardization during discussion of this [information] manual, the oncology nurses who provided the telephone social support participated in a training session and used an additional manual developed by the investigators. Each chapter in the nurses' manual matched a chapter in the participants' manual" (p. 824).

HOW IS THE CRITERION OF OPERATIONAL ADEQUACY APPLIED TO PROCEDURES FOR DATA COLLECTION?

When applied to the data collection procedures element of empirical research methods, the criterion of **operational adequacy** refers to the amount of information about the data collection procedures given in a research report and focuses attention on whether the procedures were appropriate for the theory-generating research or theory-testing research reported. The operational adequacy criterion, when applied to data collection procedures, is met when you can answer yes to two questions:

- Are the data collection procedures clearly identified and described?
- Are the data collection procedures appropriate?

Are the Data Collection Procedures Clearly Identified and Described?

All data collection procedures should be clearly identified and described. Specifically, a description of the where, when, and who of data collection should be included in the research report. Examples for descriptive, correlational, and experimental research are given in Boxes 10–8, 10–9, and 10–10.

Are the Data Collection Procedures Appropriate?

Evaluation of the appropriateness of the procedures used for data collection focuses on the extent to which those procedures are accurate for the type of theory-generating research design

BOX 10-8	Example of Description of the Data Collection Procedure for Descriptive Research

Pilkington (2005) used Parse's basic research method to guide collection of data for her descriptive study of the experience of grieving a loss: "Data were gathered through dialogical engagement, an intersubjective process in which the researcher was truly present with the participants as they described the phenomenon under study. . . . Dialogues took place in the privacy of the participants' rooms [in a long-term care facility]. After reviewing the purpose of the research, the researcher initiated the dialogue by asking the participants to describe as completely as possible their experience of grieving a loss. . . . The dialogical engagement ended when the participants indicated that they were finished. The dialogues lasted anywhere from 20 min to more than an hour" (pp. 234–235).

The description of the data collection procedure reveals that the data were collected in a naturalistic setting (participants' rooms in a long-term care facility), retrospectively (recall of the experience of grieving a loss), cross-sectionally (just once), and by the researcher herself.

| BOX 10-9 | Example of Description of the Data Collection Procedure for Correlational Research |

For her correlational study of the relation of maternal role involvement, student role involvement, and total network social support to maternal-student role stress, Gigliotti (2004) explained: "Data were collected at 11 community colleges in the New York and New Jersey area" (p. 160). She also explained that female students who volunteered to participate in the study completed the questionnaires at home and returned them via mail.

The description of the data collection procedure reveals that the data were collected in a naturalistic setting (participants' homes following sample recruitment at community colleges), retrospectively (recall of role activities and social support), and cross-sectionally (just once). Inasmuch as research assistants were not mentioned, it can be inferred that the data were collected by the researcher herself.

| BOX 10-10 | Example of Description of the Data Collection Procedure for Experimental Research |

For their experimental study of the effect of positioning on back pain, Chair, Taylor-Piliae, Lam, and Chan (2003) reported: "All participants were invited by one of the six research assistants to take part in the study. . . . Following coronary angiography, . . . frequent observations were made for bleeding and haematoma formation at the femoral catheter insertion site, and for back pain perception. Pedal pulses were evaluated each time the femoral site was assessed" (pp. 473–474).

The description of the data collection procedure reveals that the data were collected in a naturalistic setting (in a hospital following coronary angiography), prospectively (after angiography), longitudinally (a chart included in the article indicated that the data were collected at 15, 30, and 45 minutes, at 1, 2, 3, 4, 5, 6, and 7 hours, and the next morning following coronary angiography), and by six research assistants.

or theory-testing research design used, as well as the extent to which the research findings can be applied in situations that are similar to those of the study reported. Or, in other words, the appropriateness of the data collection procedures is met when you answer yes to the following three questions:

- Are the data collection procedures accurate for the type of research design being used?
- Can the research findings be applied to situations that are similar to the study reported?
- Does the design adhere to the max-min-con principle?

For theory-generating qualitative research designs, **accuracy** is assessed by considering **rigor**, and **applicability** is assessed by considering **transferability**. For theory-testing research designs, **accuracy** is determined by considering **internal validity**, and **applicability** is determined by assessing **generalizability**. Evaluation of rigor and internal validity takes into account the extent to which the procedures yielded research results that are accurate for the study sample (Macnee & McCabe, 2008). Evaluation of transferability and generalizability takes into account the extent to which the research results can be applied to samples from the same population.

Researchers may acknowledge that the accuracy and applicability of their data are limited, but they rarely provide a detailed discussion of specific threats to rigor and internal validity. They may, however, indicate that the sample was too small or too lacking in diversity for the reader to have confidence in the transferability or generalizability to other samples from the same population or to other populations. Thus, the reader must be aware of all possible factors that could influence the data and make an independent judgment about the rigor and transferability of qualitative data or the internal validity and generalizability of quantitative data.

Accuracy of the Data: Rigor and Internal Validity

Burns and Grove (2007) identified five tasks associated with collecting data—recruiting research participants, collecting data in a consistent manner, maintaining the controls specified by the research design, protecting the integrity of the research design, and solving any problems that might disrupt the research. Rigor (for qualitative research designs) and internal validity (for theory-testing research designs) draw attention to the extent to which those five tasks yield data that are accurate for the research participants.

The research design and data collection procedures should provide "confidence that the findings of a study are characteristic of the variables being studied and not the investigative procedure itself" (Sandelowski, 1986, p. 29). LoBiondo-Wood (2006) explained, "When reading research, one must feel that the results of a study are [rigorous or] valid, based on precision, and faithful to what the researcher wanted to measure" (p. 209).

Rigor refers to the accuracy of the data collection procedures used with qualitative research designs. Macnee and McCabe (2008) pointed out that although qualitative research designs are frequently flexible, the data collection procedures "still must have a function that fits the research question and provides the foundation ensuring the accuracy of the data" (p. 198).

Internal validity refers to the accuracy of the data collection procedures used with quantitative research designs. Specifically, internal validity refers to the extent to which the research design in general and the data collection procedures in particular are accurate and correct (Macnee & McCabe, 2008). When applied to correlational or experimental research designs, internal validity refers to the extent to which the independent variable, rather than some other variable or condition, influences the dependent variable (Polit & Beck, 2006).

Threats to Rigor or Internal Validity. Threats to rigor or internal validity include selection bias effects, history effects, maturation effects, testing effects, instrumentation effects, mortality effects, and statistical regression, as well as interaction between any two or more of the threats. These threats are considered alternative explanations or rival hypotheses to the explanation or hypotheses that the study findings were the result of the participants' unbiased true responses (Kerlinger & Lee, 2000).

Selection bias effects refer to the extent to which the way in which the sample was selected influenced the results. Selection bias effects are more likely to occur than any other threat to rigor or internal validity. Parahoo (2006) identified two points of potential bias in sample selection: (1) the judgment the researcher has to make about who actually meets the inclusion and exclusion criteria, regardless of type of research design—use of inclusion and exclusion criteria that are more objective than subjective can reduce selection bias; and (2) how, in experimental research designs, participants are assigned to experimental and control treatments. Selection bias in experimental research can be reduced by use of random assignment of participants to treatments. If random assignment is not possible, the characteristics of the participants in the experimental and control groups can be compared to determine whether selection bias occurred (Polit & Beck, 2008).

History effects refer to the extent to which an uncontrolled external event that occurred during data collection influenced the participants' responses. The event may be common-place, such as change of seasons of the year, or of substantial historical importance, such as a major storm with a high level of damage and fatalities. In either case, if the event is not known to the researcher or not taken into account in interpreting the data (Parahoo, 2006), the rigor or internal validity of the research is threatened. History effects should be taken into consideration with all types of descriptive, correlational, and experimental research designs. History effects are minimized, however, in qualitative research designs because those designs place participants' experiences in the context of their own and sociopolitical history (Sandelowski, 1986).

Maturation effects refer to the extent to which participants changed over time during data collection. Specifically, maturation effects refer to "the developmental, biological, or psycho-logical processes that operate within an individual as a function of time and are external to the events of the investigation" (LoBiondo-Wood, 2006, p. 218).

Maturation effects should be taken into consideration with all types of descriptive, corre-lational, and experimental research designs. As with history effects, maturation effects are minimized or offset in qualitative research designs because those designs take the context of the participants' experiences into account (Sandelowski, 1986).

Testing effects—also called **sensitization**—refer to the extent to which repeated adminis-tration of the same instruments influenced the participants' responses. The interval between repeated administrations of the instruments may be short (minutes or hours) or long (days, weeks, months, or even years). Polit and Beck (2008) noted that "the mere act of collecting data from people changes them" (p. 297). When more than one instrument is used to collect data, researchers sometimes address testing effects by administering the instruments in ran-dom order. If the order of administration is not random, the researcher-determined order of administration should be consistent. Testing effects should be considered whenever the same questions are asked at different times during a study, regardless of the research design.

Instrumentation effects refer to the extent to which any change in the instruments used to measure the same middle-range theory concept or any change in experimental conditions in a study influenced participants' responses. This threat also refers to the continued precision of data collected by means of biophysiological equipment, which is why calibration of equip-ment should be checked prior to and after data collection (LoBiondo-Wood, 2006). Moreover, instrumentation effects apply to the consistency or fidelity of data collection by dif-ferent members of the research team. Consequently, all data collectors should be carefully trained in a systematic manner and should adhere to specific data collection procedures (LoBiondo-Wood). Furthermore, instrumentation effects refer to the extent to which researchers' preferences for particular instruments without consideration of their appropriate-ness for the research may influence its rigor or internal validity (Parahoo, 2006).

The threat to rigor or internal validity associated with changes in instruments should be con-sidered in all types of descriptive, correlational, and experimental research designs. A change in experimental conditions is a threat to internal validity with experimental research designs.

Mortality effects—also called **attrition**—are the extent to which loss of participants from one data collection point in a study to another data collection point influenced the results. In experimental research, mortality also refers to differences in the attrition rates of participants in the experimental and control treatment groups. Polit and Beck (2008) commented that mortality effects are a "concern if the [attrition] rate exceeds 20%" (p. 297).

The threat to rigor or internal validity associated with attrition should be considered whenever data are collected more than one time in any type of descriptive, correlational, or experimental research design or when more than one treatment group is used in experimental research. In descriptive qualitative research designs, the threat of mortality may be minimized by the "close relationship" between the researcher and each participant (Sandelowski, 1986, p. 30).

Statistical regression—also called **regression to the mean**—refers to the extent to which high or low instrument scores move closer to the sample mean when an instrument is administered a second or subsequent time (Parahoo, 2006). Statistical regression occurs because "very high scores and very low scores [which are considered outliers] occur by chance, and the chances of this happening is lower than for scores [that] reflect the mean or average" (Parahoo, p. 240). Statistical regression is a threat to the internal validity of any quantitative research design that involves more than one administration of an instrument.

Interaction of threats can produce yet another threat, as pointed out by Campbell and Stanley (1963). Selection effects could, for example, interact with maturation effects, or history effects could interact with testing or instrumentation effects, and so on.

Determining Degree of Rigor or Internal Validity

Descriptive qualitative research designs are thought to have a **high degree of rigor** if conducted in keeping with the methods of the particular research design used by the researcher. Descriptive quantitative research designs and correlational research designs are sometimes regarded as having a **low degree of internal validity** because environmental and testing conditions may interfere with consistency in data collection procedures. That judgment, however, may be a legacy of emphasis on experimental research designs as the "best." These designs—especially true experiments and randomized controlled trials (RCTs)—are thought to have a **high degree of internal validity** because randomization to experimental treatment and control treatment is supposed to eliminate alternative explanations for the findings. In other words, true experimental research designs and RCTs are thought to avoid most, if not all, threats to internal validity (Campbell & Stanley, 1963).

Applicability of the Data: Transferability and Generalizability

In Chapter 8, we explained that **transferability** is associated with the adequacy and appropriateness of the sample for qualitative research designs, and **generalizability** is associated with the adequacy and appropriateness of the sample for quantitative research designs. We also explained that transferability is sometimes referred to as **fittingness** and that generalizability is sometimes referred to as **external validity**.

Transferability and generalizability are also relevant when evaluating data collection procedures. They draw attention to the extent to which the procedures support using the results of the theory-generating research or theory-testing research as evidence for situations external to that of the particular research that was reported. In the case of qualitative research designs, special consideration is given to the extent to which the results " 'fit' into contexts outside the study situation and [the extent to which readers view the] findings as meaningful and applicable in terms of their own experience" (Sandelowski, 1986, p. 32).

Threats to Transferability or Generalizability. Threats to transferability or generalizability are found in data collection procedures that limit the extent to which the findings of a study can be applied to other people from the same population as the study participants and to other situations or environmental conditions. In other words, the threats are questions of "under what conditions and with what types of [people and in what types of situations] the same results can be expected to occur" (LoBiondo-Wood, 2006, p. 213).

Threats to transferability or generalizability include measurement effects, novelty effects, researcher effects, interaction of history and treatment effects, and expectancy effects, as well as interaction effects of selection bias and the independent variable, multiple treatment interference, and the reactive or interaction effect of testing. Although some of the terms used for threats to transferability or generalizability are similar to those used for the threats to rigor or internal validity that we discussed in the previous section, the focus in this section is on limitations imposed by the research design and data collection procedures (Macnee & McCabe, 2008).

Measurement effects refer to the extent to which study results apply to "another group of people who are not also exposed to the same data collection (and attention-giving) procedures" (Polit & Beck, 2004, p. 219). Measurement effects should be considered a threat with any type of descriptive, correlational, or experimental research design.

Novelty effects refer to the extent to which participants and researchers reacted to new experimental conditions or unusual data collection procedures. Reactions may indicate enthusiasm for or skepticism about the treatment or procedure. Study findings "may reflect reactions to the novelty rather than to the intrinsic nature of an intervention [or procedure]; once the treatment is more familiar, results might be different" (Polit & Beck, 2004, p. 219). If the novelty is the data collection procedures, the threat should be considered with any type of descriptive, correlational, or experimental research design. If the novelty is confined to experimental conditions, this threat should be considered only with experimental research designs.

Researcher effects—also called **experimenter effects**—refer to the extent to which participants' responses were influenced by the researchers' or research assistants' characteristics, such as their appearance, gender, or age. As Polit and Beck (2008) pointed out, "To the extent possible, data collectors should match study participants with respect to such characteristics as racial or cultural background and gender. . . . The greater the sensitivity of the questions, the greater the desirability of matching characteristics" (p. 382).

Researchers' or research assistants' personalities, such as being very friendly or very distant, may also influence participants' responses. In addition, researchers' or research assistants' expectations about study results may influence participants' responses. Polit and Beck (2004) explained, "The investigators often have an emotional or intellectual investment in demonstrating that their hypotheses are correct and may unconsciously communicate their expectations to [participants]. If this is the case, the results [of] the original study might be difficult to [duplicate] in a more neutral situation" (p. 219). Furthermore, responses of participants in a study involving longitudinal data collection may be influenced by any changes in the researcher or research assistant who collects the data from each participant. Ideally, the same research team member should collect data from the same participant throughout the study (Polit & Beck, 2008). The threat to transferability or generalizability of researcher effects should be considered with any type of descriptive, correlational, or experimental research design.

Interaction of history and treatment effects refer to the possibility that events occurring during data collection (history) may interact with the data collection procedures or experimental conditions to influence the participants' responses. When the data collection procedures or experimental conditions are administered again "in the absence of the other events, different results may be obtained" (Polit and Beck, 2004, p. 219). This threat should be considered with all types of descriptive, correlational, or experimental research designs.

Expectancy effects—also called **reactivity effects**—refer to the extent to which "mere participation in a . . . study . . . could have an effect on the participant that would not occur if the participant was in a natural setting" (Kerlinger & Lee, 2000, p. 477). One aspect of the expectancy effects threat is the possibility that research participants behaved in a particular way primarily because they are aware of participating in the research. This aspect is sometimes labeled the **Hawthorne effect**, which comes from the findings of a study of working conditions conducted by Mayo (1953) at the Western Electric Hawthorne Works, located in Cicero, Illinois. The Hawthorne effect is typically considered in experimental research but should also be considered in descriptive and correlational research.

Another aspect of the expectancy effects threat is labeled the **placebo effect**. This is the possibility that research participants who were assigned to a control treatment in an experimental study—or what Polit and Beck (2008) call a **pseudointervention**—demonstrated changes or improvements primarily because they were aware of participating in the research. Still another aspect of the expectancy effects threat is the **nocebo effect**, which is the occurrence of adverse side effects experienced by participants who received the control treatment (Polit & Beck, 2004). Because the behavior of participants in a control treatment group is the focus, consideration of the placebo effect or the nocebo effect is confined to experimental research. The major issue associated with placebo and nocebo expectancy effects is that participants would not behave in the same way if the experimental or control treatment were not administered within a research context (Polit & Beck, 2004).

Interaction effects of selection bias and the independent variable refers to the extent to which generalizability is influenced by the way in which bias in participant selection interacts with the independent variable that influences the dependent variable (Campbell & Stanley, 1963; Kerlinger & Lee, 2000). More simply, this threat "indicates that selection of participants can very well affect generalization of the results" (Kerlinger & Lee, p. 477). Because of the involvement of independent and dependent variables, which are not typically parts of descriptive research designs, this threat should be considered primarily with correlational and experimental research designs.

Multiple treatment interference refers to the extent to which participants' responses to data collection procedures or experimental conditions were influenced by their responses to earlier data collection procedures or experimental conditions (Campbell & Stanley, 1963; Kerlinger & Lee, 2000). This threat should be considered whenever data are collected from each research participant more than one time, regardless of the type of descriptive, correlational, or experimental research design. The threat should especially be considered with experimental research designs that involve more than one administration of the experimental or control treatment. Campbell and Stanley explained that multiple treatment interference is "likely to occur whenever multiple treatments are applied to the same [participants], because the effects of prior treatments are not usually erasable" (p. 6).

The **reactive or interaction effect of testing** refers to the extent to which a pretest given prior to administration of experimental conditions "may decrease or increase the sensitivity of the participant to the independent variable [that is, the experimental conditions] . . . [which] would make the results for the pre-tested population unrepresentative of the treatment effect for the non-pretested population" (Kerlinger & Lee, 2000, p. 477). This threat should be considered with all pretest-posttest experimental research designs.

Max-Min-Con Principle

Procedures used to conduct a study according to the research design blueprint should adhere to the **max-min-con principle** (Kerlinger & Lee, 2000), which asserts that researchers construct efficient research designs and adhere to specific data collection procedures in an attempt to **max**imize variance, **min**imize error variance, and **con**trol the effects of extraneous factors that may affect the study variables.

Variance is the focus of the max and min components of the max-min-con principle. Variance is a statistical term that refers to how much dispersion or variability is evident in numeric data. This meaning of variance is most relevant to quantitative theory-testing research designs. Variance is also a nonstatistical term that refers to how much dispersion or variability is evident in word data. That meaning of variance is most relevant to qualitative theory-generating research designs.

In quantitative research designs, **maximizing variance** refers to the extent to which the variability in the dependent variable is due solely to the independent variable (Kerlinger & Lee, 2000). In correlational research, both the independent and the dependent variable have to exhibit some variability for a relation to be evident. In experimental research designs, variability in the independent variable occurs when the experimental treatment and the control treatment are as different as possible. In qualitative research designs, maximizing variance could be interpreted to mean that the participants' responses reflect the full range of possible responses about a particular experience.

Error variance can be minimized when instruments provide data that are sufficiently dependable (word data in qualitative research designs) or reliable (number data in quantitative research designs). When applied to quantitative research designs, error variance—or **measurement error**—is defined as "the variability of [instrument scores] due to random fluctuations whose basic characteristic is that they are self-compensating, varying now this way, not that way, now positive, now negative, now up, now down" (Kerlinger & Lee, 2000, p. 462).

An important function of a research design and the data collection procedures is "to control variance" (Kerlinger & Lee, 2000, p. 450). This **control of variance** function is the extent to which the research design and data collection procedures maximize control of extraneous or external factors that might interfere with the overall integrity of the research project (Burns & Grove, 2007; Kerlinger & Lee; Macnee & McCabe, 2008; Polit & Beck, 2006). Consideration should be given to the extent to which the researcher was able to minimize, nullify, or isolate the effects of any extraneous factors (Kerlinger & Lee). Researchers can control variance by eliminating any extraneous factors, or they can include the factor as a study variable. In quantitative research, researchers can also control variance by randomization. And in research designs with more than one group, the participants in each group can be matched on relevant characteristics.

Conclusion

A research design and data collection procedures that are adequately planned and systematically and consistently implemented foster confidence in the results; readers can, in other words, rely on the results and regard them as accurate (Kerlinger & Lee, 2000). In this chapter, you continued to learn more about how to evaluate the E component of C-T-E structures using the criterion of operational adequacy. Specifically, you learned how to determine how good the information about the data collection procedures given in a research report is.

In this chapter, we focused on two types of validity—internal and external. **Internal validity** refers to the accuracy of the data obtained from a specific research design and data collection procedures that yielded numeric data. **External validity** refers to the extent to which numeric data obtained from one sample can be applied to other people who are members of the same population. In Chapter 9, we discussed **measurement validity**, which refers to the appropriateness of instruments and experimental conditions. The three types of validity are related. Macnee and McCabe (2008) explained:

> Logically, if a study lacks internal validity, it automatically lacks external validity. If the results are not accurate within the study, they clearly will not be accurate in other samples or settings. Similarly, if a study lacks measurement validity, it will lack internal validity. However, a study can have measurement validity and not have internal validity, or it can have correct findings and thus be internally valid but not externally valid. That is, the findings of a study may be real and correct to the specific sample and setting of the study but not applicable to the general population or to other settings. (p. 199)

Although internal validity and external validity are aspects of quantitative research designs, measurement validity applies to instruments used with both qualitative and quantitative research designs. If we substitute rigor for internal validity and transferability for external validity, we can say that the relations among rigor, transferability, and measurement validity are the same as the relations Macnee and McCabe (2008) proposed for internal validity, external validity, and measurement validity. Transferability is related to rigor, and generalizability is related to internal validity, such that inadequate rigor or internal validity means that transferability or generalizability is compromised. Adequate rigor or internal validity does not, however, mean that the data collection procedures support transferability or generalizability (Macnee & McCabe, 2008).

The questions to ask and answer as you evaluate the data collection procedures are listed in Box 10–11. Application of the criterion of operational adequacy for data collection procedures should help you continue to better understand the E component of C-T-E structures. The learning activities for this chapter, found on the accompanying CD that comes with this book, will help you to continue to increase your understanding of the operational adequacy criterion and its application to the contents of research reports addressing data collection procedures.

BOX 10-11	Evaluation of Data Collection Procedures: *How Good* is the Information?

Operational Adequacy

- Are the data collection procedures clearly identified and described?
- Are the data collection procedures appropriate?

References

Full citations for all references cited in this chapter are provided in the Reference section at the end of the book.

Learning Activities

Activities to supplement what you have learned in this chapter, along with practice examination questions, are provided on the CD that comes with this book.

Chapter 11

Evaluation of Procedures for Protecting Research Participants

This chapter continues the focus on the empirical research methods (E) component of the conceptual-theoretical-empirical (C-T-E) structures for research and the criterion of operational adequacy. Specifically, this chapter focuses on procedures used to protect the human beings who participate in theory-generating research or theory-testing research.

KEYWORDS

American Nurses' Association Code of Ethics

Anonymity

Autonomy

Belmont Report

Beneficence

Certificate of Confidentiality

Code of Federal Regulations

Confidentiality

Declaration of Helsinki

Ethics Committee

Exempt from Review

Expedited Review

Family Educational Rights and Privacy Act (FERPA)

Fidelity

Full Disclosure

Full or Complete Review

Health Insurance Portability and Accountability Act (HIPAA)

Human Rights

Informed Consent

Institutional Review Board (IRB)

Justice

Nonmalfeasance

Nuremberg Code

Patient's Bill of Rights

Privacy

Respect for Persons

Self-Determination

Veracity

Voluntariness

Vulnerable Populations

Recall from Chapter 2 that the E component of a C-T-E structure encompasses five major elements—the research design, the sample, the instruments and any experimental conditions, the procedures used to collect the data and protect participants from harm, and the techniques used to analyze the data. In Chapter 3, you began to learn *where* to look for information about procedures to protect research participants in research reports (Box 11–1) and *what* information you could expect to find (Box 11–2).

In Chapter 4, you began to learn how to determine *how good* the procedures are for protecting research participants by using our framework for evaluation of the different

| BOX | Evaluation of Procedures for Protecting Research |
| 11-1 | Participants: *Where* Is the Information? |

Look in the method section of the research report.

| BOX | Evaluation of Procedures for Protecting Research |
| 11-2 | Participants: *What* Is the Information? |

• Statement of approval of the research by an institutional review board or ethics committee

• Description of procedure used to obtain informed consent from research participants

components of C-T-E structures for theory-generating research and theory-testing research.

In this chapter, we discuss the criterion of operational adequacy as it applies to procedures for protecting research participants from harm in detail and provide examples that should help you better understand how to apply the criterion as you read research reports. Application of the operational adequacy criterion will facilitate your evaluation of *how good* the information in the research report is about the procedures used to protect research participants.

WHY DO RESEARCH PARTICIPANTS NEED TO BE PROTECTED?

Research participants are human beings from or about whom data are collected for research purposes. Human beings have rights that must be protected when they are involved in research. **Human rights** may be defined as "claims and demands that have been justified in the eyes of an individual or by the consensus of a group of individuals" (Burns & Grove, 2007, p. 203). The participants need to be protected because their rights have sometimes been violated, probably since research began in ancient times. In modern times, documented violations began in the 1700s and have continued into the 21st century. Some well-known examples of violations of research participants' rights are listed in Box 11–3.

WHAT ARE THE GUIDELINES FOR PROTECTING HUMAN BEINGS WHO PARTICIPATE IN RESEARCH?

Codes, laws, and regulations to protect the rights of human beings who participate in research began to be developed in the middle of the 20th century (Oddi & Cassidy,

BOX 11-3	Examples of Documented Violations of the Rights of Research Participants

1789: Inoculation of children and other people with swinepox or cowpox against smallpox without consent and without knowledge of the safety of the swinepox and cowpox (Reich, 1995)

1932–1972: The Tuskegee Syphilis Study: Withholding of treatment of over 400 Black sharecroppers in Alabama for syphilis so that physicians could study the effects of the untreated disease (Jones, 1981)

1930s–1940s: Conduct of experiments on prisoners and others by the Nazi government in Germany to study, for example, the effects of immersion in subfreezing water, deprivation of oxygen, and injection of lethal organisms, as well as methods of sexual sterilization (Reich, 1995)

1955–1958: Administration of lysergic acid diethylamide (LSD) to an American soldier without his knowledge in an experiment conducted by the United States Army Intelligence Corps (*United States vs. Stanley,* 1987)

1950s: Administration of the drug thalidomide to pregnant women for morning sickness despite lack of testing for safety in human beings (Dally, 1998)

1960s: Injection of patients at the Jewish Chronic Disease Hospital in New York City with live cancer cells without their informed consent or any institutional board review (Bandman, 1985; Bandman & Bandman, 2002)

1999: Jesse Gelsinger, an 18-year-old boy, died as a result of unanticipated effects of gene therapy for ornithine transcarbamylase deficiency, raising questions about the safety of gene therapies (Stolberg, 1999)

2000: Administration of the drug hexamethonium without an adequate review of literature about its hazards (Perkins, 2001)

2000s: AIDS drugs tested on foster children who had no independent advocate to determine advantages and disadvantages of the drugs (Alliance for Human Research Protection, 2005); withholding of data about adverse reactions to Vioxx® (rofecoxib) by the pharmaceutical company that manufactures the drug (Consumer Affairs, 2004)

1990). The codes include the *Nuremberg Code, the Declaration of Helsinki, the Belmont Report, the Patient's Bill of Rights,* and the American Nurses' Association (ANA) *Code of Ethics.*

The Nuremberg Code

The core of the **Nuremberg Code** is protection of human beings who participate in research. The Nuremberg Code was written by the War Crimes Tribunal in 1949, soon after World War II. The Tribunal was established to address the atrocities committed against Jewish people and others by the Nazi government of Germany. These crimes against humanity included, but were not limited to, surgically removing men's and women's healthy reproductive and other organs, pouring disinfectant into wounds, and experimenting with genes.

The Declaration of Helsinki

Scientific principles, adequate research design, qualified researchers, and minimal risk to human beings who participate in research are emphasized in the Declaration of Helsinki. The Declaration was first issued in 1964; revisions have been issued periodically from 1975 through 2004 (World Medical Association, 1964–2004).

The Belmont Report

The National Commission for the Protection of Human Subjects of Biomedical and Behavioral Research (1978) was created when the National Research Act (Public Law 93-348) was signed into law on July 12, 1974. The Commission was charged with (1) identifying ethical principles derived from the Nuremberg Code and Declaration of Helsinki that would underscore the conduct of biomedical and behavioral research involving human beings and (2) developing guidelines for assuring application of the principles in research. The work of the Commission, commonly known as the Belmont Report, focused on three ethical principles that are relevant for research with human beings: respect for persons, beneficence, and justice.

Respect for persons holds the researcher accountable in two areas—the autonomy of human beings to willingly participate in research and the requirement to protect those who may be especially vulnerable to abuses in research. **Autonomy** is protected when people are able to volunteer to participate in research. **Vulnerable populations** include frail older persons; hospice patients; persons with no or little income; children; pregnant women; physically, mentally, and emotionally challenged persons; students; and prisoners. Vulnerable populations are protected when, for example, family caregivers are interviewed about a loved one's process of dying rather than the dying person who is receiving hospice care.

Beneficence requires the researcher to do no harm (or minimize the possibility of harm) and maximize possible benefits. For example, the researcher must provide the services of a mental health professional if a research participant's scores on a depression scale or responses to an interview indicate that he or she is at risk for suicide.

Justice requires the researcher to distribute the benefits and burdens of research equally to all individuals. Justice is ensured in research when an equal share is provided to each person based on individual need, individual effort, or individual merit. The Tuskegee Syphilis Study (see Box 11–3) is an egregious example of a lack of justice in research, because African American sharecroppers were denied a readily available treatment for syphilis so that physicians could study the effects of nontreatment.

The Patient's Bill of Rights

The Patient's Bill of Rights, which was developed in 1973 and revised in 1992 (American Hospital Association, 1992), lists the rights of people when they are hospitalized or otherwise under the care of health-care professionals. Most rights deal with clinical care. Some rights are also relevant for research, including those addressing informed consent, privacy, and confidentiality in such institutional settings as hospitals. The research-relevant rights emphasize patients' right to choose or not choose to participate in health-care institution-sponsored research.

American Nurses' Association Code of Ethics

The Nightingale Pledge, dating from 1893, is considered the first nursing code of ethics. The first purpose of the Nurses' Associated Alumnae of the United States and Canada (now the American Nurses' Association) was to formulate a code of ethics, which was issued in 1896 (ANA, 2001). The ANA published the most recent Code of Ethics for Nurses with Interpretive Statements (ANA Code of Ethics) in 2001. The ANA Code of Ethics was developed to guide nursing practice, but it also contains statements that are relevant for researchers. The relevance of certain sections of the ANA Code of Ethics for research underscores the close connection between the nursing practice process and the nursing research process that we discussed in Chapter 1 (see Table 1–1).

The ANA Code of Ethics has always focused on doing no harm, benefit to others, loyalty, truthfulness, and social justice. In recent versions, the Code has also addressed the changing context of health care and patient and nurse autonomy (ANA, 2001). For example, Section 1.1 addresses respect for human dignity, Section 1.4 focuses on autonomy, and Section 3.3 emphasizes protection of research participants, especially when the participants are members of a vulnerable group.

A comparison of the contents of the Nuremberg Code, the Declaration of Helsinki, the Belmont Report, and the Patient's Bill of Rights with the research-relevant content of the ANA Code of Ethics is given in Table 11–1, which is on the CD that comes with this book.

Code of Federal Regulations

The United States Department of Health and Human Services (DHHS; 2005) issued federal regulations that reflect the ethical principles of the Belmont Report in the Code of Federal Regulations Title 45 Public Welfare, Part 46 Protection of Human Subjects. The regulations are used to evaluate the ethical aspects of research conducted by researchers who reside in the United States (U.S.), as well as those residing outside of the U.S. who receive funding from or are otherwise subject to regulation by the U.S. federal government. Similar guidelines are used to regulate research in other countries.

The three areas addressed by the federal regulations are:

- General requirements for informed consent, including information to be given to potential research participants and how informed consent should be documented
- Requirements for institutional review boards (IRBs), including membership, functions, and operations
- Guidelines for reporting and dealing with scientific misconduct

The Office for Human Research Protections (www.hhs.gov/ohrp), under the DHHS, is responsible for interpretation and oversight of the regulations.

WHAT ETHICAL PRINCIPLES AND ETHICAL RULES OF CONDUCT ARE RELEVANT FOR RESEARCH?

Ethical principles and ethical rules of conduct guide researchers' treatment of the people who participate in their studies (Beauchamp & Childress, 1994). As can be seen in Table 11–2, which is on the CD that comes with this book, the ethical principles and rules of conduct are evident in the various codes we already discussed in this chapter.

Ethical Principles

Four ethical principles guide researchers' treatment of people in their studies. These are the principles of autonomy, nonmalfeasance, beneficence, and justice.

Autonomy

The principle of **autonomy**, also known as **self-determination**, means that individuals have the right to make their own decisions, free from the threat of harm or coercion by others. Autonomy includes the right to privacy and forms the philosophical basis for informed consent in health care (ANA, 2001). The principle of autonomy allows a potential participant to freely choose to participate in or withdraw from research at any time without penalty or loss of any benefits. Implicit in autonomy is full disclosure, understanding, and voluntariness.

Making an informed decision to participate in research requires **full disclosure** of any known risks and benefits of the research by the researcher to potential participants (Beauchamp & Childress, 1994). With regard to **understanding**, the researcher also must make sure that a potential research participant—especially a sick, anxious, or frightened person—understands other available alternatives to any experimental conditions and how alternatives might be better or worse than participation in the study. **Voluntariness** means that people volunteer to participate in research and that the researcher does not attempt to manipulate or coerce them to do so.

The principle of autonomy is evident in statements from the ANA Code of Ethics (2001):

- [P]atients have the moral and legal right to determine what will be done with their own person; to be given accurate, complete, and understandable information in a manner that facilitates an informed judgment; to be assisted with weighing the benefits, burdens, and available options in their treatment, including the choice of no treatment; to accept, refuse, or terminate treatment without deceit, undue influence, duress, coercion, or penalty. (p. 8)
- [E]ach individual has the right to choose whether or not to participate in research . . . [and] to refuse to participate in research or to withdraw at any time without fear of adverse consequences or reprisal. (pp. 12–13)

Nonmalfeasance

The principle of **nonmalfeasance** requires that research participants not be exposed to any foreseeable harm or risk from the research instruments, experimental conditions, or procedures for collecting the data. Levine (1981) classified risks into four categories—physical, psychological, social, and economic. A person might be at a physical risk for adverse or unexpected complications from an experimental study of the effects of a new drug; a psychological risk for stress or anxiety from talking to a researcher about the experience of being a spouse whose husband is dying from cancer; a social risk for stigmatization by society if the person's participation in a study about sexually transmitted diseases were revealed; and an economic risk for loss of work, health-care insurance, or other monetary benefits if participation in research about substance abuse were to become known to an employer.

The principle of nonmalfeasance is evident in this statement from the ANA Code of Ethics (2001):

- [T]he nurse advocates for an environment that provides for sufficient physical privacy, including auditory privacy for discussions of a personal nature and policies and practices that protect the confidentiality of information. (p. 12)

Beneficence

The principle of **beneficence** requires the researcher to examine the balance between risks and benefits for people participating in research. Potential benefits must outweigh any risks. For example, although it may be helpful to know what terminally ill people are experiencing, asking them to participate in research usually is considered excessively intrusive, especially if the same data can be collected from a family member or other caregiver. Therefore, the researcher would have to have a compelling and convincing reason for asking terminally ill people to participate in research.

The principle of beneficence is evident in this statement from the ANA Code of Ethics (2001):

- [N]urses should be cognizant of the special concerns raised by research involving vulnerable groups, including children, prisoners, students, the elderly, and the poor. (p. 13)

Justice

The principle of **justice** requires that research participants be selected equally from target or accessible populations without specific regard for their race, gender, religion, or socioeconomic status, unless particular participant characteristics are the focus of the research. For example, studies of men's experiences of caring for a loved one with Alzheimer's disease are obviously limited to males unless a comparison with women's experiences is of interest (Garity, 1999). Similarly, studies of responses to pregnancy are limited to females unless male partners' responses are of interest.

The principle of justice is evident in this statement from the ANA Code of Ethics (2001):

- The nurse practices . . . unrestricted by considerations of social or economic status, personal attributes, or the nature of health problems. (p. 7)

Ethical Rules of Conduct

The ethical rules of conduct used to guide researchers' treatment of people in their studies include rules of privacy, confidentiality, veracity, and fidelity.

Privacy

Privacy refers to individuals' right to control access to personal information about their body, thoughts, and experiences by others. Privacy also includes the degree, timing, and conditions under which personal information may be shared. For example, the **Health Insurance Portability and Accountability Act** (HIPAA; 1996) outlines conditions under which researchers can access and use private health information, and the **Family Educational Rights and Privacy Act** (FERPA; 1974) protects the privacy of student records.

Controlling access to personal information can be challenging because being listed on a welfare roll, for example, is public information, but the amount of one's personal savings is not. Similarly, unless students request that a school not provide access to their records, a great deal of information is considered part of the public record, including name, telephone number, e-mail address, major field of study, dates of attendance, degrees and awards received, full-time or part-time enrollment status, and other educational institutions attended. If students are athletes, additional public record information includes date of birth, height, and weight. There are also limitations on the right to privacy of minor children's and institutionalized individuals' information. We discuss those limitations later in this chapter, in the section on special considerations for informed consent.

Four areas of research raise privacy concerns—the methods used to identify and recruit subjects; covert observation with, for example, a concealed tape recorder or camera; use of information about a person from another person, such as adult children providing information about their parents' child-rearing practices; and questions about sensitive topics, such as domestic violence and mental illness.

The ethical rule of privacy is evident in this statement from the ANA Code of Ethics (2001):

- The nurse safeguards the patient's right to privacy[,] . . . does not justify unwanted intrusion into the patient's life[,] . . . [and] advocates for an environment that provides for sufficient physical privacy for discussions of a personal nature. (p. 12)

Confidentiality

Whereas privacy is about control of access to personal information, **confidentiality** represents an agreement between the researcher and the research participants about the ways in which personal information and other data will be used and made available to others. The researcher has an obligation to keep confidential all data collected from participants and cannot disclose any data to anyone else without participants' permission. When informing potential participants about research, the researcher must be able to provide an answer for each of the questions listed here:

- What data will be collected?
- Why are the data needed?

- When will the data be collected?
- Where will the data be stored?
- Who will have access to the data?
- How will the data be reported?

Researchers maintain confidentiality through strategies such as using a code number to identify each participant, maintaining a list of all participants' names and code numbers only if participants are to be contacted more than once for data collection, keeping any name and code number list in a locked file to which only certain research team members have access, and keeping all field notes, journals, diaries, and health records in a secure place. Researchers must also safeguard the security of all transcribed interviews and electronic data files. Maintenance of confidentiality is always important and even more so when the release of data would result in a physical, psychological, social, or economic risk to any research participant.

The ethical rule of confidentiality is evident in this statement from the ANA Code of Ethics (2001):

- The nurse has a duty to maintain confidentiality of all patient information. The patient's well being could be jeopardized and the fundamental trust between the patient and nurse destroyed by unnecessary access to data or by inappropriate disclosure of identifiable patient information. The rights, well being, and safety of the individual patient should be the primary factors in arriving at any professional judgment concerning the disposition of confidential information received from or about the patient, whether oral, written or electronic. (p. 12)

There are some **limits to confidentiality** that need to be clearly explained to potential research participants. Child, domestic-partner, or elder abuse; intent to harm oneself or others; or presence of communicable disease will be reported to authorities. In the U.S., researchers sometimes obtain a **certificate of confidentiality** from the National Institutes of Health (NIH) to protect identifiable information from forced disclosure in civil, criminal, administrative, or other legal proceedings at the federal, state, or local level. Data that can be included in a certificate of confidentiality include substance abuse; illegal behaviors; sexual attitudes, preferences, or practices; and genetic information.

Confidentiality and anonymity are not the same. In research, **confidentiality** refers to data that do not include any information that could identify a research participant to a reader of the research report. **Anonymity** refers to data from participants who are not known to the researcher or anyone else associated with the research project.

Veracity

Veracity calls for the researcher to tell the truth and not lie or deceive others (Veatch & Fry, 2006). This means that the researcher must make sure the participant understands the purpose of the research but does not, for example, have false hope about the potential effects of a new drug. Although the ANA Code of Ethics (2001) does not include an explicit statement about veracity, nurses are expected to tell patients the truth.

Fidelity

Fidelity obligates the researcher to remain faithful to commitments, including keeping promises, maintaining confidentiality, and demonstrating caring behaviors (Fry, 1991). The researcher demonstrates fidelity in research by maintaining the participant's privacy when collecting, reporting, and storing data; keeping all data confidential; obtaining each individual's consent to participate in the study; and adhering to the research design. The ANA Code of Ethics does not include an explicit statement about fidelity. However, nurses are expected to remain faithful to their commitments to patients, maintain confidentiality of all information about patients, and behave in a caring manner toward patients.

HOW IS THE CRITERION OF OPERATIONAL ADEQUACY APPLIED TO PROTECTION OF RESEARCH PARTICIPANTS?

When applied to procedures for protecting research participants from harm, the criterion of **operational adequacy** focuses attention on whether the research report includes a statement indicating that the research was approved by an IRB or ethics committee and a description of the procedure used to obtain informed consent from the human beings who participated in the research.

The operational adequacy criterion, when applied to protection of human beings as research participants, is met when you can answer yes to two questions:

- Does the research report include a statement indicating approval by an IRB or ethics committee?
- Does the research report include a description of the procedure used to obtain informed consent from participants?

Does the Research Report Include a Statement of Approval?

In Chapters 3 and 4, we pointed out that the empirical research methods section of a research report should include a statement indicating that the research was approved by an **institutional review board** or **ethics committee** if human beings participated in the research. In the U.S., institutions that receive federal funding or conduct research on drugs or medical devices, such as teaching hospitals, universities, and major pharmaceutical companies, are required by federal regulations to establish IRBs (*Federal Register*, May 30, 1974). In many other countries, similar regulations require establishment of ethics committees. The three ethical principles of the Belmont Report—respect for persons, beneficence, and justice—are now used as the basis for review of research by IRBs and ethics committees.

In the U.S., IRBs consider three categories of review—exempt from review, expedited review, and full or complete board review. Research that is **exempt from review** is permissible when there is no anticipated risk to the participants. Research that qualifies for **expedited**

review is permissible when only minimal risk to participants might occur. "Minimal risk means that the probability and magnitude of harm or discomfort anticipated in the research are not greater in and of themselves than those ordinarily encountered in daily life or during the performance of routine physical or psychological examinations or tests" (DHHS, 2005, Section 46.102i). **Full or complete review** is required when greater than minimal risk to participants is anticipated and/or when the participants are members of a vulnerable group.

The protocol for any research involving human beings as participants must be submitted to an IRB. The chairperson or other members of the IRB make the decision whether the research qualifies for a particular category. For example, a researcher may request that a study be exempt from review, but the IRB may decide that there is a potential for a risk, such as loss of confidentiality, and therefore requires expedited review. In the U.S., research with human beings that involves drugs, medical devices, biological products, dietary supplements, and electronic products must also be approved by the U.S. Food and Drug Administration (FDA; 2006).

Approval to conduct research must be received from each agency in which the data will be collected before the research can begin. Review by the IRB or ethics committee certifies that the wording in the consent form promotes autonomy of people to freely choose to participate in the research. The importance of approval to conduct research is emphasized in this statement from the ANA Code of Ethics (2001):

- [P]rior to implementation, all research should be approved by a qualified review board to ensure patient protection and the ethical integrity of the research. (p.13)

The name of the university and/or health-care organization giving IRB or ethics committee approval is not mentioned when doing so would risk the loss of confidentiality for the participants. An example of an approval statement found in research reports is given in Box 11–4; other examples are given in Table 11–3, which is on the CD that comes with this book.

Reports of research involving data collected from animals also must include a statement indicating approval by a review committee. The U.S. Public Health Service has developed guidelines on humane care and use of laboratory animals. Holtzclaw and Hanneman (2002) noted that researchers should have a compelling reason for using animals in research. For example, the use of mice to simulate the neurological changes associated with Alzheimer's disease, multiple sclerosis, or Parkinson's disease may be considered a legitimate use of the mice as research participants.

BOX 11-4	Example of Statement of Approval to Conduct Research

Camper and parent participation in follow-up surveys was approved by the Institutional Review Board (IRB) of the University of Alabama at Birmingham by expedited review procedures. (Buckner et al., 2005, p. 204)

   (Note that in this example, the name of the university is given. It is unlikely that loss of confidentiality would occur because the setting for the study was a young teen asthma camp not directly connected to the university.)

Does the Research Report Include a Description of the Procedure Used to Obtain Informed Consent from Participants?

Review by the IRB or ethics committee also ensures that the essentials of informed consent, as defined by federal regulations in the U.S. and similar legislation in other countries, are included in the consent form. In the U.S., the essential content of a consent form includes:

- Purpose of the research
- Duration of participation in the research
- Data collection procedures, including any experimental conditions
- Any appropriate alternative procedures or treatments
- Foreseeable risks or discomforts from participating in the research
- Benefits of participating in the research
- How confidentiality will be maintained
- Any financial or other compensation for time spent participating in the research
- Researcher's name and contact information
- A statement that participation is voluntary and will involve no penalty or loss of benefits and that the person can discontinue participation at any time without adverse consequences

IRBs and ethics committees must also approve all sample recruitment strategies, such as flyers, e-mail messages, and newspaper advertisements. In addition, IRBs and ethics committees review the reading level of the consent form, any language and cultural characteristics of the prospective target population that might affect potential participants' understanding of the research, and data supporting accurate translation of research instruments into one or more different languages. IRBs and ethics committees may require separate consent for different procedures for data collection, such as consent to be interviewed and to make an audio or video recording of the interview.

U.S. federal regulations allow for—but do not mandate—a waiver of any or all essential content of informed consent if four criteria are met:

1. There is minimal risk to participants.
2. The rights and welfare of participants will not be adversely affected.
3. Research cannot be carried out in any other practical way.
4. Participants will be debriefed after participation.

One example of waiver of informed consent is research in which participants' knowledge of being observed would change their behavior, such as patterns of smoking, drinking, or substance abuse. Another example is research in which participants are told that the research is about their use of e-mail when the actual purpose is to uncover the number of times participants view specific Internet sites. Still another example is research in which the researcher needs to reduce occurrence of socially desirable responses, such as number and frequency of sexual encounters.

Informed Consent

In Chapters 3 and 4, we noted that the empirical research methods section of a research report should include a description of the procedure used to obtain informed consent from the human beings who participated in the research.

Informed consent is defined as:

> [T]he knowing consent of an individual or his [or her] legally authorized representative under circumstances which provide the prospective subject or representative sufficient opportunity to consider whether to participate without undue inducement or any element of force, fraud, deceit, duress or other forms of constraint or coercion. (DHHS, 2005, pp. 9–10)

Informed consent is typically documented by each participant's signature on a written consent form or by an audio or video recording of the participant's oral consent. Individuals who cannot read or write for any reason but are capable of understanding the consent form when administered orally may document their informed consent by making a mark, such as X, on the consent form. Examples of descriptions of informed consent are given in Box 11–5 and in Table 11–3 on the CD that comes with this book.

The process of informed consent begins with the initial recruitment and screening of potential research participants and continues throughout the participants' involvement in the research. Three elements are necessary for informed consent:

1. Mental competence
2. Adequate information
3. Freedom from coercion and vulnerability

BOX 11-5	Examples of Descriptions of Informed Consent

Condon et al. (2007) described the informed consent procedure used in their descriptive qualitative study of prisoners' views about health services provided in prisons. They stated, "Participants gave written consent for audiotaping of interviews, and for direct quotations to be used in dissemination of the findings. Prisoners were advised before the interview that, if a disclosure were made about any current criminal activity, this information would be passed to the relevant authorities" (p. 218).

Tsai, Tak, Moore, and Palencia (2003) described the informed consent procedure they used for their correlational study of the test of a theory of chronic pain experienced by older people with arthritis. They explained, "If a potential participant met the inclusion criteria and agreed to participate in the study, . . . consent was obtained" (p. 162).

Headley, Ownby, and John (2004) described the informed consent procedure they used for their experimental study of the effect of seated exercise on fatigue and quality of life in women with advanced breast cancer. They stated, "[T]he researchers invited eligible subjects waiting in the outpatient chemotherapy treatment area to participate in the study and obtained written informed consent" (p. 979).

Coercion and Undue Influence. The National Commission for the Protection of Human Subjects of Biomedical and Behavioral Research (1978) distinguished coercion from undue influence. The commission explained: "**Coercion** occurs when an overt threat of harm is intentionally presented by one person to another in order to obtain compliance. **Undue influence**, by contrast, occurs through an offer of an excessive, unwarranted, inappropriate, or improper reward or other overture in order to obtain compliance. Also, inducements that would ordinarily be acceptable may become undue influence if the subject is especially vulnerable" (p. 14).

An example of coercion is telling cancer patients that they will have untoward effects or possibly die unless they agree to participate in a clinical trial of a new surgical procedure. An example of undue influence is offering several hundred dollars to people with very low incomes for their participation in a study.

The importance of informed consent for participation in research is evident in this statement from the ANA Code of Ethics (2001):

- It is imperative that the patient or legally authorized surrogate receive sufficient information that is material to an informed decision, to comprehend that information, and to know how to discontinue participation in research without penalty. Necessary information to achieve an adequately informed consent includes the nature of participation, potential harms and benefits, and available alternatives to taking part in research. (pp.12–13)

Special Considerations in Informed Consent. Several categories of research participants require special consideration when obtaining informed consent—children; mentally, emotionally, or physically challenged persons; and persons who are institutionalized. Parents or legal guardians usually give consent for children younger than 7 years (Polit & Beck, 2006). After that age, it is generally thought prudent to obtain the child's assent in additional to parental consent. Assent, which is obtained out of respect for the child's autonomy, means that the child agrees to participate in the research. Examples of parental consent and child assent are given in Box 11–6.

BOX 11-6	Examples of Parental Consent and Child Assent

Donly, Henson, Jamison, and Gerlach (2006) conducted an experimental study of the effects of two types of peroxide whitening strips on tooth color changes in a sample of 48 teens, 13 to 17 years of age. They explained that they obtained informed consent from the teens' parents and assent from the teens.

Mahon, Yarcheski, and Yarcheski (2004) conducted a correlational study of social support and health practices in a sample of 134 adolescents, 12 to 14 years of age. They stated: "In addition to University Institutional Review Board approval, school officials reviewed and approved the research protocol as appropriate for seventh and eighth grades. One week prior to testing, the researchers approached all seventh and eighth graders to inform them about the research project. The students received a packet for their parents containing an explanation about the study and a parental consent form. On the testing date 1 week later, students who had parental consent and gave informed consent [that is, assent] as well participated in the study" (pp. 223–224).

Individuals under the age of 18 do not always have to have parental consent to participate in research. **Emancipated minors**—adolescents who are considered competent adults by virtue of marriage, military service, or court approval—may give informed consent to participate in research (Smith, 2007). For example, a married female under the age of 18 who has given birth may provide informed consent to participate in a study of maternal responses to cesarean birth.

Parents or legal guardians usually give consent for mentally, emotionally, or physically challenged persons. Assent may also be obtained from such persons. For example, a parent may give informed consent for an adult child with Down syndrome to participate in a study of the effect of physical activity on body weight. The adult child may also be asked to assent—that is, agree—to participate in the study.

In the case of institutionalized individuals, a family member identified as the primary caregiver or a guardian ad litem appointed by the court may give informed consent for an individual to participate in research. For example, a family caregiver may give informed consent for a parent with Alzheimer's disease to participate in a study of the effects of a new drug.

Conclusion

This chapter has highlighted the ethical codes, ethical principles, and ethical rules of conduct that have been developed to protect research participants from harm. We have underscored the ethical requirements for protection of human beings and discussed IRB or ethics committee approval and informed consent.

If ethical codes and procedures exist and the reason for conducting research is the advancement of knowledge, why would researchers act unethically? Several plausible reasons have been proposed, such as pressure on college faculty to conduct enough research to qualify for promotion and tenure, pressure on practitioners to advance their careers through research, limited guidance and mentoring of novice researchers, and weaknesses in institutional review, particularly oversight of ongoing research. Nurses can contribute to a reduction of violations of ethical principles and ethical rules of conduct in research by following the ANA Code of Ethics (2001), which stipulates that "nurses have the duty to question and, if necessary, to report and to refuse to participate in research they deem morally objectionable" (p. 13).

The questions to ask and answer as you evaluate procedures to protect research participants are listed in Box 11–7. The learning activities for this chapter will help you increase your

BOX 11-7	Evaluation of Procedures for Protection of Research Participants: *How Good is the Information?*

Operational Adequacy

• Does the research report include a statement indicating approval of the research by an institutional review board or ethics committee?

• Does the research report include a description of the procedure used to obtain informed consent from research participants?

understanding of the criterion of operational adequacy when applied to the content of research reports addressing protection of research participants from harm.

References

Full citations for all references cited in this chapter are provided in the Reference section at the end of the book.

Learning Activities

Activities to supplement what you have learned in this chapter, along with practice examination questions, are provided on the CD that comes with this book.

Chapter 12

Evaluation of Data Analysis Techniques

This chapter completes the focus on the empirical research methods (E) component of conceptual-theoretical-empirical (C-T-E) structures for research and the criterion of operational adequacy that began in Chapter 7. In this chapter, we discuss the data analysis techniques element of E component of C-T-E structures.

KEYWORDS

Audit Trail	Measures of Effect
Bracketing	Measures of Frequency
Confirmability	Measures of Relation
Content Analysis	Measures of Variability
Data Analysis Technique	Nonparametric Statistics
Descriptive Statistics	Null Hypothesis
Distribution of Data	p Value
Inferential Statistics	Parametric Statistics
Inquiry Audit	Statistical Conclusion Validity
Level of Measurement	Type I Error
Measures of Central Tendency	Type II Error

Recall from Chapter 2 that the E component of a C-T-E structure encompasses five major elements—the research design, the sample, the instruments and any experimental conditions, the procedures used to collect data and protect research participants from harm, and the techniques used to analyze the data. In Chapter 3, you began to learn *where* to look for the data analysis techniques in research reports (Box 12–1), and *what* information you could expect to find (Box 12–2). In Chapter 4, you began to learn how to determine *how good* the data analysis techniques are by using our framework for evaluating C-T-E structures for research.

In this chapter, we discuss in detail the criterion of operational adequacy as it applies to data analysis techniques and provide examples that should help you better understand how to apply the criterion as you read research reports. Application of the operational adequacy criterion will facilitate your evaluation of *how good* the information is about the data analysis techniques provided in the research report.

BOX 12-1	Evaluation of Data Analysis Techniques: *Where* Is the Information?

- Look in the data analysis subsection of the method section of the research report.
- Look in the results section of the research report.

BOX 12-2	Evaluation of Data Analysis Techniques: *What* Is the Information?

- Techniques used to analyze qualitative (word) data
- Techniques used to analyze quantitative (number) data

WHAT ARE DATA ANALYSIS TECHNIQUES?

Recall from Chapter 1 that data are words or numbers. Qualitative theory-generating studies typically yield hundreds or even thousands of pages of words provided by participants in response to interview questions. Quantitative theory-generating studies or theory-testing studies may yield hundreds, thousands, or even millions of numbers the participants provided in response to questionnaire items.

Data analysis techniques are specific procedures used to summarize the words or numbers and create a meaningful structure for their interpretation (Polit & Beck, 2006). Without an analysis, the researcher would be able to present only meaningless words or numbers.

Although data analysis techniques are needed to interpret the words or numbers, each technique imposes some restrictions on how questions are asked and the answers that are obtained (Pedhazur, 1982). Suppose, for example, that a researcher wants to know exactly how many people responded "strongly agree" to an item on a survey questionnaire. Suppose also that the researcher selects a data analysis technique that provides the percentage of people who rated the item as "strongly agree." The question must then be stated as "What percentage of all people who responded to the questionnaire item rated the item as 'strongly agree'?" The answer obviously is a percentage, not the absolute number of people who rated the item as "strongly agree." A researcher who was really interested in the absolute number of people would have to select a data analysis technique that provided the absolute number rather than a technique that provided the percentage.

Relation of Data Analysis Techniques, Conceptual Models, Theories, and Research Designs

The C-T-E structure for the research should always be considered when evaluating data analysis techniques. The close connection between data analysis techniques and middle-range theories was highlighted by Pedhazur (1982), who explained that the middle-range theory that is generated or tested "determines . . . the choice of the analytic technique, the manner in which it is to be applied, and the interpretation of the results" (p. 11). In turn, data analysis techniques "shed light on [the] theory" (Pedhazur, p. 11). Data analysis techniques also shed light on the conceptual model that guided the research. In other words, analysis of the data provides a concrete view of the more abstract concepts and propositions of the conceptual model (C) and theory (T) components of the C-T-E structure.

WHAT ARE THE DIFFERENT DATA ANALYSIS TECHNIQUES?

Different data analysis techniques are used with different theory-generating and theory-testing research designs. In general, word data obtained from qualitative theory-generating research designs are analyzed using a content analysis procedure, whereas number data from quantitative theory-generating research and -testing research designs are analyzed using a statistical procedure.

Qualitative Research Designs and Content Analysis

Content analysis refers to a general data analysis technique used to identify similarities and differences in word data. The goal of content analysis is to create a comprehensive "word picture that is as multifaceted and complicated as life in today's world" (Kearney, 2007, p. 299). A meaningful structure of themes or categories is created as the content analysis reveals similarities and differences in words. As the content analysis continues, the themes or categories may be further organized into subthemes or subcategories.

The organizing structure identified by the content analysis may be discovered in the data, or it may reflect the concepts or concept dimensions of a conceptual model that was used to guide the study. For example, DeSanto-Madeya (2006a) discovered seven themes in the word data collected for her study of the meaning of living with spinal cord injury. Knipp (2006), in contrast, used the Roy Adaptation Model modes of adaptation—physiological, self-concept, role function, and interdependence—to organize the word data collected for her theory-generating study of teens' perceptions of attention deficit/hyperactivity disorder and medications. She explained, "Transcripts were analyzed using content analysis. . . . Within each sentence the essence of thought was isolated. . . . Emergent repetitive subthemes were identified within the four modes [of the Roy Adaptation Model]. The main theme was derived from the four modes' subthemes" (p. 121).

Approaches to Content Analysis

Various approaches to content analysis of word data are used, because each qualitative theory-generating research design requires a specific approach. The content analysis approach used with each qualitative theory-generating research design we identified in Chapter 7 is given in Table 12–1, which is on the CD that comes with this book.

Some qualitative theory-generating research designs may be associated with more than one content analysis approach. For example, each of the different approaches to phenomenology, developed by Colaizzi (1978), Giorgi (1985), van Kaam (1959, 1966), and van Manen (1984), is associated with a different approach to content analysis of the word data. Bournes and Ferguson-Paré (2005), for example, used van Kaam's approach (see Table 12–1 on the CD).

Bracketing

The close relationship that can develop between the researcher and each participant in qualitative research can reduce the number of participants who withdraw from a study, but it can also create a problem when the data are analyzed. Sandelowski (1986) explained:

> Paradoxically, the closeness of the [researcher/participant] relationship both enhances and threatens the truth value of a qualitative study. The researcher in qualitative inquiry is more likely to have direct access to [participants'] experiences, but may also be unable to maintain the distance from those experiences required to describe or interpret them in a meaningful way. (p. 31)

Consequently, some content analysis approaches require the researcher to bracket his or her ideas about the topic of the theory-generating research. **Bracketing** means that researchers set aside their personal feelings or experiences or what they already know about the research topic (Creswell, 1998). For example, Leininger's (1991) Ethnonursing Research Methodology requires the researcher to withhold, suspend, or control personal biases, prejudices, and opinions as the words are analyzed. Analysis of data obtained from phenomenology research designs also involves bracketing. Bultemeier (1997), for example, explained that she used bracketing to avoid biasing the analysis with her own ideas about the attributes—or characteristics—of perceived dissonance.

Coding Word Data

Content analysis of word data can be accomplished with manual coding or with a computer software program. Some examples of computer programs are Atlas.ti, ETHNOGRAPH, HyperQUAL, HyperRESEARCH, NUD*IST (Non-numerical Unstructured Data Indexing Searching and Theorising), NVivo, and WinMax. For example, Radwin (2000) used the HyperRESEARCH computer program, and Carboni (1998) used the NUD*IST program (see Table 12–1 on the CD).

Quantitative Research Designs and Statistical Procedures

Statistical procedures is a term that refers to data analysis techniques used to organize and interpret numbers. Statistics are used to describe and summarize number data and to identify associations between the numbers that represent various concepts (Munro, 2005). As we explained in Chapter 2, associations between concepts take the form of the relation between two or more concepts or the effect of one concept on another. Serlin (1987) emphasized the reciprocal relationship between statistics and theory when he declared, "Statistics and theory inform each other" (p. 371). Elaborating, Kerlinger and Lee (2000) explained that statistics help researchers to make decisions to accept or reject hypothesized theoretical associations between concepts.

Statistics and Word Data

Statistics can also be used to analyze word data if numbers are assigned to the words. Burns and Grove (2007) noted that assigning numbers by counting is required if a researcher wants to make judgments about the relative importance of a theme or category discovered in word data. Although Weber (1990) pointed out, "The best content-analytic studies use both qualitative and quantitative operations on texts" (p. 10), only a few researchers assign numbers to the results of their analysis of word data. Breckenridge (1997), for example, reported the number of participants in her study whose responses to open-ended interview questions reflected each theme.

Types of Statistical Procedures

The five basic types of statistical procedures used to analyze number data are:

- Measures of the frequency of the occurrence of a concept
- Measures of the central tendency of a concept
- Measures of the variability of a concept
- Measures of the relations between concepts
- Measures of the effect of one concept on one or more other concepts

Measures of frequency, central tendency, and variability are considered **descriptive statistics**. Measures of relations and effects are considered **inferential statistics**. The specific type of descriptive and inferential statistics used is determined by the level of measurement of the data and their distribution.

Distributions and Levels of Measurement of Data. The **distribution of data** for the scores for a concept may be normal or non-normal. Descriptions of normal and non-normal distributions and associated terms are given in Box 12–3.

BOX 12-3	Terms Associated With the Distribution of Data

Normal distribution: The plot of the distribution—or spread—of scores for a variable is a symmetrical bell-shaped curve. (The scores are plotted on the x-axis, and the frequency of each score is plotted on the y-axis.)
Non-normal distribution: The plot of the distribution—or spread—of scores for a variable is not a symmetrical bell-shaped curve. (The scores are plotted on the x-axis, and the frequency of each score is plotted on the y-axis.)

Continued

BOX 12-3	Terms Associated With the Distribution of Data—cont'd

Skew: One aspect of a distribution that is not normal; the extent of asymmetry of a curve depicting the distribution of scores for a variable

    Positive skew indicates that most scores are low but many are high; referred to as *skewed to the right* because a long tail of the plot of the distribution is on the right side of the distribution curve.

    Negative skew indicates that most scores are high but many are low; referred to as *skewed to the left* because a long tail of the plot of the distribution is on the left side of the distribution curve.

Transformation of data: Various techniques used in an attempt to transform the scores for a variable that are skewed into a normal distribution, including square root transformation, logarithmic (log) transformation, and inverse transformation

Kurtosis: One aspect of a distribution that is not normal. The extent of flatness or peakedness of a curve depicting the plot of the distribution of scores for a variable

Outlier: A score that is extremely low or extremely high relative to the other scores for the variable

    Level of measurement refers to the type of scale the number data form. The four levels of measurement—nominal, ordinal, interval, and ratio (Stevens, 1946)—reflect "the fact that numerals can be assigned . . . to objects or events . . . under different rules" (Stevens, 1951, p. 1). The description of each level of measurement is given in Box 12–4.

BOX 12-4	Terms Associated With Levels of Measurement

Nominal: Numbers are assigned by the researcher to represent categories, which are artificially created for research participants' responses or characteristics. The categories must be exhaustive and mutually exclusive. Categories may also be created from word data. Examples: religious denomination, gender, socioeconomic status, experimental or control treatment group membership

Ordinal: Numbers represent rank order, which is based on the standing of each research participant's score relative to the other research participants' scores. Examples: rank order of scores from low to high; Likert scale ratings of level of agreement, such as strongly agree, agree, disagree, strongly disagree

Interval: Numbers are separated by a meaningful interval, and each interval between any two numbers is equal to every other interval between two numbers. Examples: age, years of education, Scholastic Aptitude Test (SAT) scores, Fahrenheit scale of temperature

Ratio: Numbers represent an absolute value or score and are relative to a possible and *meaningful* zero value. Examples: vital signs (pulse rate, respiratory rate, blood pressure), weight, Celsius (centigrade) scale of temperature

Categorical data: Numbers at the nominal and ordinal levels of measurement; categorical data that form two categories are considered dichotomous; categorical data that form three categories are considered trichotomous

Continuous data: Numbers at the interval and ratio levels of measurement

Specific statistics and their functions for each basic type of statistical procedure are listed in Tables 12–2 to 12–9, which are on the CD that comes with this book. Examples of the use of specific statistical procedures for quantitative theory-generating research and theory-testing research designs are given in Tables 12–10 and 12–11 on the CD.

Descriptive Statistics

Descriptive statistics—that is, measures of frequency, central tendency, and variability of a concept—summarize numbers (see Tables 12–2, 12–3, and 12–4 on the CD). Descriptive statistics are used to summarize the demographic characteristics of research participants, such as age, gender, education, and occupation. Hurst, Montgomery, Davis, Killion, and Baker (2005), for example, reported the number and percentage—which are measures of frequency—for the age categories of the 62 women with HIV who participated in their study. The researchers also reported the participants' mean and median ages—which are measures of central tendency—as well as the age range and standard deviation—which are measures of variability.

Descriptive statistics are also used to summarize research participants' health-related characteristics, such as number of pregnancies, severity of illness, and number of comorbid health conditions. For example, Hurst et al. (2005) reported the number and percentage of HIV-associated symptoms for the participants, along with the mean and standard deviation for length of time of HIV infection.

In addition, descriptive statistics are used to summarize the scores for the research instruments used to measure each concept. For example, Hurst et al. (2005) reported the means and standard deviations of the scores for the instruments used to measure social support, self-care agency, and self-care practices.

Finally, descriptive statistics are used to test descriptive theories focused on development of research instruments. For example, Lancaster (2004) developed the Coping With Breast Cancer Threat (CBCT) instrument to measure the middle-range theory concept of primary prevention coping behaviors used by women who have a family history of breast cancer. Lancaster proposed that the concept encompasses three dimensions—dietary factors, chemical agents, and early detection. She conducted an exploratory factor analysis (see Table 12–5 on the CD) to test her theory of a three-dimension concept and found that 10 of the 11 CBCT items formed subscales reflecting the three dimensions. Lancaster then reported the means and standard deviations for each item, as well as for all items within each CBCT subscale.

Inferential Statistics

Inferential statistics—that is, measures of the relations between concepts and the effect of one concept on one or more other concepts—are used to test hypotheses about data obtained from a sample (see Tables 12–6 to 12–9 on the CD). More specifically, inferential statistics are tests of conjectures about population characteristics based on number data from a sample selected from the population.

Inferential statistical tests require some variation in the numbers that represent each concept. In other words, scores for measures of variability must be greater than zero, and concepts must be variables if inferential statistical tests are to be used. If every participant in a study used exactly the same number to rate each questionnaire item, no variation would be evident, and inferential statistics could not be used.

The result of use of an inferential statistic is the numerical value of the statistic and its probability, or p value. The p **value** is the level of statistical significance, or more precisely, the probability that the numerical value of the statistic represents chance alone (Rempher & Urquico, 2007). If, for example, the p value for a statistic is 0.01, the probability that the numerical value of the statistic occurred by chance is 1%. Even more precisely, the p value is the probability of incorrectly rejecting a **null hypothesis**—that is, a hypothesis asserting no relation between concepts or no effect of one concept on another. When a null hypothesis is incorrectly rejected, a **Type I error** is said to occur. A **Type II error** is said to occur when a false null hypothesis is accepted as true.

Types of Inferential Statistics. Two broad types of inferential statistics are nonparametric statistics and parametric statistics. **Nonparametric statistics** are typically used when the distribution of data is not normal or the level of measurement of the numbers is nominal or ordinal. Specific nonparametric statistics are listed in Tables 12–6 and 12–8 on the CD. **Parametric statistics** are typically used when the data are normally distributed and the level of measurement of the numbers is interval or ratio. Specific parametric statistics are listed in Tables 12–7 and 12–9. Because most parametric statistics are considered **robust**, they may also be used with data at the ordinal level of measurement. Much more information about many parametric and some nonparametric statistical procedures can be found in most statistics textbooks. Detailed information about nonparametric statistics can be found in Siegel's (1956) classic textbook.

Nonparametric and parametric inferential statistics are used to test explanatory and predictive middle-range theories. Tests of explanatory theories require a statistic that measures the relation between two or more concepts (see Tables 12–6 and 12–7 on the CD). For example, Scordo (2007) used a nonparametric measure of relations—Cramer's V—to test her explanatory theory of the relation between level of medication use and frequency of symptoms of mitral valve prolapse syndrome. In contrast, Hurst et al. (2005) used a parametric measure of relations—the Pearson product moment correlation coefficient—to test their explanatory theory of the relations between social support and self-care agency and between social support and self-care practices.

Tests of predictive theories require a statistic that measures the effects of a concept on one or more other concepts (see Tables 12–8 and 12–9 on the CD). For example, Steele, French, Gatherer-Boyles, Newman, and Leclaire (2001) used a nonparametric measure of effects—the Mann-Whitney U statistic—to test their predictive theory of the effects of continuous acupressure on nausea and vomiting. In contrast, Melancon and Miller (2005) used a parametric measure of effects—analysis of variance—to test their predictive theory of the effects of massage therapy on pain and disability for people with low back pain.

Analyzing Number Data

Computer software programs are now almost always used to analyze number data. Two of the most frequently used computer programs for most statistical procedures are SPSS (Statistical Package for the Social Sciences) and SAS (Statistical Analysis System). Other computer software programs are sometimes used for complex statistics. For example, LISREL (estimation of LInear Structural RELationships), AMOS (Analysis of MOment Structures), and EQS are used for structural equation modeling. As can be seen in Tables 12–10 and 12–11 on the CD, several researchers used SPSS and one used SAS as well as STATA, which is similar to SPSS.

HOW IS THE CRITERION OF OPERATIONAL ADEQUACY APPLIED TO DATA ANALYSIS TECHNIQUES?

When applied to the data analysis techniques element of empirical research methods, the criterion of **operational adequacy** refers to the amount of information about the data analysis techniques given in a research report and focuses attention on whether the techniques were appropriate for the theory-generating research or theory-testing research reported. The operational adequacy criterion, when applied to data analysis techniques, is met when you can answer yes to two questions:

- Are the data analysis techniques clearly identified and described?
- Are the data analysis techniques appropriate?

Are the Data Analysis Techniques Clearly Identified and Described?

All data analysis techniques should be clearly identified and described. A description of exactly how the word data or number data were analyzed and interpreted should be included in the research report. Examples of descriptions of data analysis techniques for various types of qualitative theory-generating research designs and quantitative theory-generating and theory-testing research designs are given in Tables 12–1, 12–10, and 12–11, on the CD that comes with this book.

Are the Data Analysis Techniques Appropriate?

The criterion of operational adequacy requires that the data analysis techniques be appropriate for the type and amount of data collected. Evaluating appropriateness of data analysis techniques involves determining whether the correct data analysis technique was used and whether the results of using the data analysis techniques were interpreted correctly.

Using the Correct Data Analysis Technique

The middle-range theory that is generated or tested and the specific research design determine "the choice of the analytic technique, the manner in which it is to be applied, and the interpretation of the results" (Pedhazur, 1982, p. 11). The analysis of both qualitative and quantitative data should also be consistent with the research methods guidelines of the conceptual model or grand theory that guided the study (see Tables 5–5 and 5–6 on the CD).

Selecting the correct content analysis approach depends on the type of qualitative theory-generating research design. For example, if a phenomenological research design is based on van Kaam's (1966) approach to data collection, the analysis of the word data should be based on van Kaam's approach to content analysis of the data. The contents of Table 12–1, on the CD, encompass many different approaches to content analysis that are used with various qualitative research designs.

Selecting the correct inferential statistics depends, in part, on the distribution of the data for each concept (see Box 12–3) and the level of measurement of each concept (see Box 12–4). In general, if the data are not normally distributed, nonparametric statistics are used. Conversely, if the data are normally distributed, parametric statistics are used. Ravesloot, Seekins, and White (2005), for example, initially used analysis of variance (ANOVA), which is a parametric statistic, to analyze the data for their study of the effects of a health promotion program. However, inasmuch as their data were not normally distributed, they also used a nonparametric statistic and obtained a different result. They explained:

> The health care cost outcomes variables were very positively skewed . . . [and] the costs of health care were accrued largely by less than 25% of the sample. . . . Although repeated-measures ANOVA results were statistically significant, these data clearly do not meet assumptions of multivariate normality. . . . [G]iven the high percentage of zero values in the data, transformations were ineffective for approximating a normal distribution. . . . [Therefore,] we computed the Friedman nonparametric repeated-measures test [which was not statistically significant]. (p. 243)

Selecting the correct inferential statistic also depends on the theory-testing research design. In general, data obtained from correlational research designs are analyzed using a measure of relation (see Tables 12–6 and 12–7 on the CD). Data obtained from a specific correlational research design are analyzed using a specific statistic that is a measure of relation. For example, normally distributed interval level data obtained from a path model research design are analyzed using a special type of multiple regression called path analysis (see Table 12–7).

Similarly, data obtained from experimental research designs are analyzed using a measure of effect, and data from a specific experimental research design are analyzed using a specific statistic that is a measure of effect. For example, ANOVA with a multiple comparison procedure (see Table 12–9 on the CD) is the correct statistical procedure for an experimental research design that involves one experimental and two control treatment groups and normally distributed interval level dependent variable data.

Interpreting the Results of the Data Analysis Techniques Correctly

Correct interpretation of the results of analysis of word data is known as confirmability. Correct interpretation of the results of analysis of number data is known as statistical conclusion validity. In this chapter, we briefly discuss confirmability and statistical conclusion validity. We discuss the correct interpretation of the results of data analysis in more detail in Chapter 13, which addresses evaluation of the research findings.

Confirmability

Confirmability refers to the extent to which the word data were analyzed objectively, such that analysis of the same data by another researcher would yield the same results (Lincoln & Guba, 1985). In other words, the analysis should reflect a neutral interpretation of the data rather than the researcher's personal views about the topic (Lincoln & Guba; Sandelowski, 1986).

Confirmability is assessed by means of an **audit trail** which consists of documents about procedures used for and results of data collection, data analysis, and interpretation of the data. Documents that make up an audit trail may include the actual data; transcripts of interviews with research participants; records of observations; a methodological log or process notes about the methods used to analyze the data and the rationale for the methods; personal notes, such as a personal diary of reflections on the researcher's own values, interests, and insights about the study and the data; and the final report of themes or categories discovered in the data (Lincoln & Guba, 1985). Lou and Dai (2002), for example, explained that the audit trail for their theory-generating study of nurses' experiences of caring for delirious patients included "transcripts, detailed notes, and a written record of an analytic decision trail" (p. 282). The purpose of an audit trail is to clearly and objectively document the data and thought processes that led to the themes or categories (Speziale & Carpenter, 2003).

The **inquiry audit** used to estimate dependability, which we discussed in Chapter 9, is the process used by another researcher to examine the audit trail for the study. For example, Renker (2006) explained that confirmability of her analysis of data about teenagers' experiences of violence during the perinatal period was accomplished by an "audit of the paper trail by two doctorally prepared nurse researchers who had conducted qualitative research" (p. 59).

The overlap between estimating dependability using an inquiry audit and evaluating confirmability is evident in Lin, Hsu, and Tasy's (2003) report of their qualitative theory-generating study of how to teach students about clinical judgment. They stated:

> To enhance dependability and confirmability, a nursing expert in both clinical judgment and qualitative research was consulted concerning the analyzed and coded interview data. The researchers and the nursing expert discussed the results of the data analysis from all interviews, in order to reach 100% agreement on the themes and representative statements. (p. 161)

Statistical Conclusion Validity

Statistical conclusion validity refers to the correct interpretation of statistical tests of number data (Higgins & Straub, 2006). This means that the researcher can conclude that a hypothesis is supported only if the statistical test is significant at the preset level of probability, such as $p < 0.05$ or $p < 0.01$.

The level of statistical significance can be thought of as an absolute cutoff point for accepting or rejecting a hypothesis. Absolute, as Burns and Grove (2007) explained, means that even if the obtained p value is a fraction greater than the preset level of $p = 0.05$, for example, such as $p = 0.051$, the hypothesis must be rejected. As we explain in more detail in Chapter 13, an interpretation that a *p* value "approached significance" or that a hypothesis was "partially supported" is incorrect.

The level of statistical significance should not be confused with the practical value or meaningfulness of the results of analysis of number data. For example, a *p* value of 0.0001 should not be regarded as more practically valuable than a *p* value of 0.05. We discuss the practical value of the results of data analysis in Chapter 14.

Conclusion

This chapter presented only an overview of data analysis techniques. Readers who are interested in more detail are referred to statistics textbooks and books and journal articles about specific data analysis techniques used with specific qualitative and quantitative research designs.

In this chapter, we added **statistical conclusion validity** to our discussion of types of validity for number data. We discussed **external validity** (the extent to which data obtained from one sample can be applied to other people who are members of the same population) in Chapters 8 and 10. We discussed **internal validity** (the accuracy of the data obtained from a specific research design and data collection procedures) in Chapter 10. And, we mentioned **measurement validity** (the appropriateness of instruments and experimental conditions) in Chapter 10. All four types of validity—internal, external, measurement, and statistical conclusion—can be considered broad categories of **study** or **design validity**, which refers to "the evaluation of a researcher's design (blueprint) of a study" (Higgins & Straub, 2006, p 25). Evaluation of each type of validity provides a comprehensive evaluation of the E component of C-T-E structures for research that involves number data and represents a comprehensive application of the criterion of operational adequacy.

The questions to ask and answer as you evaluate data analysis techniques are listed in Box 12–5. Application of the criterion of operational adequacy for data analysis techniques should help you continue to better understand the E component of C-T-E structures. The learning activities for this chapter will help you to continue to increase your understanding of the operational adequacy criterion and its application to the contents of research reports.

BOX 12-5	Evaluation of Data Analysis Techniques: *How Good* Is the Information?

Operational Adequacy

- Are the data analysis techniques clearly identified and described?
- Are the data analysis techniques appropriate?

References

Full citations for all references cited in this chapter are provided in the Reference section at the end of the book.

Learning Activities

Activities to supplement what you have learned in this chapter, along with practice examination questions, are provided on the CD that comes with this book.

Part Four

Evaluation of the Adequacy and Utility of Theories and Conceptual Models

Chapter 13

Evaluation of the Research Findings

This chapter returns our attention to the theory (T) component of conceptual-theoretical-empirical (C-T-E) structures for research.

KEYWORDS

Alternative Methodological Explanation

Alternative Substantive Explanation

Empirical Adequacy

Hypothesis

Research Findings

Recall from Chapter 2 that the T component of a C-T-E structure is the middle-range theory that was generated or tested by research. In that chapter, we defined a theory as a set of relatively concrete and specific concepts and propositions that are derived from the concepts and propositions of a conceptual model. In Chapter 3, we explained *where* to look for information about the theory in research reports (Box 13–1), and in Chapters 3, 4, and 6, we explained *what* information about the middle-range theory should be included in a research report (Box 13–2).

BOX 13-1	Evaluation of the Research Findings: *Where Is* the Information?

Look in the results and discussion sections of the research report.

BOX 13-2	Evaluation of the Research Findings: *What Is the* Information?

- The results of the data analysis
- For theory-generating research, the names and descriptions of the concepts and propositions of the middle-range theory that emerged from the analysis of data
- For theory-testing research, the results of statistical tests that summarize scores for variables and the results of tests of hypotheses

Recall that in Chapter 4 you began to learn how to determine *how good* the information is about the middle-range theory, and we presented a framework for evaluation of C-T-E structures for theory-generating research and theory-testing research. In this chapter, we help you learn more about how to determine *how good* the information is about the T component of C-T-E structures for theory-generating and theory-testing research. We discuss in detail the criterion used to evaluate the research findings—namely, empirical adequacy—and provide examples that should help you better understand how to apply the empirical adequacy criterion as you read research reports. Application of the empirical adequacy criterion will facilitate your evaluation of *how good* the information is about the research findings.

WHAT ARE RESEARCH FINDINGS?

Research findings, which may be referred to simply as "results" or "findings" in research reports, are the results of a study that was designed to generate or test a middle-range theory. Although the grounded theory qualitative research design, which we discussed in Chapter 7, explicitly emphasizes the importance of using data to develop theories (Glaser & Strauss, 1967), all qualitative and quantitative research designs provide data that are used to generate or test middle-range theories. Consequently, all middle-range theories are grounded in—or based on—data. The name of the theory may be explicit (that is, clearly stated) or implicit (implied). As we explained in Chapter 6, if the name of the theory is implicit, the reader can make up a label from the statement of the purpose of the research.

HOW IS THE CRITERION OF EMPIRICAL ADEQUACY APPLIED TO RESEARCH FINDINGS?

Empirical adequacy refers to the amount of information about the findings given in the research report and the extent to which the data agree with the middle-range theory that was generated or tested. The empirical adequacy criterion is met when you can answer yes to two questions:

- Does the research report include sufficient information about the research findings?
- Is the middle-range theory consistent with the research findings?

Does the Research Report Include Sufficient Information About the Research Findings?

The research findings should be presented as the results of the analysis of the word data or the number data. A well-organized research report includes a detailed presentation of the results of the data analysis for each research question or specific aim the study was designed to answer, as well as specific conclusions about any hypotheses that were tested. The report should present data for every middle-range theory concept and any dimensions—or components—of each concept, as well as for every proposition of the theory.

Findings From Theory-Generating Research

The product of theory-generating research is a description of one or more concepts, which we consider a descriptive middle-range theory. In reports of theory-generating qualitative research, researchers frequently refer to the middle-range theory concepts as themes or categories, and to the dimensions of the concepts as subthemes or subcategories. Propositions found in reports of theory-generating research are usually definitions or descriptions of the concepts. The example of findings from theory-generating research given in Box 13–3 is from DeSanto-Madeya's (2006a) phenomenological study of the meaning of living with a spinal cord injury. The product of her research is a descriptive middle-range theory of the meaning of living with a spinal cord injury. Other examples of findings from theory-generating research are given in Tables 13–1 and 13–2 on the CD that comes with this book.

BOX 13-3   Example of a Report of Findings From Theory-Generating Qualitative Research

DeSanto-Madeya (2006a) reported: "Seven themes and several subthemes emerged from the stories of the day-to-day life of living with spinal cord injury" (p. 272). Each theme is a middle-range theory concept, and the subthemes are the dimensions of the concepts. The description of each theme is a middle-range theory proposition.

The theme of looking for understanding of a life that is unknown, described as the "quest for their own understanding of the injury, the process of day-to-day life living with spinal cord injury, and the unknown future" (p. 272), has three subthemes: family's lack of understanding, society's lack of understanding, and health care's lack of understanding.

The theme of stumbling along an unlit path, described as "in an instant, their dreams and goals were replaced with uncertainty" (p. 275), has two subthemes: struggling through the day and worrying about the future.

The theme of viewing self through a stained glass window, described as "When an unexpected event causes paralysis, the injured person and others view the person as different. Many times, this image is distorted as if viewing self through a stained-glass window" (p. 276), has two subthemes: devaluing of personal self and being perceived as different.

The theme of challenging the bonds of love, described as the "bond or connection with others can be affected when a family member has a spinal cord injury" (p. 277), has two subthemes: strengthening the relationship and straining the relationship.

The theme of being chained to the injury is described as the discovery "that the most frustrating aspects of having a spinal cord injury were the loss of their independence and freedom" (p. 279). No subthemes were identified.

The theme of moving forward in a new way of life, described as "learning to 'see life differently' and coming to terms with 'that's the way it is' as necessary steps" (p. 280), has two subthemes—gaining a new perspective on life and learning to live with a changed life.

The theme of reaching normalcy is described as "focusing on the injured person's abilities" (p. 282). No subthemes were identified.

In this example, each theme is a concept and each subtheme is a dimension of a concept.

Findings From Qualitative Theory-Generating Research Designs.

Reports of theory-generating qualitative research should include enough word data, usually presented as quotations from research participants, for the reader to understand how the researcher identified each middle-range theory concept and any dimensions of each concept. The example in Box 13–4 is from DeSanto-Madeya's (2006a) phenomenological study of the meaning of living with spinal cord injury.

BOX 13-4	Example of Participants' Quotations in a Report of Findings From Theory-Generating Qualitative Research

DeSanto-Madeya (2006a) provided quotations that reflected each of the seven themes (concepts) that emerged from the analysis of word data from people who had spinal cord injuries and their family members. Two quotations that reflected one theme are given here.

A quotation from a spinal cord–injured man that reflected the theme, being chained to the injury, is: "It's not that freedom of being able to jump in the car and go wherever you want to go; you have to rely on public transportation. Also, just living around personal care, now I have time-frames when I need to be home. I don't have the freedom of doing a lot of the spur of the moment, spontaneous things" (p. 279).

A quotation from the mother of a spinal cord–injured woman that also reflected the theme of being chained to the injury is: "It's not always good to be the primary caregiver. You are depended upon by that person so much. You are afraid to leave her alone. I was afraid to go to the grocery store or the bank. If I did run out, I flew right home because I was afraid she might fall forward in her wheelchair and not be able to get up. So I felt locked in at times" (p. 280).

Some qualitative research designs, especially phenomenology, rely on "the phenomenological nod" to determine whether the theory that was generated is an accurate description of a particular lived experience. "The phenomenological nod occurs when participants from the respective research population[s] read or hear the interpretations and nod in agreement" (DeSanto-Madeya, 2006a, p. 271). For example, DeSanto-Madeya explained that the "phenomenological nod by the spinal cord injured persons and their family members indicated that a true representation of the essence of the phenomenon had been captured" (p. 271) by the themes and subthemes given in Box 13–3.

It is unclear whether a phenomenological nod indicates that all, most, or only a few of the research participants agreed that the theory clearly represents their lived experience. More precise information comes from inclusion of measures of frequency for the number and percent of research participants whose responses reflected each concept or for the number and percent of responses for each concept or concept dimension in reports of theory-generating qualitative research. Although many researchers who conduct qualitative research do not include measures of frequency in their reports, we agree with Weber (1990), who declared: "The best content-analytic studies use both qualitative and quantitative operations on texts" (p. 10). (Recall that in Chapter 12, we explained that content analysis is the basic data analysis technique used with all qualitative research designs.) Measures of frequency help the reader to understand whether every participant or only some participants provided data that reflect each concept or concept dimension. Specifically, information about the number or percent of participants whose data reflect each concept or concept dimension helps the reader to determine the extent of transferability of the findings to people from the same population who did not participate in the research.

The example of reported measures of frequency data from theory-generating research given in Box 13–5 was extracted from a qualitative study of women's responses to cesarean childbirth (Fawcett, Aber, & Weiss, 2003). Content analysis of the word data from women's

BOX 13-5	Example of Presentation of Measures of Frequencies: For Positive and Negative Feelings During Cesarean Delivery (N = 123 responses)			
THEME SUBTHEMES	**POSITIVE FEELINGS**		**NEGATIVE FEELINGS**	
	n	(%)	*n*	(%)
Feelings during cesarean delivery	57	(46.4)	66	(53.6)
Physical feelings	21	(17.1)	20	(16.3)
Feelings about self	20	(16.3)	33	(26.8)
Feelings about being a mother	8	(6.5)	10	(8.1)
Feelings about need for contact with partner and baby	8	(6.5)	3	(2.4)

responses to the question "How did you feel during the cesarean birth?" revealed one theme (concept) with four subthemes (concept dimensions). The theme is feelings about cesarean delivery. The subthemes are positive and negative physical feelings, positive and negative feelings about self, positive and negative feelings about being a mother, and positive and negative feelings about need for contact with partner and baby. Figure 13–1 is a diagram of the theme and subthemes as a concept and concept dimensions.

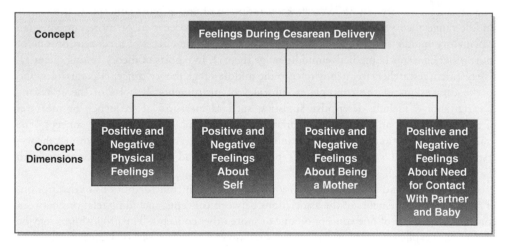

Figure 13-1. Diagram of a concept and its dimensions.

Findings From Quantitative Theory-Generating Research Designs.

Reports of theory-generating quantitative research should include enough number data for the reader to understand how the researcher identified each middle-range theory concept and any dimensions of the concepts. The results of the analysis of the number data from a status survey, for example, could be presented as measures of frequency (n, %), as can be seen in Box 13–5, as well as in two of the examples in Table 13–2, which is on the CD that comes with this book. Or the results could be presented as measures of central tendency (M, median, or mode) and measures of variability (SD, range) for each item or for clusters of items making up a status survey (Box 13–6).

BOX 13-6	Means and Standard Deviations for Perception of the Birth Experience and Adaptation to Cesarean Birth for Women Who Had Unplanned and Planned Cesarean Births					
VARIABLE	UNPLANNED CESAREAN BIRTH			PLANNED CESAREAN BIRTH		
	n	*M*	(SD)	*n*	*M*	(SD)
Perception of the birth experience	41	3.41	(0.53)	49	3.41	(0.40)
Adaptation to cesarean birth	42	44.13	(25.58)	49	67.07	(21.61)

Findings From Theory-Testing Research

The product of theory-testing research is a description of one or more concepts (a descriptive middle-range theory), an explanation of the relations between two or more concepts (an explanatory middle-range theory), or a prediction about the effects of a concept on one or more other concepts (a predictive middle-range theory). In reports of theory-testing quantitative research, researchers frequently refer to the middle-range theory concepts as variables, and to the dimensions of the concepts as subscales of instruments. Reports of theory-testing research should include descriptive statistics, such as measures of frequency or measures of central tendency and measures of variability, for each middle-range theory concept. The example of presentation of means and standard deviations given in Box 13–6 is from a theory-testing correlational study of women's perceptions of and adaptation to cesarean birth (Fawcett, Myers, Hall, & Waters, 2007).

Propositions found in reports of theory-testing research include definitions or descriptions of concepts and statements of the associations between concepts, including relations between concepts and effects of one concept on one or more other concepts. The propositions may be presented as explicit or implicit hypotheses that assert the dimensions of a concept, the relation between two or more concepts, or the effect of one concept on another, expressed as a difference in the scores for a concept between two or more groups. Recall that in Chapter 2, we explained that a hypothesis is a conjecture or tentative statement about one concept or the association between two or more concepts. In Chapter 12, we explained that inferential statistics are tests of hypotheses based on data from a sample. Thus, every inferential statistical test represents the test of a hypothesis. The general forms of hypotheses for theory-testing descriptive, correlational, and experimental research designs are given in Box 13–7.

BOX 13-7	Types of Theory-Testing Research Designs and General Forms of Hypotheses

Research Design: Quantitative Descriptive

Hypothesis: There is a (high, moderate, low) amount of x.

Research Design: Descriptive, Instrument Development

Hypothesis: Concept x is made up of n dimensions.

Research Design: Correlational

Hypothesis: There is a relation between x and y.

Research Design: Experimental

Hypothesis: There is a difference between the experimental and control treatment groups (x) in y.

The example of findings from theory-testing research given in Box 13–8 is from Headley, Ownby, and John's (2004) experimental study of the effects of exercise on fatigue and quality of life, a predictive middle-range theory that was the product of their research. Other examples of findings from theory-testing research are given in Table 13–3 on the CD.

Theory-testing research reports should include the results of inferential statistical tests for each research question, specific aim, or hypothesis. The results of Headley et al.'s (2004) study, given in Box 13–8, include their conclusions for the results of the tests of five hypotheses—one for fatigue and one for each of the four components of quality of life—physical well-being, social well-being, emotional well-being, and functional well-being.

BOX 13-8	Example of a Report of Findings From Theory-Testing Quantitative Research

Headley, Ownby, and John's (2004) Roy Adaptation Model–based experimental study was designed to determine the effects of an experimental seated exercise treatment and a control usual physical activity treatment on fatigue and the physical, social, emotional, and functional well-being components of quality of life (QOL) for women with metastatic breast cancer who were receiving chemotherapy.

Headley et al. referred to fatigue and the components of QOL as variables, which are the middle-range theory concepts. Based on the Roy Adaptation Model, they explicitly "hypothesized that the intervention of a seated exercise program would alter subjects' coping mechanisms aimed at the focus stimulus, which would result in adaptive responses (decreased fatigue and improved QOL) [physical well-being, social well-being, emotional well-being, and functional well-being]" (p. 978). The hypotheses are middle-range theory propositions asserting the difference between the experimental and control groups in fatigue and each component of QOL.

The results of the data analysis revealed that "[a]lthough both groups demonstrated increases in fatigue and decreases in physical well-being, the [experimental] group experienced significantly less increase in fatigue . . . $t(49) = 2.78$, $p = 0.0078$) . . . and less decrease in physical well-being . . . $t(49) = 2.31$, $p = 0.0252$. No significant differences existed between groups for the social, functional, or emotional well-being subscale scores" (p. 980).

The name, degrees of freedom, value of each statistical test, and level of statistical significance (p) should be given in the research report. As can be seen in Box 13–8, Headley et al. (2004) reported the numerical values of the t-tests they used to test two hypotheses as 2.78 and 2.31, with p values for 49 degrees of freedom of 0.0078 and 0.0252, respectively.

As can be seen in Box 13–9, Fawcett et al. (2007) reported numerical values of –0.001, 0.257, and 0.431 for Pearson correlation coefficients (r) testing hypotheses of the relations for type of cesarean birth, perception of the birth experience, and adaptation to cesarean birth, for which the levels of statistical significance are $p = 0.995$, $p = 0.015$, and $p < 0.0005$, respectively. Although the degrees of freedom are not reported, that value can be determined using the formula $df = N - 2$. Using the example in Box 13–9, with a sample size of 90, the degrees of freedom for the correlation coefficients are 88 ($df = 90 - 2 = 88$).

BOX 13-9	**Example of a Correlation Matrix: Correlations for Type of Cesarean Birth, Perception of the Birth Experience, and Adaptation to Cesarean Birth ($N = 90$)**			
VARIABLE	**PERCEPTION OF THE BIRTH EXPERIENCE**		**ADAPTATION TO CESAREAN BIRTH**	
	r	*p*	*r*	*p*
Type of childbirth	−.001	0.995	0.431	< 0.0005
Perception of the Birth Experience	−		0.257	0.015
Adaptation to Cesarean Birth	0.257	0.015	−	

Subtracting the level of statistical significance from 1 ($1 - p$) tells the researchers and the readers of research reports how much confidence they can have in the generalizability of the hypothesis from the sample to the population. For example, if the level of statistical significance was reported to be $p = 0.01$, the researcher and readers could have 99% confidence in the finding. In Box 13–8, the p values of 0.0078 and 0.0252 indicate a high level of confidence—99.22% and 97.48%, respectively. In Box 13–9, the p values of 0.0005 and 0.015 also indicate a high level of confidence that a relation between variables exists for the population—99.95% and 98.5%, respectively. The p value of 0.995, in contrast, indicates a very low level of confidence that any relation between the variables exists for the population, namely 0.005%.

Is the Theory Consistent With the Research Findings?

The criterion of empirical adequacy requires that the middle-range theory be consistent with the research findings.

Theory-Generating Research Designs

In theory-generating research, the middle-range theory concepts and propositions that emerge from the data analysis should clearly reflect the data that were collected. The empirical adequacy criterion is applied to the results that make up the new theory. The data that are presented as research participants' direct quotations should clearly reflect each concept and proposition of the new theory (see Box 13–4 for an example).

Theory-Testing Research Designs

In theory-testing research, the empirical adequacy criterion is applied to a comparison of the version of the middle-range theory that was tested and the version that was retained after testing. The repeated application of the criterion yields an informative judgment about what was proposed versus what was actually found. For example, Headley et al. (2004) tested a predictive theory proposing that the experimental treatment group would have less fatigue and greater physical, emotional, functional, and social quality of life than the control treatment group; but after testing, the theory was limited to less fatigue and greater physical quality of life (see Box 13–8). The result, therefore, was a more parsimonious theory; that is, the theory was more concise (see Chapter 6 for discussion of parsimony). Specifically, the theory that was tested included fatigue and four dimensions of quality of life, whereas the theory that emerged from the research included fatigue and only one dimension of quality of life.

Tests of Hypothesis and Interpretation of the Results. Hypotheses may be as simple as a conjecture that one concept is related to another concept or that there is a difference between two groups for a concept. Complex hypotheses include conjectures about direction (positive, negative), magnitude or strength (weak, moderate, strong), and level of statistical significance ($p = 0.05$, $p = 0.01$, or some other level). Two examples of complex hypotheses are given here.

- The relation between physical energy and functional status will be positive (direction), moderate (magnitude), and statistically significant at the p 5 0.05 level (level of statistical significance).
- There will be a large difference (magnitude) in fatigue between the experimental and control treatment groups at the $p = 0.01$ level (level of statistical significance), such that the experimental treatment group will have less fatigue than the control treatment group (direction).

The logic of scientific inference dictates that if the empirical data are consistent with the conjecture stated in the hypothesis, it is appropriate to conclude that the hypothesis is supported. Conversely, if the empirical data are not consistent with the hypothesis, it is appropriate to conclude that the hypothesis is not supported. Consideration of the empirical adequacy of a middle-range theory must take into account all conjectures included in each hypothesis. If, for example, a hypothesis asserts that there will be a negative, strong, and statistically significant relation at the $p = 0.01$ level between number of physical symptoms and functional status, the

hypothesized direction and magnitude must be evident at the required level of statistical significance. If the hypothesized level of statistical significance is not attained, or if the direction
and/or magnitude are not as hypothesized, the correct conclusion is that a relation does
not exist. It is *not correct* to say, for example, that the relation is *positive but nonsignificant;* that
there is a *tendency* for the experimental treatment group to have higher scores than the control
treatment group; or that the hypothesis was *partially supported.*

For example, Williams and Schreier (2005) incorrectly stated that an increase in use of
self-care behaviors "was greater, but not statistically significant, in the experimental group"
(p. 142). If the increase was not statistically significant, it is incorrect to indicate that there is
any increase (or decrease). In contrast, Bournaki (1997) correctly rejected her hypothesis
because all conjectures were not supported (see Table 13–3 on the CD that comes with this
book). She stated, "Inasmuch as all variables did not enter the analysis, the study hypothesis
was not supported" (p. 151).

An example of acceptance of a hypothesis with multiple conjectures comes from Smith's
(2001) experimental study, which is included in Table 13–3 on the CD. Her data supported
a single hypothesis with multiple conjectures, including a difference between the experimental and control groups for two outcomes—cultural self-efficacy and cultural knowledge—as
well as maintenance of the group differences at the end of the experimental culture school or
control informatics class and 3 weeks later.

Guidelines for accepting and rejecting hypotheses are:

- **Accept** the hypothesis *if and only if every conjecture* in the hypothesis is supported.
- **Reject** the hypothesis *if just even one conjecture* in the hypothesis is not supported.

Consideration of the empirical adequacy of a middle-range theory must also take into
account every hypothesis that is tested. If every hypothesis is supported by the data, the entire
theory can be considered empirically adequate. If, however, one or more hypotheses are not
supported by the data, the theory must be considered empirically inadequate. As can be seen
in Box 13–8, Headley et al.'s (2004) theory must be considered empirically inadequate
because three of the five hypotheses were not supported. Several other examples of the results
of hypothesis testing are given in Table 13–3 on the CD.

The finding that a hypothesis is statistically significant "does not give unequivocal support
to the . . . hypothesis" (Phillips, 1987, pp. 14–15). It is always possible that an exception could
occur or that some other concept that was not included in the theory could have influenced the
results. For example, if the findings of an experimental study revealed a statistically significant
difference in body weight between an experimental treatment group who was very physically
active for 6 weeks and a control treatment group who performed very little physical activity for
6 weeks, the researcher should wonder whether some other concept, such as the age or
physical health of the participants, could account for the findings. Other concepts could also
account for a finding of no statistically significant difference in body weight between the two
groups. Consequently, the empirical adequacy of theories tested using quantitative research
designs always is based on probability rather than certainty (Hoyle, Harris, & Judd, 2002).

Competing Hypotheses

Platt (1964) maintained that every theory-testing study should include multiple competing
hypotheses derived from alternative substantive theories. He claimed that this approach

eliminates errors in interpreting findings that are due to the researcher's intellectual or emotional investment in one particular theory.

Yarcheski, Mahon, and Yarcheski (1997), for example, tested two competing hypotheses for an explanatory middle-range theory of positive health practices in adolescents. One hypothesis proposed that age, gender, self-esteem, social support, and *future time perspective* were related to adolescents' positive health practices. The other hypothesis proposed that age, gender, self-esteem, social support, and *perceived health status* were related to adolescents' positive health practices.

The Value of Empirically Inadequate Middle-Range Theories

A middle-range theory that is not empirically adequate is not necessarily useless and may be just as informative as one that is empirically adequate. It is equally important to learn "what is" and "what is not" for as Glanz (2002) pointed out, "There is as much to learn from failure as there is to learn from success" (p. 546). Knowing "what is not" advances theory development by eliminating a false line of reasoning before much time and effort are invested. We agree with Popper (1965) that the results of testing a middle-range theory should be used to refine the theory so that each remaining concept and proposition can be judged to be empirically adequate or inadequate in another study. As Barry (1997) explained, "Science [that is, empirical research] . . . does not compromise. Instead, science forces ideas to compete in a dynamic process. This competition refines or replaces old hypotheses, gradually approaching a more perfect representation of the truth, although one can reach truth no more than one can reach infinity" (p. 90).

Alternative Methodological and Substantive Explanations

A middle-range theory may be a barrier or may act as blinders to researchers (Chinn & Kramer, 2004). When analyzing qualitative data, it can be difficult for researchers to bracket—that is, to suspend judgments and their own ideas about what the word data mean. It also can be difficult when analyzing quantitative data, for researchers may pay attention to number data that are not consistent with what they expected to find. The difficulties can be overcome by identifying alternative explanations for the findings.

Alternative explanations for findings of theory-generating research and theory-testing research should be taken into account regardless of whether the theory was found to be empirically adequate or inadequate. **Alternative methodological explanations** attempt to account for the research findings by examining each element of the empirical research methods. One methodological explanation is that the findings can be attributed to errors in use of a research design; a faulty sampling strategy; use of instruments that lack dependability and credibility or reliability and validity; data collection procedures that are not rigorous or internally valid; use of unethical procedures involving deception or coercion; use of incorrect data analysis techniques; or interpretations of data analysis that lack confirmability or statistical conclusion validity. Another methodological explanation is that the findings were produced by many small errors of measurement, such as errors due to participants' lack of understanding of instrument items, or errors made in recording their responses to items, as well as errors made by researchers when coding the data or entering the data into a computer file. In the case of tests of predictive theories, the experimental research design may not provide a sufficiently strong "dose" of the treatment to produce the expected effect (Brooten & Youngblut, 2006).

McGahee and Tingen (2000), for example, offered an alternative methodological explanation for the lack of support for two of the three hypotheses they tested (see Table 13–3 on the CD). They explained:

> Although children in the intervention [experimental] groups reported more negative subjective norms and more positive perceptions of refusal skills on the post-tests than children in the control groups, the difference was not statistically significant (Hypotheses II and III). There are a number of possible explanations for this. The subjective norms subscale had the lowest reliability of all the subscales. It may simply be that this variable was not adequately measured. In addition, this variable concerns parents, siblings, friends, popular classmates, and many other people important to the child. This variable is not one for which the intervention was targeted to change, at least for the questions related to beliefs about what others think. The smoking prevention classes had no influence on what others think, and thus, would not be sensitive to change on the questionnaire. The lack of significant effect on refusal skills may be a developmental issue. The subjects in this study all indicated fairly strong perceptions of their refusal skills related to smoking at both pre- and post-test times in both control and intervention groups. Children at this age may feel that they are strong enough to withstand the pressure to smoke. . . . The measures of refusal skills may need to be improved not only with better self-report items, but also with alternative measures such as observational techniques. (pp. 21–22)

Flaws in the empirical research methods are not always the reason why a middle-range theory is empirically inadequate. It may be that the theory is flawed. **Alternative substantive explanations** attempt to account for the research findings by identifying the flaws in the theory and then recommending an entirely different middle-range theory to account for the findings. An alternative substantive explanation may also include a recommendation to refine the theory by eliminating some concepts, adding other concepts, and/or proposing different linkages between concepts. For example, Nuamah, Cooley, Fawcett, and McCorkle (1999) explained that social support, when defined as presence of a caregiver for the patient, was not an adequate representative of the Roy Adaptation Model interdependence response mode. They stated, "The data failed to support the [Roy Adaptation Model] proposition that all four response modes are interrelated. . . . [The quality of] social support or interpersonal relationships, rather than the mere presence of a caregiver, should have been used" (p. 239).

Conclusions About Research Findings

Downs (1984) pointed out that conclusions about the findings of theory-generating research and theory-testing research should take into account four possibilities:

1. The data are inaccurate and cannot be relied upon for theory development.
2. The data are accurate but have no relevance to the theory.
3. The data are accurate, but the theory is faulty and should be refined or abandoned.
4. The data are accurate, and the theory should be regarded as empirically adequate.

The conclusions about theory-generating research or theory-testing research should not include claims that are not consistent with the findings—that is, the conclusions should not incorrectly go beyond the data. For example, if a researcher concluded that the experimental treatment was effective because the mean score for severity of symptoms was higher in the control treatment group, although no statistically significant difference between the experimental treatment group and the control treatment group was found for severity of symptoms the conclusion would be incomplete.

Multiple Tests of a Middle-Range Theory

It is unlikely that any one study will provide enough information to establish the empirical adequacy of a middle-range theory. Researchers, however, do not always conduct repeated studies if the findings from the first study support the empirical adequacy of the theory. Researchers may also be reluctant to abandon a theory if findings from one study do not support the theory. Decisions about empirical adequacy should take the findings of several related studies into account; the more studies that yield findings in support of the theory, the more confident researchers and readers can be that a theory is empirically adequate. No matter how many times a study about a particular theory is conducted, the theory should never be considered absolute truth, for it is always possible that additional studies will yield different findings or that other theories will provide a better fit with the data (Hoyle et al., 2002).

Conclusion

The purpose of research is not to determine the absolute truth of middle-range theories, but rather to determine the degree of confidence warranted by the best research design, the best sampling strategy, the best instruments and experimental conditions, the best procedures for data collection and protection of research participants, and the best data analysis techniques. If confidence is high, the theory may be retained and should be subjected to continued development. If, however, confidence is low, the researcher must be prepared to abandon the theory and search for a better one (Serlin, 1987).

Inasmuch as research findings are the results of theory-generating research or theory-testing research, research findings and middle-range theory can be considered synonymous terms. In Box 13–10, we emphasize this point by rearranging the content of Box 1–1 and expanding it

BOX 13-10	Research, Theory, Research Findings, Evidence, and Practice

- Practice = Research
- Research = Theory development
- Research findings = Theory
- Theory = Evidence
- Evidence-based practice = Theory-based practice

by adding the equivalence of research findings with theory. We can, therefore, conclude that **evidence-based practice actually is theory-based practice.**

The questions to ask and answer as you evaluate the research findings are listed in Box 13–11. Application of the criterion of empirical adequacy should help you to better understand the T component of C-T-E structures. The learning activities for this chapter will help you to continue to increase your understanding of the empirical adequacy criterion and its application to the contents of research reports.

BOX 13-11	Evaluation of Research Findings: *How Good Is the Information?*

Empirical Adequacy

- Does the research report include sufficient information about the research findings?
- Is the middle-range theory consistent with the research findings?

References

Full citations for all references cited in this chapter are provided in the Reference section at the end of the book.

Learning Activities

Activities to supplement what you have learned in this chapter, along with practice examination questions, are provided on the CD that comes with this book.

Chapter 14

Evaluation of the Utility of the Theory for Practice

This chapter continues our attention on the theory (T) component of conceptual-theoretical-empirical (C-T-E) structures for research. In Chapter 13, we focused on the empirical adequacy of middle-range theories—that is, the extent to which the data agree with the theory that was generated or tested. Evaluation of the utility of the theory—the focus of this chapter—takes into account what is required to translate the concepts and propositions of an empirically adequate middle-range theory into practice activities.

KEYWORDS

Best Practices	Metasummary
Clinical Significance	Metasynthesis
Compatibility	Narrative Review
Effect Sizes	Practice Guidelines
Feasibility	Pragmatic Adequacy
Integrated or Systematic Reviews	Statistical Significance
Knowledge Translation	Translational Research
Meta-Analysis	

In Chapters 3, you began to learn *where* to look for information about the utility of the theory for practice in research reports (Box 14–1), and in Chapters 3 and 4, you learned *what* information about the utility of the theory for practice should be included in a research report (Box 14–2).

BOX 14-1	Evaluation of the Utility of the Theory: *Where* Is the Information?

- Look in the discussion section of the research report.
- Look for separate "Implications for Practice" and/or "Implications for Research" sections.

BOX 14-2	Evaluation of the Utility of the Theory: *What* Is the Information?

Implications for the use of the theory in practice

Recall that in Chapter 4, you began to learn how to determine *how good* the information about the middle-range theory is, and we presented a framework for evaluation of C-T-E structures for theory-generating research and theory-testing research. Recall also from Chapter 13 that research findings actually are middle-range theories.

In this chapter, we help you learn more about how to determine *how good* the information is about the utility of the T component of C-T-E structures for theory-generating research and theory-testing research for practice. We discuss in detail the criterion used to evaluate the utility of middle-range theories for practice—namely, pragmatic adequacy—and provide examples that should help you better understand how to apply the pragmatic adequacy criterion as you read research reports. Application of the pragmatic adequacy criterion will facilitate your evaluation of *how good* the information is about the utility of the theory provided in the research report.

HOW DOES A THEORY GUIDE PRACTICE?

Nursing is a professional discipline, which means that nurses have an obligation to not only develop and disseminate knowledge but also to *use* that knowledge in practice (Donaldson & Crowley, 1978). Accordingly, the ultimate goal of nursing research, as well as the goal of research conducted by members of other professional disciplines, is translation of theories into useful practice activities.

Emphasis on the translation of theories into practice activities, such as assessment of health-related experiences and interventions used to promote positive responses to those experiences, has increased in recent years. In the United States, for example, some funding by the National Institutes of Health (NIH) is targeted to translational research (Office of Portfolio Analysis and Strategic Initiatives, 2007). **Translational research,** also called **knowledge translation,** is a research process used to determine what conditions, costs, and resources are required to progress from theory generation and testing to theory utilization, or evidence-based practice. Canada has also begun to emphasize translational research—the Canadian Institutes of Health Research (2004) were created in 2000 to "excel in the creation of new knowledge and to translate that knowledge from the research setting to real-world applications" (p. 1).

The goal of translational research is to speed the translation of empirically adequate middle-range theories into use as practice tools and intervention protocols that will improve people's health and quality of life and strengthen health-care systems.

We explained in Chapters 1 and 13 that theory is equivalent to evidence. Therefore, using a theory in practice means that evidence is used in practice. Box 14–3, which expands Box 13–10 in Chapter 13, highlights the equivalence of using theory and using evidence, so that evidence-based practice is the same as theory-based practice.

Developing Theory Versus Using Theory

We agree with Glanz (2002) that "[i]t is important not to confuse *using* or *applying* theory with testing theory or developing theory" (p. 546). In other words, using a theory in practice

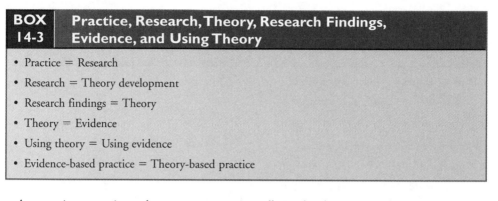

BOX 14-3 | **Practice, Research, Theory, Research Findings, Evidence, and Using Theory**

- Practice = Research
- Research = Theory development
- Research findings = Theory
- Theory = Evidence
- Using theory = Using evidence
- Evidence-based practice = Theory-based practice

and generating or testing a theory are two separate albeit related activities. Although "[n]othing is quite so practical as a good theory" (Lewin, as cited in Van de Ven, 1989, p. 486), and theories are "the most important influence on practice" (Kerlinger, 1979, p. 296), their influence is indirect rather than direct. The indirect influence is best appreciated when it is understood that the concepts and propositions that make up theories must first be translated into innovative practice tools and intervention protocols that then are used in practice.

Types of Practice Activities and Types of Theories

We believe that evidence, in the form of middle-range theories, is needed for every step of the nursing practice process—assessment, planning, implementation, and evaluation (Box 14–4). Specifically, evidence in the form of findings from descriptive theory-generating research can be used to construct new tools for the assessment, planning, and evaluation steps of the nursing process. Evidence in the form of findings from tests of explanatory middle-range theories can be used for construction of more comprehensive tools. Evidence in the form of findings from tests of predictive middle-range theories can be used to develop new intervention protocols for the implementation step of the nursing process.

Although most researchers agree that findings from tests of predictive middle-range theories can be used to develop intervention protocols, few researchers identify the practical uses of findings from tests of explanatory middle-range theories, and even fewer cite the practical uses of findings from generation and testing of descriptive middle-range theories. Kearney (2001) pointed out that construction of assessment tools is a legitimate mode of application of the findings of theory-generating research. Such findings "can be extremely valuable in changing nursing practice inasmuch as [the] goal [of theory-generating research] is to yield understanding" (Cohen, Kahn, & Steeves, 2002, p. 466).

HOW ARE THEORIES TRANSLATED INTO PRACTICE ACTIVITIES?

Translation of theory concepts and propositions into practice tools and intervention protocols occurs in three stages—awareness, adoption, and implementation. Each stage is identified and

BOX 14-4	The Nursing Practice Process, Practical Activities, and Types of Middle-Range Theories Used as Evidence for the Practical Activities

Nursing Practice Process: Assessment

Practical activities: Assessment tools

Types of middle-range theories: Descriptive, explanatory

Nursing Practice Process: Planning

Practical activities: Tool to prioritize planning

Types of middle-range theories: Descriptive, explanatory

Nursing Practice Process: Implementation

Practical activities: Intervention protocols

Type of middle-range theory: Predictive

Nursing Practice Process: Evaluation

Practice activities: Assessment tools

Types of middle-range theories: Descriptive, explanatory

described in Box 14–5. The translation of theories into new tools and protocols is usually slow to occur because people need time to think about a change in the way they practice and then to actually implement the change. The time taken to translate theory into practice activities may, however, be shortened by public media attention. Celebrities sometimes use public media in an attempt to shorten the translation time (Lerner, 2007). For example, actor Michael J. Fox has used the public media to advocate for new treatments for Parkinson's disease, and television newsperson Katie Couric has used the public media to advocate for colorectal cancer screening.

WHAT ARE IMPLICATIONS FOR PRACTICE?

Discussion of the utility of a middle-range theory for practice and what is required to translate the theory into a particular practice tool or intervention protocol is usually found in the implications section of a research report. **Implications for practice** are researchers' recommendations for use of middle-range theories in practice. Researchers' may recommend immediate use of a theory in practice or they may emphasize the need for further research prior to such a recommendation. **Implications for research** are researchers' recommendations for research that will extend middle-range theory development. Researchers may recommend testing a descriptive theory that was generated, testing an explanatory theory that extends a descriptive theory by linking two or more concepts, or testing a predictive theory by deriving an intervention from the explanatory theory. Researchers may also recommend refinement of an explanatory or predictive theory by further testing. Examples of implications for practice

BOX 14-5	Description of Stages of Translation of Theories to Practice Activities

First Stage: Awareness

- Become aware of a new practice tool or new intervention protocol through printed or electronic media, workshops, or conferences.
- Become aware of a new tool or protocol through external change agents, such as government agencies, professional associations, or researchers.
- Identify advantages of the new tool or protocol over the currently used tool or protocol.
- Consider the compatibility of the new tool or protocol with a specific setting and population.
- Consider the complexity of the new tool or protocol.

Second Stage: Adoption

- Be persuaded by peers who have experience implementing other new practice tools or intervention protocols to adopt the new tool or protocol
- Reinforce belief that use of the new tool or protocol will lead to favorable outcomes.
- Decide to adopt the new tool or protocol.

Third Stage: Implementation

- Learn more about the theory that guided development of the new practice tool or intervention protocol.
- Learn how to implement the new tool or protocol.
- Make a partial or total commitment to implement the new tool or protocol.
- Implement the new tool or protocol.
- Use a reminder system to sustain use of the new tool or protocol.
- Appoint a leader to monitor and reinforce use of the new tool or protocol.

Constructed from Brett (1987); Leeman, Jackson, and Sandelowski (2006); Leeman, Baernholdt, and Sandelowski (2007); MacGuire (1989/2006); and Rogers (2003).

and research are given in Box 14–6. Other examples are given in Tables 14–1, 14–2, and 14–3 on the CD that comes with this book.

When discussing implications for practice, researchers frequently emphasize interventions even though the research was not designed to test a predictive theory of the effects of the proposed intervention. As can be seen in Box 14–6, Burns (2004), who discussed the findings of her correlational theory-testing research, mentioned how the findings could be used as the basis for nursing interventions.

The information included in the research report about practical uses of the theory should allow readers to determine whether the theory is ready for use in practice. The challenge for researchers "is to interpret the findings in light of their clinical or practical significance without over[stating] or understating their importance" (Fawcett, 1998, p. 1). Beyond a requirement to include practice implications and research implications, however, little

BOX 14-6	Examples of Implications for Practice and Research

Example From a Qualitative Theory-Generating Study of the Meaning of Living With Spinal Cord Injury

The four modes of adaptation in the Roy [adaptation] model were used to classify the themes of meaning of living with spinal cord injury. The findings revealed that living with spinal cord injury reflects all four modes of adaptation [physiological, self-concept, role function, interdependence]. This secondary analysis gives evidence that the Roy adaptation model can be used as a comprehensive framework for the assessment of living with spinal cord injury . . . [and] provides the foundation for further exploration of the relationships between the focal and contextual stimuli and living with spinal cord injury. The finding that time since injury could be regarded as the focal stimulus suggests that studies designed to describe and compare the spinal cord injured persons' experiences of adaptation at various time intervals following the initial injury are needed. (DeSanto-Madeya, 2006b, pp. 245–246)

Example From a Quantitative Correlational Theory-Testing Study of the Relations of Demographic Variables to Perceived Problems and Coping, and the Relations of Perceived Problems and Coping to Blood Pressure, Body Weight, Potassium Levels, Self-Esteem, Work Status, and Interactions With Family

Nurses who work at dialysis centers do not limit their practice to performing technical skills and managing complicated equipment. Rather, they engage in ongoing patient assessment and have the opportunity to provide emotional support that is based on recognition of stressors that accompany this treatment that patients experience as an illness. . . . Research is needed to develop and test specific nursing interventions that are efficacious in assisting hemodialysis patients to cope with these stressors and improve their quality of life. (Burns, 2004, pp. 123–124)

Example From a Quantitative Experimental Theory-Testing Study of the Effects of a Seated Exercise Program on Fatigue and Quality of Life

Women with metastatic breast cancer often have existing exercise regimens. Participation in some form of exercise can reduce fatigue associated with chemotherapy treatment. The role of nurses in assessment and implementation of care is crucial to addressing patients' exercise preferences and tolerance and potential effects on symptom control. . . . The researchers suggest that future studies address alternate ways of measuring exercise intensity, closer subject follow-up and monitoring, and factors that relate to adherence to exercise programs. (Headley, Ownby, & John, 2004, p. 982)

guidance is found in the printed or online author guidelines or manuscript specifications for most nursing journals. Consequently, the "Implications for Practice" and "Implications for Research" sections of many research reports contain no more than a sentence or two. For example, Leeman, Jackson, and Sandelowski's (2006) analysis of 46 reports of studies of diabetes self-management interventions revealed that the reports "do not include all of the information needed to help clinicians adopt and implement evidence-based changes in practice" (p. 175).

HOW IS THE CRITERION OF PRAGMATIC ADEQUACY APPLIED?

Pragmatic adequacy refers to the extent to which the theory should serve as the basis for practice guidelines and policies regarding ways to assess patients and deliver care.

The pragmatic adequacy criterion is met when you can answer yes to the six questions listed here. The answers to those questions can help you evaluate the extent to which a middle-range theory should be used as the basis for development of new practice tools or intervention protocols:

- Is the social meaningfulness of the theory evident?
- Is use of the theory appropriate for a specific practice situation?
- Is use of the theory in a particular practice setting feasible?
- Is use of the theory consistent with the public's expectations?
- Does the practitioner have legal control of use of the theory in practice?
- Is the theory ready for use in practice?

Is the Social Meaningfulness of the Theory Evident?

The first question asked when evaluating pragmatic adequacy is answered by determining the social meaningfulness of the theory. Evaluating social meaningfulness requires reconsideration of the social significance of the theory, which we discussed in Chapter 6. Social meaningfulness is essentially the same as social significance (see Box 6-4), but when used as part of the evaluation of pragmatic adequacy, emphasis is on the extent to which translation of the theory into a new practice tool or intervention protocol would yield desired outcomes. Desired outcomes include comprehensive assessments of health-related experiences and positive effects of interventions, such as reduction in the incidence of physical or psychological symptoms and improved quality of life. Radwin, Washko, Suchy, and Tyman (2005), for example, identified five desired outcomes of oncology nursing care:

- Sense of well-being—"the patient's positive emotional state"
- Trust—"the patient's confidence that care was appropriate and reliable and would be as successful as possible"
- Fortitude—"the patient's strength and willingness to bear the effects of cancer treatments and the symptoms of the disease"
- Optimism—"the patient's belief that he or she had made appropriate choices regarding treatment and the patient's feelings of hopefulness about treatment outcomes"
- Authentic self-representation—"the patient's sense of genuine self-portrayal" (Radwin et al., p. 93)

In reports of qualitative research, the discussion should focus on how confident the researcher is that the findings are meaningful for practice and can be translated into a new practice tool. In reports of quantitative research, the discussion should include the statistical significance of the findings as well as their clinical—or practical—significance. **Statistical significance** is determined by the *p* value. However, as Slakter, Wu, and Suzuki-Slakter (1991) pointed out, "Statistical significance does not guarantee clinical significance and more to the point, the magnitude of the *p* value . . . is no guide to clinical significance" (p. 249). Instead, **clinical significance** is determined by the magnitude of the findings, which is calculated as an effect size.

As we explained in Chapter 8, **effect sizes** for different statistical tests can be classified as a small, medium, or large frequency of occurrence of a phenomenon, relation between variables, or difference between groups (Cohen, 1992). Newman (2005), for example, reported effect sizes for the relations of self-esteem and personal health to various dimensions of functional status. The effect sizes, which ranged from small to large, allow the reader to decide what to include in a comprehensive assessment of the caregivers of children in body casts and whether the time and effort required to develop and implement a new assessment tool would be worthwhile.

Social meaningfulness can also be evaluated by considering the advantages of the new practice tool or intervention protocol in terms of its effects on utilization of health care and its cost-effectiveness (Leeman et al., 2006). For example, Mock and colleagues (2005) pointed out that a home-based walking exercise intervention was "low-cost . . . and well received" by women receiving treatment for breast cancer (p. 475).

Is Use of the Theory Appropriate for a Specific Practice Situation?

The second question asked when evaluating pragmatic adequacy is answered by determining whether the study findings are compatible with the particular practice situation for which a new practice tool or intervention protocol is sought. Information needed to evaluate **compatibility** of the theory with the practice situation includes a detailed description of the characteristics of the sample of participants used to generate or test the theory, a description of the setting in which the research took place, the procedures used to generate or test the theory, the expertise of the researchers, and the context of the "broader healthcare policy environment" (Leeman et al., 2006, p. 176). In essence, the study findings should be compatible with a particular practice specialty, particular problems, and/or particular ages or developmental phases of the people for whom the new practice tool or intervention protocol is intended. For example, Mock et al. (2005) claimed that the findings of their study of the effects of a home-based walking exercise program on fatigue were "widely applicable . . . to many women with breast cancer" (p. 475).

Although this aspect of pragmatic adequacy may seem self-evident, sometimes a proposal for a new practice tool or intervention protocol is based on a theory that is unrelated to a practice problem and patient population of interest. Suppose, for example, that a nurse wants to design an intervention that will reduce postpartum depression. Suppose also that the intervention protocol is to be based on tests of a theory using samples of older adult men who experience depression. In this fictitious example, the study sample was selected from an entirely different population (older men) than that for which the intervention protocol is being designed (women of childbearing age). Clearly, additional research would be needed to determine if the theory of depression experienced by older men is the same as or different from a theory of depression experienced by women following childbirth.

Is Use of the Theory in a Particular Practice Setting Feasible?

The third question asked when evaluating pragmatic adequacy is answered by determining the feasibility of translating the theory into practical activities in a particular practice setting. Evaluation of **feasibility**, which is a central feature of translational research, involves identifying the complexity of the new practice tool or new intervention protocol derived from the theory in terms of the resources needed to implement the new tool or protocol (Leeman et al., 2006).

Complexity is evaluated by considering:

- The type of training and the time needed to learn how to use the new practice tool or intervention protocol
- The number, type, and expertise of personnel required for all aspects of the design and implementation of the new practice tool or intervention protocol
- The number of contacts and amount of time for each contact required for use of the new tool or to deliver and evaluate the new intervention
- The cost of in-service or other continuing education, salaries, and equipment

Feasibility also requires determining the **willingness of those who control resources to utilize those resources** If they are not willing to utilize those resources to implement the new tool or protocol, its complexity does not matter. However, it may be easier to convince whoever controls the resources to allocate them if the new practice tool or intervention protocol requires little training and a short time to learn how to use it, few personnel to implement it, few contacts of short duration, and minimal cost.

Finally, feasibility requires determining the **willingness of nurses or other health-care personnel to use a new tool or protocol** Making time to locate and read reports of research and using the research findings to develop new tools or protocols can be especially difficult given heavy workloads and the current "fast-paced, high risk [health-care] environment" (Farrell, 2006, p. 119).

Is Use of the Theory Consistent With the Public's Expectations?

The fourth question asked when evaluating pragmatic adequacy is answered by determining the extent to which a practice tool or intervention protocol derived from the theory is consistent with the public's expectations about practice. For example, Mock et al. (2005) noted that a home-based walking exercise program was "acceptable" to many women with breast cancer (p. 475). Their comment, coupled with their finding that almost three quarters (72%) of the women in the experimental treatment group adhered to the walking exercise intervention, implies that walking exercise was consistent with the women's expectations about nursing practice.

If the new practice tool or intervention protocol is not consistent with existing expectations, either it should not be used or people should be helped to change their expectations for practice. As Johnson (1974) pointed out more than 30 years ago, "Current . . . practice is not entirely what it might become and [thus the public] might come to expect a different form of practice, given the opportunity to experience it" (p. 376). Suppose, for example, that a researcher found that listening to music the day before surgery reduced patients' anxiety the morning of the surgery and that perioperative nurses decided to implement the music intervention as part of routine preoperative preparation. Some patients might be receptive to the music intervention, whereas others might indicate that they did not expect to be asked to listen to music the day before their surgery. The perioperative nurses would then have to explain the research results and why they decided to adopt the music intervention.

Does the Practitioner Have Legal Control of Use of the Theory in Practice?

The fifth question asked when evaluating pragmatic adequacy is answered by determining whether the practitioner has legal control over implementation of the new practice tool or intervention protocol and measurement of its effectiveness. Control of practice may be problematic because practitioners are not always able to carry out legally sanctioned responsibilities due to the resistance of others. Sources of resistance include attempts by physicians to control nursing practice, financial barriers imposed by health-care organization administrators and third-party payers, and skepticism by other health professionals about the ability of nurses to carry out the proposed interventions (Funk, Tornquist, & Champagne, 1995). Additionally, some health-care systems do not permit nurses to implement independent interventions but rather require a physician order to carry out nursing interventions (Hasseler, 2006). The cooperation of and collaboration with others may therefore have to be secured.

Leeman, Baernholdt, and Sandelowski (2007) noted that "the extent to which the actions of individuals and/or units are closely interrelated in the process of delivering of care" (p. 192) needs to be evaluated. In general, the greater the extent of interrelationships, the greater the amount of coordination required to implement the new tool or protocol. For example, implementation of an intervention protocol to manage the symptoms associated with chemotherapy may be opposed by physicians who are concerned that patients might be distressed by knowledge about the symptoms or even develop certain symptoms due to their expectation that those symptoms actually will occur. Implementation of the symptom management intervention protocol may also be opposed by health-care system administrators who are concerned about the cost of the resources needed to implement the protocol. And a physician order may be required to implement the symptom management intervention protocol in some practice settings.

Is the Theory Ready for Use in Practice?

The sixth question asked when evaluating pragmatic adequacy is answered by determining whether the theory is ready to be translated into practice activities, such as a new tool to assess patients' pain or a new intervention protocol to decrease patients' pain. Leeman et al. (2006) pointed out that inclusion of detailed information about a tool or protocol that could be developed from the research findings in the research report will help the reader to decide whether the theory that was generated or tested should be translated into practice. In her research report, for example, DeSanto Madeya (2006b) included a tool that can be used to assess patients' adaptation to spinal cord injury, which was based on the findings of her theory-generating study.

When considering the readiness of a theory for use in practice, the answers to the previous five questions need to be considered. In addition, what needs to be studied, as well as the operational adequacy and empirical adequacy of what has already been studied, must be determined (Hunt, 1981). The decision tree shown in Figure 14–1 may help you reach a conclusion regarding the utility of any middle-range theory for practice. The conclusion can be a need for additional research (**What Needs Additional Study**), advocating adoption of a new practice tool or intervention protocol (**What Should Be Done**), or conducting a trial of a new tool or protocol in a practice setting (**What Could Be Tried**), as well as discontinuing a currently used tool or protocol or not developing a new tool or protocol (**What Should NOT Be Done**).

If the decision is to translate the theory into practice activities—What Should Be Done or What Could Be Tried—the how, when, and where of implementation of the new tool or protocol also need to be considered. **How** refers to the procedures to follow to actually use the tool or protocol. **When** refers to the time during an individual's experience in the health-care system the tool or protocol is used, such as when the person initially seeks treatment, during the time that treatment is being received, or at the end of treatment. **Where** refers to the location in which the new tool or protocol will be used, such as in a hospital or people's homes.

When making a decision about the readiness of a theory for use in practice, all research designed to generate or test the theory should be considered. If more than one study has been conducted, the findings of all studies must be integrated and evaluated before a final decision is made, using all of the criteria we have already discussed in Chapters 5 through 13 of this book, as well as the criterion of pragmatic adequacy.

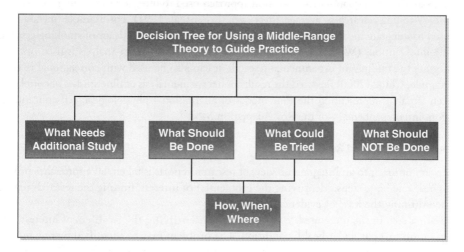

Figure 14-1. Decision tree for using a theory to guide practice.

Integrated Reviews of Research

Research findings are integrated by means of **integrated or systematic reviews** of available research reports. There are several approaches to integrated reviews, but all basically follow the same steps.

Approaches to Integrated Reviews of Research Reports. Narrative review is one approach to integrating research findings. A narrative review is a written report of a review and integration of two or more research reports about a topic. For example, Skalski, DiGerolamo, and Gigliotti (2006) used the narrative approach to integrate the findings of several Neuman Systems Model–based studies of client system stressors. Many different guidelines for integrated or systematic narrative reviews of research are available. See, for example, the *Journal of Advanced Nursing* guidelines for review papers (http://www.journalofadvancednursing.com/default.asp?file= guidereview), as well as guidelines offered by Cooper (1989). Templates for writing integrated reviews of research that take into account the C-T-E structure of each research report are included on the CD that comes with this book (see "Evidence-Based Practice Paper Template–Practice Tools" and "Evidence-Based Practice Paper Template–Intervention Protocols").

Metasynthesis and metasummary are two special approaches used to integrate the findings of theory-generating research. **Metasynthesis** is a qualitative approach that involves integrating the findings of two or more qualitative theory-generating studies of the same phenomenon that are reported as themes or categories (Finfgeld, 2003; Sandelowski, 2006). Mitchell, Beck, and Erickson (2007), for example, used metasynthesis to integrate the findings of 29 studies of the experience of fatigue during and after treatment for cancer.

Metasummary is a quantitative approach that involves integration of the findings of two or more qualitative or quantitative theory-generating studies of the same phenomenon that are reported as simple descriptions of an experience or lists of the frequency of responses, rather than as themes or categories (Sandelowski, Barroso, & Voils, 2007). For example, Sandelowski et al. used metasummary to integrate the findings of 19 studies of factors that favor antiretroviral adherence and factors that favor nonadherence in HIV-positive women.

Meta-analysis is a quantitative, statistical approach used to integrate the findings of quantitative theory-testing research as average effect sizes (Rosenthal, 1991). For example, meta-analysis was used to integrate the findings of 29 experimental studies of the efficacy of smoking cessation nursing interventions (Wewers, Sarna, & Rice, 2006). Although meta-analysis is used primarily to integrate the findings of experimental research, it can also be used with correlational research. For example, Chiou (2000) reported the results of her meta-analysis of nine studies of correlations between variables representing the four modes of adaptation—physiological, self-concept, role function, interdependence—of the Roy Adaptation Model.

Steps in the Integrated Review Process

Whatever approach to an integrated review of research reports is taken, all approaches proceed through several basic steps: identifying the problem(s) of interest, finding the research reports, and determining the level of evidence.

The first step in the integrated review process is **identifying the problem** of interest, such as adaptation to a particular health condition. The problem may be identified by one nurse or a group of nurses. If a group of nurses is involved in identifying the problem, a survey questionnaire, a focus group, or the Delphi technique could be used to achieve consensus about the most pressing problem (see Chapter 7).

Finding the research reports is the next step. All integrated reviews of research continue with a search for relevant literature. A **literature search** involves an actual search for relevant journal articles, books, book chapters, doctoral dissertations, and master's theses. Literature searches can now be done relatively easily through the use of **electronic databases,** including electronic library card catalogs and citation indexes. Journal articles and some books can be located in citation indexes, many of which are electronic versions of print indexes, such as the *Cumulative Index to Nursing and Allied Health Literature* (CINAHL), in which are listed some nursing doctoral dissertations; *Index Medicus* (Medline or PubMed); *Psychological Abstracts (PsycInfo); Sociological Abstracts;* and *Dissertation Abstracts International* or Dissertation Abstracts Online, in which are listed doctoral dissertations and master's theses. Books can be located in WorldCat, which is an electronic catalog of books and other materials from before 1000 B.C. to the present in the collections of libraries throughout the world. Most electronic databases can be accessed by computer through subscriptions held by college, university, and some public libraries and by health-care organizations.

Computers and electronic databases have greatly facilitated literature searches in the past 15 or 20 years. A comprehensive search of literature, however, still takes a considerable amount of time. Parker (2006) explained,

> If you are new to computer searching of nursing literature, be prepared to spend many, many hours searching for information. When first becoming acquainted with the electronic world, be prepared to accept that you will forget where you are on this electronic highway. It takes practice and intense focus to remain on the elusive information trail. (p. 31)

Although we have emphasized searches of electronic databases, we recognize the value of manual searches of journals and books in which research reports can be found. A **manual search** involves actually looking through the tables of contents of journals and books in which research reports are usually published for relevant articles and chapters. Manual searches may also extend to the print versions of electronic databases, especially if the electronic version is not as comprehensive as the print version.

Manual searches are limited to the journals, books, and indexes that are available in university, college, or public libraries to which a nurse has access or are in a nurse's personal library. Electronic databases typically include citations to many more journals and books than any one library or individual is likely to have, but many databases are limited by the number of years of publications included. For example, the electronic version of CINAHL starts in 1982 and continues to the present, whereas the print version (until its demise in 2007 [D. Pravikoff, personal communication, June 28, 2007]) included citations from 1956 to 2007.

When the relevant literature is located and retrieved, each article, book, or book chapter must be evaluated. Use of the framework for evaluation of C-T-E structures that we presented in Chapter 4 will provide a comprehensive evaluation of all aspects of empirical research. Evaluation of each article, book, and book chapter is followed by integration of the various publications. The decision tree depicted in Figure 14–1 then can be applied to the integrated research findings, and if the integrated findings are deemed ready to use or could be tried, a practice tool or intervention protocol can be developed and used in practice.

Many integrated reviews of research about a particular topic are published in nursing theory and research journals, such as the *Journal of Advanced Nursing,* the *Journal of Nursing Scholarship,* and *Worldviews on Evidence-Based Practice.* Integrated research reviews are also beginning to be published in nursing clinical specialty journals, such as the *Clinical Journal of Oncology Nursing.* Many other reports of the integration of research findings are available on the Internet, such as:

- Cochrane Database of Systematic Reviews (www.thecochranelibrary.com)
- Database of Abstracts of Reviews of Effects (www.york.ac.uk/inst/crd/crddatabases. htm#DARE)

- Campbell Collaboration (www.campbellcollaboration.org)
- Registered Nurses' Association of Ontario
  (www.rnao.org/Page.asp?PageID=861&SiteNodeID=133)

Highlights or summaries of integrated research reviews are available in various general and specialty nursing journals. Two general journals are the *Journal of Advanced Nursing* and *Evidence-Based Nursing;* two specialty journals are the *Journal of Obstetric, Gynecological, and Neonatal Nursing* and the *Journal of Midwifery and Women's Health.*

A major shortcoming of many integrated research reviews is lack of attention to the implicit or explicit conceptual model that guided the research and the implicit or explicit middle-range theory that was generated or tested. Another shortcoming of integrated research reviews is an overemphasis on experimental research designed to test predictive middle-range theories about interventions. Little attention is given to integrating the findings of descriptive or correlational research, which could be translated into practice tools.

Determining the levels of evidence is the third step. The overemphasis on experimental research, especially randomized controlled clinical trials (RCTs), is evident in various schemas for levels of evidence (West et al., 2002). Levels-of-evidence schemas usually include ratings for various types of research designs and even expert opinion, although the best ratings are typically assigned to integrated reviews of experimental research, especially RCTs. For example, Melnyk and Fineout-Overholt (2004) include both descriptive and experimental research in their schema. However, they place integrated reviews of experimental research at the highest level (level 1) and integrated reviews of quantitative and qualitative descriptive research at level 5 in their seven-level schema; only findings from a single descriptive study and expert opinion are at lower levels. An example of an eight-level evidence schema is given in Box 14–7. Both examples of levels of evidence, as well as others, ignore the different contributions of each type of research—descriptive, correlational, experimental—to practice (see Box 14–4).

Relation of Integrated Reviews of Research, Practice Guidelines, and Best Practice Guidelines

Integrated reviews of research may be translated into **practice guidelines,** which are "systematically developed statements to assist health care practitioners' decisions about appropriate health care for specific clinical circumstances" (Wallin, 2005, pp. 248–249). The Conduct and Utilization of Research in Nursing (CURN) publications of the early 1980s are among the first formal practice guidelines based on integrated research reviews available to nurses (Horsley, Crane, Crabtree, & Wood, 1983). The CURN project staff developed guidelines in the form of protocols for the nursing interventions listed here:

- Clean intermittent catheterization (Horsley, Crane, & Reynolds, 1982a)
- Closed urinary drainage systems (Horsley, Crane, Haller, & Bingle, 1981a)
- Deliberative nursing interventions for pain (Horsley, Crane, & Reynolds, 1982b)
- Distress reduction through sensory preparation (Horsley, Crane, Reynolds, & Haller, 1981a)
- Intravenous cannula change (Horsley, Crane, & Haller, 1981a)
- Mutual goal setting in patient care (Horsley, Crane, Reynolds, & Haller, 1982)

BOX 14-7	Example of Levels of an Evidence Schema

1++: High-quality meta-analyses, systematic reviews of randomized controlled trials (RCTs), or RCTs with a very low risk of bias

1+: Well-conducted meta-analyses, systematic reviews of RCTs, or RCTs with a low risk of bias

1−: Meta-analyses, systematic reviews of RCTs, or RCTs with a high risk of bias

2++: High-quality systematic reviews of case control or cohort studies; high-quality case control or cohort studies with a very low risk of confounding or bias and a high probability that the relationship is causal

2+: Well-conducted case control or cohort studies with a low risk of confounding or bias and a moderate probability that the relationship is causal

2−: Case control or cohort studies with a high risk of confounding or bias and a significant risk that the relationship is not causal

3: Non-analytic studies (e.g., case reports, case series)

4: Expert opinion

Source: Scottish Intercollegiate Guidelines Network (SIGN) (2003, July). *Cutaneous melanoma. A national clinical guideline.* Edinburgh: Author (SIGN Publication No. 72). Retrieved July 14, 2007, from http://www.guideline.gov/summary/summary.aspx?doc_id=3877&nbr=003086&string=cutaneous+AND+melanoma

- Preoperative sensory preparation to promote recovery (Horsley, Crane, Reynolds, & Haller, 1981b)
- Prevention of decubitus ulcers (Horsley, Crane, Haller, & Bingle, 1981b)
- Reduction of diarrhea in tube-fed patients (Horsley, Crane, & Haller, 1981b)
- Structured preoperative teaching (Horsley, Crane, Reynolds, & Bingle, 1981)

Some or all of the CURN practice guidelines most likely have to be revised to account for more recent research findings, but they serve as a starting point for contemporary practice guideline development. Contemporary practice guidelines that may be of interest to nurses and other members of the health-care team are available from the National Guideline Clearinghouse, at www.guideline.gov.

A practice guideline may sometimes be referred to as *best practice*. **Best practice** or **best practices** refers to "the organizational use of evidence to improve practice" (Driever, 2002, p. 593). Best practice involves the use of evidence-based practice guidelines by health-care personnel and typically ■ emphasizes the best way to use human resources and equipment to attain the best possible patient outcomes.

Information about best practices is available online from the Joanna Briggs Institute (JBI). The JBI staff work with researchers, clinicians, and managers in nursing, medicine, nutrition and dietetics, physical therapy, occupational therapy, and podiatry to prepare **Best Practice Information Sheets,** which are easy-to-read summaries of best practice based on the results of systematic reviews of research. Best Practice Information Sheets can be downloaded from www.joannabriggs.edu.au/pubs/best_practice.php. Just a few of the many available JBI Best Practice Information Sheets are listed here:

- Effective dietary interventions for overweight and obese children
- Removal of Short-term Indwelling Urethral Catheters

- Solutions, Techniques and Pressure in Wound Cleansing
- Management of Asymptomatic Hypoglycaemia in Healthy Term Neonates for Nurses and Midwives
- Nurse Led Cardiac Clinics for Adults with Coronary Heart Disease
- Oral Hygiene Care for Adults with Dementia in Residential Aged Care Facilities

Conclusion

The outcome of the evaluation of pragmatic adequacy not only is a thorough understanding of the theoretical and empirical base for various practical activities but is also a catalyst for the development of health policies. Cohen et al. (1996) emphasized the importance of translating empirically and pragmatically adequate theories into policies for the public's good. For example, on the basis of the findings of her study of correlates of functional status of caregivers of children in body casts, Newman (2005) declared, "At the policy level, nurses can advocate for insurance coverage for alternate caregiver services . . . [such as] home health aide service to provide respite for caregivers" (p. 421).

Health policies formulated by health-care organizations, such as hospitals and home-care agencies, as well as by professional nursing specialty organizations, such as the American Association of Critical Care Nurses and the Association of periOperative Registered Nurses (AORN), are presented in the form of practice guidelines. For example, the AORN developed a practice guideline called the Correct Site Surgery Tool Kit (www.aorn.org/PracticeResources/ToolKits/CorrectSiteSurgeryToolKit) to help nurses and other health-care team members to better understand and implement a protocol to prevent wrong site surgery.

Health policies formulated by local, state, or federal governments are typically derived from legislation that is translated into regulations, such as those in the United States for Medicare and Medicaid. Health policies may address the quality or cost of or access to health care (Russell & Fawcett, 2005). Ideally, health policies should lead to provision of high-quality, cost-effective care that is equally accessible to all people.

Application of the criterion of pragmatic adequacy is needed perhaps more than ever before in the history of modern health care, given the current mandate for evidence-based practice. As LaPierre, Ritchey, and Newhouse (2004) pointed out, nurses "need to prepare themselves with the skills needed to review current findings and determine if they are applicable for their setting" (p. 7). The content of this chapter addresses the required skills for readers of research reports to accomplish this.

The questions to ask and answer as you evaluate the utility of a middle-range theory for practice are listed in Box 14–8. Application of the criterion of pragmatic adequacy should help you to better understand the T component of C-T-E structures. The learning activities for this chapter will help you to continue to increase your understanding of the pragmatic adequacy criterion and its application to the contents of research reports.

BOX 14-8	Evaluation of the Utility of the Theory · for Practice: *How Good* Is the Information?

Pragmatic Adequacy

- Is the social meaningfulness of the theory evident?
- Is the theory relevant for a specific practice situation?
- Is use of the theory in a particular practice setting feasible?
- Is use of the theory congruent with the public's expectations?
- Does the practitioner have legal control of use of the theory in practice?
- Is the theory ready for use in practice?

References

Full citations for all references cited in this chapter are provided in the Reference section at the end of the book.

Learning Activities

Activities to supplement what you have learned in this chapter, along with practice examination questions, are provided on the CD that comes with this book.

Chapter 15

Evaluation of the Utility and Soundness of the Conceptual Model

This chapter returns our attention to the conceptual model (C) component of conceptual-theoretical-empirical (C-T-E) structures for research. Recall from Chapter 2 that the C component of a C-T-E structure is the conceptual model that guided all aspects of the theory-generating research or theory-testing research. In that chapter, we defined a conceptual model as a set of relatively abstract and general concepts and propositions that address phenomena—things—that are of central interest to a discipline. In this chapter, we focus on the utility and soundness of the conceptual model.

KEYWORD

Legitimacy

In Chapter 3, you began to learn *where* to look for information about the utility and soundness of the conceptual model in research reports (Box 15–1), and then in Chapters 3, 4, and 5, you learned *what* information about the utility and soundness of the conceptual model should be included in a research report (Box 15–2).

BOX 15-1	Evaluation of the Utility and Soundness of the Conceptual Model: *Where* Is the Information?

Look in the discussion section of the research report.

BOX 15-2	Evaluation of the Utility and Soundness of the Conceptual Model: *What* Is the Information?

- Discussion of the extent to which the conceptual model was a useful guide for the research
- Conclusions about the extent to which the research findings are consistent with the content of the conceptual model

Recall also that in Chapter 4, we presented a framework for evaluation of C-T-E structures for research, and you began to learn how to determine *how good* the information is about the utility and soundness of the conceptual model.

In this chapter, we help you learn more about *how good* the information is about the C component of C-T-E structures for theory-generating research and theory-testing research as we discuss a criterion called legitimacy in detail and provide examples that should help you better understand how to apply it as you read research reports. Application of the legitimacy criterion will facilitate your evaluation of *how good* the information is about the utility and soundness of the conceptual model provided in the research report.

In the past, the criterion of legitimacy was referred to as *credibility* (Fawcett, 1996, 1999). We changed the label to *legitimacy* to avoid confusion with *credibility* as applied to the trustworthiness of qualitative data. The idea of legitimacy of knowledge comes from Cowling (2001), who noted that development of research methods "that are grounded in nursing's uniqueness . . . [requires attention to] 'legitimate' knowledge and 'credible' research" (p. 44). Although Cowling went on to discuss legitimacy in the context of research methods, we regard it as appropriate for evaluation of knowledge in the form of conceptual models.

WHY IS EVALUATION OF THE LEGITIMACY OF A CONCEPTUAL MODEL NECESSARY?

Evaluation of the utility and soundness of the conceptual model that guided the theory-generating research or theory-testing research is necessary to avoid the danger of uncritical acceptance and adoption of conceptual models, which could easily lead to their use as ideologies. Critical reviews of the utility and soundness of each conceptual model must be encouraged, and acceptance of work that is "fashionable, well-trodden, or simply available in the nursing library" must be avoided (Grinnell, 1992, p. 57). Conceptual models benefit from evaluation of their utility and soundness; they should not be regarded as static, but rather as dynamic and modifiable.

All conceptual models may not be appropriate for all situations and for all populations in various cultures. The ultimate aim of evaluation of conceptual model utility and soundness, therefore, is to ascertain which conceptual models are appropriate for use as guides for research and practice with which populations and in which cultures. Inasmuch as the abstract and general nature of a conceptual model precludes direct empirical testing, the concepts and propositions of the conceptual model are instead tested indirectly through the generating and testing of middle-range theories. Thus, the information needed to evaluate the utility and soundness of a conceptual model comes from the design and findings of theory-generating research or theory-testing research.

Some discussion of the utility and soundness of the conceptual model that guided the theory-generating research or theory-testing research should be included in the discussion section of the research report. One example is from an exploratory descriptive study of women's responses to a vaginal birth after a cesarean birth (VBAC) (Fawcett, Tulman, & Spedden, 1994). Content analysis was used to classify the women's responses as adaptive and ineffective within the four Roy Adaptation Model modes of adaptation—physiological, self-concept, role function, and interdependence. A statistically significant difference was found between type of delivery (VBAC versus previous cesarean birth) and the women's responses to VBAC, with a greater proportion of adaptive responses to the VBAC than to the previous cesarean. The information about conceptual model legitimacy given in the research report was:

The Roy Adaptation Model proved to be a useful framework for the study of women's responses to VBAC, especially for the content analysis. Of interest are the findings of no adaptive responses in the physiological and interdependence modes and no needs within the self-concept mode for this sample. Those empty cells contrast with the findings from studies of cesarean birth, where both adaptive and ineffective responses and needs were identified for all four modes. (Fawcett et al., 1994, p. 258)

Another example is from a correlational study of women's adaptation to childbirth (Tulman & Fawcett, 2003). Correlational statistics were used to analyze the relations of several physical health, psychosocial health, and family relationships variables to functional status during pregnancy and the postpartum. The study findings revealed a much more parsimonious—that is, concise—theory than originally proposed, in that only some of the several variables were related to functional status. The information about conceptual model legitimacy given the research report was:

> The Roy Adaptation Model provided a useful structure for our review of the literature and led to the identification of the study variables. . . . We tested the [legitimacy] of the Roy Adaptation Model by examining evidence for the proposition that the response modes are interrelated. . . . [T]he physiological mode was represented by the physical health variables. . . . The self-concept mode was represented by psychosocial health variables. . . . The role function mode was represented by functional status. The interdependence mode was represented by family relationships variables. . . . During pregnancy, all modes were interrelated except the role function and interdependence modes. . . . During the postpartum, all modes were interrelated at 3 and 6 weeks and 3 months; at 6 months, all but the role function and interdependence modes were interrelated. . . . Collectively, the findings of our study add to the accumulating evidence supporting the [legitimacy] of the Roy Adaptation Model. The magnitude of statistically significant correlations between variables representing the four response modes indicated that the modes are interrelated but also independent components of adaptation to environmental stimuli. (Tulman & Fawcett, 2003, pp. 158–160)

Still another example is from a quasi-experimental study of the effects of information on adaptation to cesarean birth (Fawcett et al., 1993). The control treatment group, who received a standard childbirth education curriculum, reported a slight decline in pain intensity from 1–2 days to 6 weeks postpartum. In contrast, the experimental treatment group, who received a standard childbirth education curriculum plus a booklet of detailed information about cesarean birth, showed no change over time. No other differences between the two groups were found. The lack of substantial differences between the groups was thought to be due to the normalizing effect of the high cesarean birth rate and the attention given to this method of childbirth by expectant parents and childbirth educators. The information about conceptual model legitimacy given in the research report was:

> The hypotheses [for the study of the effects of information on adaptation to unplanned cesarean birth] were based on the Roy Adaptation Model proposition that management of contextual stimuli promotes adaptation. The study findings provide no support for this proposition and, therefore, raise a question regarding the [legitimacy] of the model. However, the study may not have been a sufficient test of the proposition because the

contextual stimul[us], in the form of the experimental and control treatments, did not differ sufficiently [for the experimental and control groups]. (Fawcett et al., 1993, p. 52)

Other examples are given in Tables 15–1, 15–2, and 15–3 on the CD that comes with this book. All too frequently, however, researchers do not provide any information about the utility and soundness of the conceptual model that guided the research, as can be seen in Table 15–3.

HOW IS THE CRITERION OF LEGITIMACY APPLIED TO CONCEPTUAL MODELS?

Legitimacy refers to the extent to which the design and findings of theory-generating or theory-testing research support the usefulness and soundness of the conceptual model that guided the research. The legitimacy criterion is met when you can answer yes to two questions:

- Was the conceptual model a useful guide for the research that was conducted?
- Is the content of the conceptual model sound and believable?

The criterion can also be applied to nursing grand theories (Leininger's Theory of Expanding Consciousness, Newman's Theory of Health as Expanding Consciousness, Parse's Theory of Human Becoming).

Was the Conceptual Model a Useful Guide for the Research That Was Conducted?

The legitimacy criterion can be applied only if the criteria of specification adequacy and linkage adequacy, which we discussed in Chapter 5, have been met. Determination of legitimacy may then proceed by comparing the research findings with the concepts and propositions of the conceptual model. If the specification adequacy and linkage adequacy criteria were not met, not enough information was given in the research report to understand how the conceptual model guided the research and, therefore, it is not possible to determine how useful a guide for the research it was and how sound and believable its content is.

Judgments about the legitimacy of a conceptual model may proceed in different ways for theory-generating and theory-testing research.

Theory-Generating Research

In theory-generating research, the judgment about legitimacy may be limited to the utility of the conceptual model to guide the selection of empirical research methods and the success of those methods in generating a new theory. Specifically, the conceptual model could be considered a useful guide for selection of the research design, sample, research instruments, data collection procedures, and data analysis techniques, and for interpretation of the data.

The conceptual model guides selection of the empirical research methods through application of its research methods guidelines, which we identified in Chapter 5. The research focus guidelines of the conceptual model are used to select a topic for study and to provide a structure for analysis and interpretation of the data. One or more concepts of the conceptual model may serve as pre-existing categories for content analysis of the data, and the findings can be compared with one or more conceptual model concepts.

For example, Fawcett et al. (1994) noted that the concepts of the Roy Adaptation Model were a useful guide for their content analysis of women's responses to VBAC. DeSanto Madeya (2006b) concluded that the Roy modes of adaptation provided a "comprehensive framework" for her content analysis of themes about the meaning of living with breast cancer (p. 244). Several other examples of conceptual model utility for theory-generating research are given in Tables 15–1 and 15–2, on the CD that comes with this book.

Theory-Testing Research

In theory-testing research, the judgment about legitimacy can be extended to the utility of the conceptual model as a guide for selection of the middle-range theory concepts and propositions. Through operationalization of the middle-range theory concepts and propositions, the conceptual model also serves as a guide for selection of the empirical research methods, including the research design, sample, research instruments and any experimental conditions, data collection procedure, and data analysis techniques.

The conceptual model guides *direct* selection of middle-range theory concepts through application of its research focus guidelines, which we identified in Chapter 5. For example, Tulman and Fawcett (2003) commented that the "Roy Adaptation Model provided a useful structure for our review of the literature and led to the identification of the study variables" (p. 158).

The conceptual model guides *indirect* selection of the empirical research methods through application of its research methods guidelines, which we identified in Chapter 5. For example, Samarel, Tulman, and Fawcett (2002) explicitly linked the self-concept and interdependence modes of adaptation to middle-range theory concepts, and then linked those concepts to the instruments they used in their Roy Adaptation Model–based experimental study of the effects of social support and education on adaptation to breast cancer. They also explained how the content of the social support and education experimental and control treatment protocols was based on the self-concept and interdependence modes of adaptation. Several other examples of conceptual model utility for theory-testing research are given in Table 15–3, on the CD.

Is the Content of the Conceptual Model Sound and Believable?

An effective way to determine whether the content of the conceptual model is sound and believable is to carefully read the narrative research report to determine whether the conceptual model concepts and propositions are supported by the design and findings of the theory-generating research or theory-testing research or whether any major flaws in the conceptual model concepts or propositions were uncovered by the research findings. Many examples of comments about the soundness and believability of the conceptual model are given in Tables 15–1, 15–2, and 15–3 on the CD that comes with this book. The approach to determining the soundness and believability of the content of the conceptual model may differ slightly when dealing with theory-generating research or theory-testing research.

Theory-Generating Research

In theory-generating research, if the concepts of the conceptual model served as pre-existing categories for data analysis, the judgment about legitimacy can be extended beyond the utility of empirical research methods to the comprehensiveness of the conceptual model content. If the middle-range theory that was generated is consistent with the conceptual model concepts that guided the research, it is appropriate to conclude that the conceptual model content is sound and believable. For example, Breckenridge (1997) used five concepts from Neuman's Systems Model as the pre-existing categories for a secondary content analysis of interview transcripts. She reported that all of the interview data could be categorized within those five concepts—namely, physiological variables, psychological variables, sociocultural variables, developmental variables, and spiritual variables. In this example, Neuman's Systems Model can be regarded as legitimate because data from Breckenridge's study represented the five concepts from the Neuman Systems Model.

If the middle-range theory that was generated *is not* consistent with the conceptual model concepts that guided the study, the appropriate conclusion is that the conceptual model content *may not be* or *is not* sound and believable and that one or more concepts or propositions of the conceptual model should be modified or eliminated, or the entire conceptual model should be rejected. Suppose, for example, that the data from Breckenridge's (1997) study were found to represent only three of the five concepts or that some of her data did not represent any of the five concepts. In this instance, the legitimacy of Neuman's Systems Model would have to be questioned, and modifications in the conceptual model concepts would be needed. Suppose further that none of Breckenridge's data represented any of the five concepts. In that instance, the appropriate conclusion may be that the conceptual model should be rejected.

Theory-Testing Research

In theory-testing research, if the theory is found to be empirically adequate, the appropriate conclusion is that the conceptual model is sound and believable. For example, a test of a predictive middle-range theory of the effects of walking exercise on physical functioning, exercise level, emotional distress, and symptom experience of women with breast cancer who were receiving radiation yielded research findings supporting the empirical adequacy of the theory. Inasmuch as the study was guided by Roy's Adaptation Model, the investigators' conclusions indicated that the conceptual model was sound and believable (Mock et al., 1997).

If the research findings *do not* support the empirical adequacy of the theory, it is appropriate to conclude that the conceptual model content *may not be* or *is not* sound and believable and that one or more concepts or propositions of the conceptual model should be modified or eliminated, or the entire conceptual model should be rejected. For example, Samarel, Fawcett, and Tulman (1997) tested a predictive middle-range theory of the effects of different amounts of social support and education on outcomes representing the four modes of adaptation—physiological mode, represented by symptom distress; self-concept mode, represented by emotional distress; role function mode, represented by functional status; and interdependence mode, represented by relationship quality. They found that the theory was not empirically adequate because the only differences between the experimental and control treatment groups were in relationship quality. Inasmuch as the theory was directly derived from Roy's Adaptation Model, the investigators concluded that the study findings "raise questions about the [credibility] of the Roy Adaptation Model and its utility for research dealing with the effects of social support and education on adaptation to breast cancer" (Samarel et al., 1997, p. 24).

Just as it is sometimes difficult to reach a definitive conclusion about the pragmatic adequacy of a middle-range theory on the basis of one study, it may be difficult to reach a definitive conclusion about the legitimacy of a conceptual model on the basis of the findings of just one or two studies. Researchers may state that the research results "raise questions" (Samarel et al., 1997, p. 24) about the utility and soundness of the conceptual model rather than recommend its rejection. For example, Samarel and colleagues (2002) continued to use the Roy Adaptation Model to guide the test of a predictive middle-range theory of the effects of social support on adaptation to breast cancer by changing the protocols for the experimental and control treatments and limiting the outcomes to variables representing the self-concept mode of adaptation—cancer-related worry, well-being, mood disturbance—and the interdependence model of adaptation—loneliness, relationship quality. They found that the middle-range theory was not empirically adequate because the only differences between the experimental and control treatment groups were in loneliness, mood disturbance, and relationship quality. They concluded, "The findings of some group differences for mood disturbances, loneliness, and relationship quality indicate that Roy adaptation model–based interventions of support and education can have some effect on adaptation to a diagnosis of breast cancer in both the self-concept and the interdependence modes, although the effects were not as wide-ranging as was hypothesized" (p. 468).

A few investigators have integrated the findings of research based on a specific conceptual model. Chiou (2000), for example, reported the results of a meta-analysis of the relations between variables representing the four modes of adaptation of the Roy Adaptation Model as reported in nine studies. She found small ($r = 0.10$) to medium ($r = 0.30$) average effect sizes (Cohen, 1992) for the relations of the physiological mode with the self-concept and role function modes, the self-concept mode with the role function and interdependence modes, and the role function mode with the interdependence mode. The relation between the physiological and interdependence modes, however, was lower than a small average effect size ($r = 0.04$). Chiou concluded, "The findings propose that the establishment of the [legitimacy] of the [Roy Adaptation] model is still in an early stage, and additional investigations are needed. The present study . . . indicates a need for further study to explore the relationships among all . . . modes [of adaptation] to impart a clearer understanding of the [legitimacy] of Roy's model" (p. 257).

Conclusion

This chapter completes evaluation of all three components of C-T-E structures for theory-generating research and theory-testing research. Although you may not yet feel completely confident about how to apply each criterion, you will gain confidence as you continue to read research reports and use the framework for evaluation of C-T-E structures presented in Chapter 4.

The questions to ask and answer as you evaluate the utility and soundness of a conceptual model are listed in Box 15–3. Application of the criterion of legitimacy should help you to better understand the C component of C-T-E structures. The learning activities for this chapter will help you continue to increase your understanding of the legitimacy criterion and its application to the contents of research reports.

BOX 15-3	Evaluation of the Utility and Soundness of the Conceptual Model: *How Good Is the Information?*

Legitimacy

• Was the conceptual model a useful guide for the research that was conducted?

• Is the content of the conceptual model sound and believable?

References

Full citations for all references cited in this chapter are provided in the Reference section at the end of the book.

Learning Activities

Activities to supplement what you have learned in this chapter, along with practice examination questions, are provided on the CD that comes with this book.

Part Five

Integrating Research
and Practice

Chapter 16

Strategies for Integrating Nursing Research and Nursing Practice

Most nurses and other health-care professionals agree that high-quality care is attained only if practice is based on evidence, which, as we have explained throughout this book, is equivalent to theory. In Chapter 14, we pointed out that nurses need to translate the empirical theories developed through theory-generating research and theory-testing research into practice tools and intervention protocols. Nurses also need to combine empirical theories with what they learn from aesthetic, ethical, personal knowing, and sociopolitical theories, which we discussed in Chapter 1, to create practice that is individualized and holistic.

KEYWORDS

Apply Existing Practice Guidelines	Evidence-Based Nursing
Combine Practice Activities with Research Activities	Evidence-Based Practice
	Evidence-Informed Practice
Evidence-Based Care	Integration
Evidence-Based Health-Care	Praxis
Evidence-Based Medicine	Theory-Based Practice

Recall from Chapter 1 that evidence-based practice is the use of evidence—that is, theory—to guide nursing practice. Evidence-based practice is essential if nurses and other health-care professionals are to meet society's mandate for high-quality and affordable health care that is effective and efficient (American Nurses' Association, 1997; Higgs & Jones, 2000; International Council of Nurses, 2007). We believe that all nurses are ultimately committed to evidence-based practice through the use of theory-based practice tools and intervention protocols. Many nurses are, however, so busy taking care of patients that little time is available for them to think critically and reflect on ways to translate theories into evidence-based tools and protocols (Pravikoff, Tanner, & Pierce, 2005). In this final chapter, we discuss strategies that all nurses can use to bring evidence-based practice to life by integrating nursing research and nursing practice.

WHAT IS INTEGRATION?

Integration refers to bringing together, mixing, combining, uniting, or balancing separate parts to form a larger whole (Oxford English Dictionary, 2007; Whittemore, 2005). Integration can also be thought of as the merger or interaction of two or more discrete entities—or separate things—to form a new unified entity (Westra & Rodgers, 1991).

BOX 16-1	Equivalence of Research/Practice Integration and Evidence-Based Practice

- Research = Theory
- Theory = Evidence
- Practice = Research
- Integration of research and practice = Evidence-based practice
- Evidence-based practice = Theory-based practice

The result of the integration of research and practice is the new, balanced, and unified entity of **evidence-based practice** that we regard as equivalent to **theory-based practice** (Box 16–1). Evidence-based practice is also referred to as **evidence-based nursing, evidence-based care, evidence-based health-care, evidence-informed practice**, or in the case of medicine, **evidence-based medicine** (Nieswiadomy, 2008; Rempher, 2006).

Integrating research and practice has resulted in elimination of any gap between the two entities, and because research is equivalent to theory development, it also eliminates the gap between theory and practice. Practice that eliminates any gaps between theory, research, and practice is sometimes called **praxis**. Rolfe (2006) explained that praxis is a "coming together of practice and research as . . . the same act" (p. 43). The integration of research and practice, evidence-based practice, theory-based practice, and praxis are, therefore, equivalent.

The Outcome of Integrating Research and Practice

When research and practice are integrated, practice is no longer based solely on the traditions and routines that come from using tenacious beliefs, authority, and *a priori* as sources of knowledge (see Table 1–2 in Chapter 1). The natural outcome of integrating research and practice is nurses' continual questioning of their observations of what is happening as they practice. Three questions to ask about what is happening in practice are:

- What works well?
- What could work better?
- What is missing?

HOW ARE NURSES' OBSERVATIONS CONVERTED TO EVIDENCE-BASED PRACTICE?

All nurses have opportunities to turn their observations of what works well, what could work better, and what is missing into evidence-based practice. We have identified two strategies for integrating research and practice by converting observations into evidence-based practice—namely, combining practice and research and applying existing practice guidelines.

Combining Practice and Research

There are various approaches to combining practice and research, all of which require consideration of ethical and practical issues.

Approaches to Combining Practice and Research

One strategy that can be used to convert observations into evidence-based practice is to **combine practice activities with research activities**. Single-case research (such as the *N*-of-1, single subject, and case study research designs discussed in Chapter 7) is an effective and relatively easy approach to combining practice and research. Another effective and relatively easy approach is to conduct audits of information that is routinely gathered in practice.

Single-case research (Rolfe, 2006) can be conducted when each encounter between a nurse and a patient is viewed as research as well as practice. When single-case research is done as a specific project, the data from many single cases can be aggregated. Each nurse may want to aggregate his or her own single cases, or several nurses may pool their single cases.

Single-case research involves use of a practice tool or an intervention protocol that was translated from research findings that met the criterion of pragmatic adequacy, which we discussed in Chapter 14. In other words, research instruments can be translated into practice tools, and experimental treatments can be translated into intervention protocols.

For example, for one single-case research project, nursing students and staff nurses used two research instruments—the Perception Of Birth Experience Scale (POBES) and the Cesarean Birth Experience Questionnaire (CBEQ)—as practice tools to assess women's perceptions of and responses to unplanned and planned cesarean birth (Fawcett, Aber, & Weiss, 2003; Fawcett et al., 2005). The impetus for this project was nurses' observations that some women had negative perceptions and responses to cesarean childbirth, whereas others had neutral or positive perceptions and responses. The observations were supported by a series of Roy Adaptation Model–based theory-generating and -testing studies that involved use of psychometrically sound research instruments (the POBES and the CBEQ) as practice tools (Fawcett, 1981; Fawcett & Burritt, 1985; Fawcett, Pollio, & Tully, 1992; Fawcett & Weiss, 1993; Reichert, Baron, & Fawcett, 1993).

Each undergraduate student and each staff nurse assessed one woman using the POBES and the CBEQ. The assessment information obtained from each woman was then coded and entered into a database by faculty researchers, who analyzed the data and prepared reports of the aggregate data. The example of a research report, in the Chapter 3 files on the CD that comes with book, includes an analysis of the perceptions and responses of the women who participated in this project at one of the several locations used.

Audits of information gathered while caring for patients are rarely thought of as an approach to converting nurses' observations into evidence-based practice. Instead, audits are frequently done within the context of quality improvement projects, which involve evaluating health-care services to determine if they are consistent with particular outcome standards and identifying how the services can be improved (Macnee & McCabe, 2008). An example of an audit done within a research context is Tomlinson's and Gibson's (2006) evaluation of the quality of an intervention protocol for treatment of obstructive sleep apnea syndrome. They explained, "The information was gathered as part of routine clinical care. . . . [T]his was essentially an audit of clinical practice" (p. 394).

Ethical Issues in Use of Practice Information as Research Data

When information gathered in practice is to be used as research data, ethical and practical issues must be considered. **Ethical issues** concern obtaining approval for the project by an institutional review board (IRB) or ethics committee and obtaining informed consent from the people from whom the information is to be gathered. Single-case research typically requires IRB or ethics committee approval and informed consent for use of the practice information as research data. For example, IRB or ethics committee approval and informed consent by the women participants at each of four sites in the United States and sites in Finland and Australia was required for the single-case research project conducted by Fawcett et al. (2005).

Nurses who plan to use practice information as research data have an ethical obligation not to coerce patients to participate in the project. Bell (2007) explained the ethical aspects of recruiting patients into her own research projects while practicing as a nurse-midwife. She stated, "As a [researcher], I must not erode a woman's autonomy by communicating subtle expectations for her to join my study. Recognition of vulnerabilities toward unethical conduct requires honesty and integrity in both professional roles" (p. 73).

Audits may or may not require IRB or ethics committee approval, and they do not usually require informed consent. However, some institutions in some countries may require the audit project to be submitted to an IRB or ethics committee to determine if it is exempt from review. Other institutions and other countries may not require submission of the audit project to an IRB or ethics committee. For example, Tomlinson and Gibson (2006), who conducted their evaluation of a sleep apnea intervention protocol in the United Kingdom, stated, "As this was essentially an audit of clinical practice, ethical approval was not sought" (p. 394).

Practical Issues in Use of Practice Information as Research Data

Practical issues concern the appropriateness of using a research instrument as a practice tool and the quality of the information. If a research instrument is to be used to gather information in practice, the length of the instrument, the reading level, and the ease with which it can be completed need to be considered, as does the relevance of the instrument items for the target cultural group (Garity, 2000). In general, short instruments made up of culturally relevant items are preferable to longer ones, as are instruments that are easy to complete by either the nurse or the patient. In addition, the reading level of the instrument should be consistent with the literacy ability of the people with whom it will be used.

The quality of the information depends on the extent to which the information was documented in a systematic and usable manner (Dalton, 2004; Jairath & Fain, 1999). Every step of the nursing process has to be carefully documented if the information gathered by practicing nurses, including students and staff nurses, is to be used as research data. The quality of the information will most likely be increased if the information is gathered using a research instrument that is appropriate for use as a practice tool. Information quality also depends on the trustworthiness—that is, the dependability and credibility—of instruments that provide qualitative data and the psychometric properties—that is, the reliability and validity—of instruments that provide quantitative data. If a research instrument is not used as the practice tool, and if the trustworthiness or psychometric properties of the practice tool have not been estimated, "the best method of measuring the variable may not be available" (Dalton, 2004, p. 450).

Applying Existing Practice Guidelines

Another strategy that can be used to convert observations into evidence-based practice is to **apply existing practice guidelines**. Evidence-based practice occurs when practice guidelines, which provide recommendations for practice in a concise format, are applied in specific health-care situations with particular populations (Scott-Findlay, 2005; Wallin, 2005). For example, Winfield, Davis, Schwaner, Conaway, and Burns (2007) described their review and application of a practice guideline for an effective dressing to cover and stabilize intravenous lines. In recent years, many other practice guidelines have been made available on the Internet by professional nursing and other organizations, as we discussed in Chapter 14.

Evaluating Use of Practice Guidelines

Any plan for application of a practice guideline should include an evaluation of the result. A comprehensive evaluation encompasses examination of outcomes for patients, health-care providers, and the health-care agency (Burns & Grove, 2007). Patient outcomes to be evaluated include effectiveness of the guideline in improving health, ease of access to care, and satisfaction with care. Health-care provider outcomes to be evaluated include perceptions of the positive and negative aspects of changes required in usual practice, resources needed to learn any new skills required to implement the guidelines, and barriers to use of the guidelines. Health-care agency outcomes to be evaluated include the cost of educating providers to use the guideline, the cost of any new equipment needed, and long-term cost savings from more effective health care.

Evaluation of the outcomes of applying a practice guideline is necessary to avoid the guideline becoming a routine that is not questioned and to continue the emphasis on evidence-based practice. Evaluation can be done by means of single-case research with each person with whom the guideline was used, or by means of an audit of the documentation of the outcomes.

WHAT ARE THE REQUIREMENTS FOR INTEGRATING RESEARCH AND PRACTICE?

The basic requirement for integrating research and practice is a commitment to do so. Several barriers to evidence-based practice have been identified (Adib-Hajbaghery, 2007; Gerrish et al., 2007; LaPierre, Ritchey, Newhouse, 2004; Pravikoff et al., 2005), such as lack of knowledge of the meaning and value of evidence-based practice, limited access to research reports, lack of administrative support, lack of time, and lack of ability to change practice activities. Each barrier can, however, be overcome when practicing nurses and nursing leaders work together.

All nurses who are sufficiently committed to the goal of evidence-based practice can integrate research and practice. Integration is easier, however, if strong support is given by the nurse leaders in a health-care organization, such as the chief nursing officer and the nurse managers. Nurse leaders can demonstrate their support by advocating the development of organizational policies that foster evidence-based practice, creating an environment emphasizing the highest quality of nursing care, being accessible to staff nurses, and addressing the concerns of each staff nurse (Scott-Findlay, 2007). Provision of the educational resources and time required by staff nurses to learn any new clinical skills that may be required to apply a practice guideline, engage in single-case research, or conduct an audit is crucial. Staff nurses also need access to computer hardware and software for searching the Internet and library databases for practice guidelines.

Nurses who provide direct nursing care have to do more than support evidence-based practice. They have to assume responsibility and be accountable for integrating research and practice by engaging in single-case research, conducting audits, and applying practice guidelines.

Conclusion

Evidence-based practice is considered a complex process that involves the three stages we identified in Chapter 14: becoming aware of a new practice tool or intervention protocol, deciding to adopt the new tool or protocol, and implementing the new tool or protocol (see Box 14–4). We agree that when evidence-based practice requires changing the culture of an entire profession—such as nursing—or an entire health-care agency, the process is indeed complex. We believe, however, that all readers of this book can carry out single-case research, conduct audits of their own practice, and apply practice guidelines with relative ease.

The integration of research and practice occurs when thinking about evidence-based practice becomes a habit. Kearney (2002) explained, "The goal is to make a habit of considering the evidence. When something you regularly do to or for patients carries risks or discomforts, be sure you have adequate evidence of its benefits" (p. 499). We believe that each nurse should have adequate evidence of the benefits of *everything* that is done to or for patients, not just risky or uncomfortable procedures. We also believe that the habit of considering the evidence should be extended to the habit of thinking of evidence-based practice as theory-based practice.

Opportunities to integrate research and practice, as well as the challenges of doing so, "are available to every professional nurse and provide pathways to embrace the journey of nursing with enthusiasm and anticipation" (Sanares & Heliker, 2006, p. 31). The learning activities for this chapter will help you continue to increase your understanding of how research and practice can be integrated.

References

Full citations for all references cited in this chapter are provided in the Reference section at the end of the book.

Learning Activities

Activities to supplement what you have learned in this chapter, along with practice examination questions, are provided on the CD that comes with this book.

References

Abraham, I. L., & Wasserbauer, L. I. (2006). Experimental research. In J. J. Fitzpatrick & M. Wallace (Eds.), *Encyclopedia of nursing research* (2nd ed., pp. 185–187). New York: Springer.

Adib-Hajbaghery, M. (2007). Factors facilitating and inhibiting evidence-based nursing in Iran. *Journal of Advanced Nursing, 58*, 566–575.

Ajzen, I. (1991). The theory of planned behavior. *Organizational Behavior and Human Decision Processes, 50*, 179–211.

Allen, D. (1995). Hermeneutics: Philosophical traditions and nursing practice research. *Nursing Science Quarterly, 8*, 174–182.

Alliance for Human Research Protection. (2005, May 4). *A national scandal: AIDS drug experiments on foster care children*. Retrieved May 28, 2007, from http://www.ahrp.org/infomail/05/05/04.php

Alligood, M. R. (1991). Testing Rogers' theory of accelerating change. The relationships among creativity, actualization, and empathy in persons 18 to 92 years of age. *Western Journal of Nursing Research, 13*, 84–96.

Alligood, M. R. (2002). A theory of the art of nursing discovered in Rogers' science of unitary human beings. *International Journal for Human Caring, 6*(2), 55–60.

Alligood, M. R. (2006). Introduction to nursing theory: Its history, significance, and analysis. In A. Marriner Tomey & M. R. Alligood (Eds.), *Nursing theorists and their work* (6th ed., pp. 3–15). St. Louis: Mosby Elsevier.

Alligood, M. R., & Fawcett, J. (1999). Acceptance of the invitation to dialogue: Examination of an interpretive approach for the Science of Unitary Human Beings. *Visions: The Journal of Rogerian Nursing Science, 7*, 5–13.

Alligood, M. R., & Fawcett, J. (2004). An interpretive study of Martha Rogers' conception of pattern. *Visions: The Journal of Rogerian Nursing Science, 12*, 8–13.

Alligood, M. R., & May, B. A. (2000). A nursing theory of personal system empathy: Interpreting a conceptualization of empathy in King's interacting systems. *Nursing Science Quarterly, 13*, 243–247.

Alligood, M. R., & McGuire, S. L. (2000). Perception of time, sleep patterns, and activity in senior citizens: A test of Rogerian theory of aging. *Visions: The Journal of Rogerian Nursing Science, 8*, 6–14.

Almost, J. (2006). Conflict within nursing work environments: Concept analysis. *Journal of Advanced Nursing, 53*, 444–453.

American Association of Colleges of Nursing. (2005). Position statement on nursing research (Draft 9-21-05). Washington, DC: Author.

American Hospital Association. (1992). *A patient's bill of rights*. Chicago: Author.

American Nurses' Association. (1997). Position statements: Education for participation in nursing research. Retrieved June 29, 2007, from http://www.nursingworld.org/readroom/position/reaserch/rseducat.htm

American Nurses' Association. (2001). *Code of ethics for nurses with interpretive statements*. Silver Spring, MD: ANA Publications. Retrieved February 21, 2007, from http://nursingworld.org/ethics/code/protected_nwcoe303.htm

ANA's Code of Ethics Project Task Force. (2000). A new code of ethics for nurses. *American Journal of Nursing, 100*(7), 70–72.

Anders, R., Daly, J., Thompson, D., Elliott, D., & Chang, E. (2005). Research in nursing. In J. Daly, S. Speedy, D. Jackson, V. A. Lambert, & C. E. Lambert (Eds.), *Professional nursing: Concepts, issues, and challenges* (pp. 153–174). New York: Springer.

Andrews, T., & Waterman, H. (2005). Packaging: A grounded theory of how to report physiological deterioration effectively. *Journal of Advanced Nursing, 52*, 473–481.

Arndt, M. J., & Horodynski, M. A. O. (2004). Theory of dependent–care in research with parents of toddlers: The NEAT project. *Nursing Science Quarterly, 17*, 345–350.

Aschen, S. R. (1997). Assertion training therapy in psychiatric milieus. *Archives of Psychiatric Nursing, 11*, 46–51.

Atkinson, P., & Hammersley, M. (1994). Ethnography and participant observation. In N. K. Denzin & Y. S. Lincoln (Eds.), *Handbook of qualitative research* (pp. 248–261). Thousand Oaks, CA: Sage.

Avant, K. C. (2000). The Wilson method of concept analysis. In B. L. Rodgers & K. A. Knafl (Eds.). *Concept development in nursing: Foundations, techniques, and applications* (2nd ed., pp. 55–76). Philadelphia: Saunders.

Babbie, E. (1990). *Survey research methods* (2nd ed.). Belmont, CA: Wadsworth.

Babbie, E. (1998). *The practice of social research* (8th ed.). Belmont, CA: Wadsworth.

Backman, C. L., & Harris, S. R. (1999). Case studies, single–subject research, and N of 1 randomized trials: Comparisons and contrasts. *American Journal of Physical Medicine and Rehabilitation, 78*, 170–176.

Bandman, E. L. (1985). Protection of human subjects. *Topics in Clinical Nursing, 7*, 115–123.

Bandman, E. L., & Bandman, B. (2002). *Nursing ethics through the life span* (4th ed.). Upper Saddle River, NJ: Prentice–Hall.

Bandura, A. (1997). *Self-efficacy: The exercise of control.* New York: Freeman Impact Publishers.

Barnum, B. J. S. (1998). *Nursing theory: Analysis, application, evaluation* (5th ed.). Philadelphia: Lippincott.

Barrett, E. A. M. (1986). Investigation of the principle of helicy: The relationship of human field motion and power. In V. M. Malinski (Ed.), *Explorations on Martha Rogers' science of unitary human beings* (pp. 173–188). Norwalk, CT: Appleton–Century–Crofts.

Barrett, E. A. M. (2000). The theoretical matrix for a Rogerian nursing practice. *Theoria: Journal of Nursing Theory, 9*(4), 3–7.

Barrett, E. A. M., Cowling, W. R., III, Carboni, J. T., & Butcher, H. K. (1997). Unitary perspectives on methodological practices. In M. Madrid (Ed.), *Patterns of Rogerian knowing* (pp. 47–62). New York: National League for Nursing Press.

Barry, J. M. (1997). *Rising tide: The great Mississippi flood of 1927 and how it changed America.* New York: Touchstone/Simon and Schuster.

Bauer, M. (2006). Collaboration and control: Nurses' constructions of the role of family in nursing home care. *Journal of Advanced Nursing, 54*, 45–52.

Baumann, S. L. (2003). The lived experience of feeling very tired: A study of adolescent girls. *Nursing Science Quarterly, 16*, 326–333.

Beanlands, H., Horsburgh, M. E., Fox, S., Howe, A., Locking-Cusolito, H., Pare, K., & Thrasher, C. (2005). Caregiving by family and friends of adults receiving dialysis. *Nephrology Nursing Journal, 32*, 621–631.

Beauchamp, T. C., & Childress, J. F. (1994). *Principles of biomedical ethics* (4th ed.). New York: Oxford University Press.

Beck, A. T. (1976). *Cognitive therapy and emotional disorders.* New York: International Universities Press.

Beck, C. T., Bernal, H., & Froman, R. D. (2003). Methods to document semantic equivalence of a translated scale. *Research in Nursing and Health, 26*, 64–73.

Becker, M. H. (Ed.).(1974). *The health belief model and personal health behavior.* Thorofare, NJ: Charles B. Slack.

Bell, A. F. (2007). Nurse–midwife and scientist: Stuck in the middle? *Journal of Obstetric, Gynecologic, and Neonatal Nursing, 36,* 71–73.

Bengtson, V. L., Acock, A. C., Allen, K. R., Dilworth-Anderson, P., & Klein, D. M. (2005). Theory and theorizing in family research: Puzzle building and puzzle solving. In V. L. Bengtson, A. C. Acock, K. R. Allen, P. Dilworth-Anderson, & D. M. Klein (Eds.), *Sourcebook of family theory and research* (pp. 3–33). Thousand Oaks, CA: Sage.

Bent, K. N., Burke, J. A., Eckman, A., Hottmann, T., McCabe, J., & Williams, R. N. (2005). Being and creating caring change in a healthcare system. *International Journal for Human Caring, 9*(3), 20–25.

Bernstein, B. (Producer). (1994). *Armchair fitness: Gentle exercise* [Motion picture]. (Available from CC-M Productions, 8512 Cedar St., Silver Spring, MD 20920.)

Beyer, J. E., Turner, S. R., Jones, L., Young, L., Onikul, R., & Bobaty, B. (2005). The alternate forms of the Oucher pain scale. *Pain Management Nursing, 6*(1), 10–17.

Boas, F. (1948). *Race, language and culture.* New York: Macmillan.

Bournaki, M.-C. (1997). Correlates of pain-related responses to venipunctures in school-age children. *Nursing Research, 46,* 147–154.

Bournes, D. A., & Ferguson-Paré, M. (2005). Persevering through a difficult time during the SARS outbreak in Toronto. *Nursing Science Quarterly, 18,* 324–333.

Bowen, M. (1985). *Family therapy in clinical practice.* New York: Jason Aronson.

Breckenridge, D. (1997). Decisions regarding dialysis treatment modality: A holistic perspective. *Holistic Nursing Practice, 12*(1), 54–61.

Brett, J. L. L. (1987). Use of nursing practice research findings. *Nursing Research, 36,* 344–349.

Brillhart, B. (2005). Pressure sore and skin tear prevention and treatment during a 10-month program. *Rehabilitation Nursing, 30,* 85–91.

Brink, P. J. (2001). Representing the population in qualitative research. *Western Journal of Nursing Research, 23,* 661–663.

Brooks, E. M., & Thomas, S. (1997). The perception and judgment of senior baccalaureate student nurses in clinical decision making. *Advances in Nursing Science, 19*(3), 50–69.

Brooten, D., & Youngblut, J. M. (2006). Nurse dose as a concept. *Journal of Nursing Scholarship, 38,* 94–99.

Brown, J. (Ed.). (1992). *A promise to remember: The NAMES project book of letters.* New York: Grolier.

Brown, S., North, D., Marvel, M. K., & Fons, R. (1992). Acupressure wristbands to relieve nausea and vomiting in hospice patients: Do they work? *American Journal of Hospice and Palliative Care, 7,* 26–29.

Brown, S. J. (1999). *Knowledge of health care practice: A guide to using research evidence.* Philadelphia: Saunders.

Browne, A. J. (2001). The influence of liberal political ideology on nursing science. *Nursing Inquiry, 8,* 118–129.

Browne, A. J. (2004). Response to critique of "The influence of liberal political ideology on nursing science." *Nursing Inquiry, 11,* 122–123.

Buckner, E. B., Hawkins, A. M., Stover, L., Brakefield, J., Simmons, S., Foster, C., Payne, S. L., Newsome, J., & Dubois, G. (2005). Knolwedge, resilience, and effectiveness of education in a young teen asthma camp. *Pediatric Nursing, 31,* 201–207, 210.

Bultemeier, K. (1993). Photographic inquiry of the phenomenon premenstrual syndrome within the Rogerian derived theory of perceived dissonance. *Dissertation Abstracts International, 54,* 2531A.

Bultemeier, K. (1997). Photo-disclosure: A research methodology for investigating unitary human beings. In M. Madrid (Ed.), *Patterns of Rogerian knowing* (pp. 63–74). New York: National League for Nursing Press.

Bunkers, S. S. (2003). Comparison of three Parse method studies on feeling very tired. The lived experience of feeling very tired: A study using the Parse research method. *Nursing Science Quarterly, 16*, 340–344.

Burns, D. (2004). Physical and psychosocial adaptation of Blacks on hemodialysis. *Applied Nursing Research, 17*, 116–124.

Burns, N., & Grove, S. K. (2007). *Understanding nursing research: Building an evidence-based practice* (4th ed.). Philadelphia: Saunders Elsevier.

Butcher, H. K. (1996). A unitary field pattern portrait of dispiritedness in later life. *Visions: The Journal of Rogerian Nursing Science, 4*, 41–58.

Butcher, H. K. (2006). Part Two: Applications of Rogers' science of unitary human beings. In M. E. Parker (Ed.), *Nursing theories and nursing practice* (2nd ed., pp. 167–186). Philadelphia: F. A. Davis.

Butcher, H. K. (1993). Kaleidoscoping in life's turbulence: From Seurat's art to Rogers' nursing science. In M.E. Parker (Ed.), *Patterns of nursing theories in practice* (pp. 183–198). New York: National League for Nursing.

Butcher, H. K. (1996). A unitary field pattern portrait of dispiritedness in later life. *Visions: The Journal of Rogerian Nursing Science, 4*, 41–58.

Butcher, H. K. (2003). Aging as emerging brilliance: Advancing Rogers' unitary theory of aging. *Visions: The Journal of Rogerian Nursing Science, 11*, 55–66.

Callaghan, D. (2005). The influence of spiritual growth on adolescents' initiative and responsibility for self-care. *Pediatric Nursing, 31*, 91–95, 115.

Campbell, D. T., & Fiske, D. W. (1959). Convergent and discriminant validation by the multitrait–multimethod matrix. *Psychological Bulletin, 56*, 81–105.

Campbell, D. T., & Stanley, J. C. (1963). *Experimental and quasi-experimental designs for research.* Chicago: Rand-McNally.

Canadian Institutes of Health Research. (2004). Knowledge translation strategy 2004–2009. Retrieved July 2, 2007, from http://www.cihr-irsc.gc.ca/e/26574.html#defining.

Carboni, J. T. (1995). A Rogerian process of inquiry. *Nursing Science Quarterly, 8*, 22–37.

Carboni, J. T. (1998). Coming home: An investigation of the enfolding–unfolding movement of human environmental energy field patterns within the nursing home setting and the enfoldment of health–as–wholeness–and-harmony by the nurse and client. *Dissertation Abstracts International, 58*, 4136B. (UMI No. 9805231)

Carmines, E. G., & Zeller, R. A. (1979). *Reliability and validity assessment.* Beverly Hills, CA: Sage.

Caron, C. D., & Bowers, B. J. (2000). Methods and application of dimensional analysis: A contribution to concept and knowledge development in nursing. In B. L. Rodgers & K. A. Knafl (Eds.), *Concept development in nursing: Foundations, techniques, and applications* (2nd ed., pp. 285–319). Philadelphia: Saunders.

Caroselli, C., & Barrett, E. A. M. (1998). A review of the power as knowing participation in change literature. *Nursing Science Quarterly, 11*, 9–16.

Carper, B. A. (1978). Fundamental patterns of knowing in nursing. *Advances in Nursing Science, 1*(1), 13–23.

Casalenuovo, G. A. (2002). Fatigue in diabetes mellitus: Testing a middle-range theory of well-being derived from the Neuman's theory of optimal client system stability and the Neuman systems model. *Dissertation Abstracts International, 63*, 2301B.

Cha, E.-S., Kim, K. H., & Erlen, J. A. (2007). Translation of scales in cross-cultural research: Issues and techniques. *Journal of Advanced Nursing, 58*, 386–395.

Chair, S. Y., Taylor-Piliae, R. E., Lam, G., & Chan, S. (2003). Effect of positioning on back pain after coronary angiography. *Journal of Advanced Nursing, 42*, 470–478.

Chan, M. F., Wong, H. L., Fong, M. C., Lai, S. Y., Wah, C., Ho, S. M., Ng, S. Y., & Leung, S. K. (2006). Effects of music on patients undergoing a C-clamp procedure after percutaneous coronary intervention. *Journal of Advanced Nursing, 53*, 669–679.

Chinn, P. L. (2001). Toward a theory of nursing art. In N. L. Chaska (Ed.), *The nursing profession: Tomorrow and beyond* (pp. 287–297). Thousand Oaks, CA: Sage. [Reprinted in Andrist, L. C., Nicholas, P. K., & Wolf, K. A. (2006). *A history of nursing ideas* (pp. 73–183). Boston: Jones and Bartlett.]

Chinn, P. L., & Kramer, M. K. (2004). *Theory and nursing: Integrated knowledge development* (6th ed.). St. Louis: Mosby.

Chiou, C.-P. (2000). A meta-analysis of the interrelationships between the modes of Roy's adaptation model. *Nursing Science Quarterly, 13*, 252–258.

Cipriano, P. (2007). On the record with Pamela Cipriano, Editor-in-Chief. *American Nurse Today, 2*(4), 26–27.

Cody, W. K. (1995). Of life immense in passion, pulse, and power: Dialoguing with Whitman and Parse—A hermeneutic study. In R. R. Parse (Ed.), *Illuminations: The human becoming theory in practice and research* (pp. 269–307). New York: National League for Nursing.

Cohen, J. (1988). *Statistical power analysis for the behavioral sciences* (2nd ed.). Hillsdale, NJ: Lawrence Erlbaum.

Cohen, J. (1992). A power primer. *Psychological Bulletin, 112*, 155–159.

Cohen, J., & Cohen, P. (1975). *Applied multiple regression/correlation analysis for the behavioral sciences.* Hillsdale, NJ: Lawrence Erlbaum Associates.

Cohen, M. R., & Nagel, E. (1934). *An introduction to logic and scientific method.* New York: Harcourt, Brace.

Cohen, M. Z. (2006). Introduction to qualitative research. In G. LoBiondo-Wood & J. Haber, *Nursing research: Methods and critical appraisal for evidence-based practice* (6th ed., pp. 131–147). St. Louis: Mosby Elsevier.

Cohen, M. Z., Kahn, D. L., & Steeves, R. H. (2002). Making use of qualitative research. *Western Journal of Nursing Research, 24*, 454–471.

Cohen, R., Ehrlich-Jones, L., Burns, K., Frank-Stromborg, M., Flanagan, J., & Askins, D. L. (2005). The nursing shortage: Can we look to teachers as a source of support? *Nursing Forum, 40*(3), 88–95.

Cohen, S. S., Mason, D. J., Kovner, C., Leavitt, J. K., Pulcini, J., & Stolchalski, J. (1996). Stages of nursing's political development: Where we've been and where we ought to go. *Nursing Outlook, 44*, 259–266.

Colaizzi, P. F. (1978). Psychological research as the phenomenologist views it. In R. Valle & M. King (Eds.), *Existential phenomenological alternative for psychology* (pp. 48–71). New York: Oxford University Press.

Coleman, E. A., Tulman, L., Samarel, N., Wilmoth, M. C., Rickel, L., Rickel, M., & Stewart, C. B. (2005). The effect of telephone social support and education on adaptation to breast cancer during the year following diagnosis. *Oncology Nursing Forum, 32*, 822–829.

Colling, J., Owen, T. R., McCreedy, M., & Newman, D. (2003). The effects of a continence program on frail community-dwelling elderly persons. *Urologic Nursing, 23*, 117–131.

Comfrey, A. L., & Lee, H. B. (1992). *A first course in factor analysis.* Hillsdale, NJ: Lawrence Erlbaum.

Condon, L., Gill, H., & Harris, F. (2007). A reivew of prison health and its implications for primary care nursing in England and Wales: The research evidence. *Journal of Clinical Nursing, 16*, 1201–1209.

Consumer Affairs. (2004, September 30). Merck withdraws Vioxx after negative reactions among patients in study. Retrieved May 28, 2007, from http://www.consumeraffairs.com/news04/vioxx.html

Cook, A. M., Pierce, L. L., Hicks, B., & Steiner, V. (2006). Self-care needs of caregivers dealing with stroke. *Journal of Neuroscience Nursing, 38*, 31–36.

Cook, T. D., & Campbell, D. T. (1979). *Quasi-experimentation: Design and analysis issues for field settings.* Boston: Houghton Mifflin.

Cooper, H. M. (1989). *Integrating research: A guide for literature reviews* (2nd ed.). Newbury Park, CA: Sage.

Copnell, B., & Bruni, N. (2006). Breaking the silence: Nurses' understandings of change in clinical practice. *Journal of Advanced Nursing, 55,* 301–309.

Cowen, M. (2005). Use of modeling parties to enhance research. *Journal of Nursing Scholarship, 37,* 298–299.

Cowling, W. R., III. (2001). Unitary appreciative inquiry. *Advances in Nursing Science, 23*(4), 32–48.

Cowling, W. R., III. (2004). Despair: A unitary appreciative inquiry. *Advances in Nursing Science, 27,* 287–300.

Creswell, J. W. (1998). *Qualitative inquiry and research design: Choosing among five traditions.* Thousand Oaks, CA: Sage.

Creswell, J. W. (2003). *Research design: Qualitative, quantitative, and mixed methods approaches* (2nd ed.). Thousand Oaks, CA: Sage.

Creswell, J. W., & Tashakkori, A. (Eds.). (2006). Journal of Mixed Methods Research: Definition of mixed methods research. Retrieved April 16, 2006, from http://www.sagepub.com/journal.aspx?pid=11777

Croteau, A., Marcoux, S., & Brisson, C. (2006). Work activity in pregnancy, preventive measures, and the risk of delivering a small-for-gestational-age infant. *American Journal of Public Health, 96,* 846–855.

Cumulative Index of Nursing and Allied Health Literature. (2005). Scope notes for nursing–practice-evidence-based. Retrieved December 27, 2005, from http://www.cinahl.com/wcgis/dsplscopre.p?term=nursing-practice-evidence-based

Currie, P. M. (2005). Balancing privacy protections with efficient research: Institutional review boards and the use of certificates of confidentiality. *IRB: Ethics and Human Research, 27*(5), 7–13.

Daiski, I. (2004). Response to "The influence of liberal political ideology on nursing science." *Nursing Inquiry, 11,* 117–121.

Dally, A. (1998). Thalidomide: Was the tragedy preventable? *Lancet, 351,* 1197–1199.

Dalton, J. M. (2004). Designing a project to evaluate a home care diabetes disease management program. *Diabetes Educator, 30*(3), 432, 434, 437–440, 442, 444, 449–450.

Dalton, J., Garvey, J., & Samia, L. W. (2006). Evaluation of a diabetes disease management home care program. *Home Health Care Management and Practice, 18,* 272–285.

Dennis, C.-L., & Faux, S. (1999). Development and psychometric testing of the Breastfeeding Self-Efficacy Scale. *Research in Nursing and Health, 22,* 399–409.

De Oliveira, E. A. A., & Hoga, L. A. K. (2005). The process of seeking and undergoing surgical contraception: An ethnographic study in a Brazilian community. *Journal of Transcultural Nursing, 16,* 5–14.

DeSanto-Madeya, S. (2006a). The meaning of living with spinal cord injury 5 to 10 years after the injury. *Western Journal of Nursing Research, 28,* 265–289.

DeSanto Madeya, S. (2006b). A secondary analysis of the meaning of living with spinal cord injury using Roy's adaptation model. *Nursing Science Quarterly, 19,* 240–246.

DeVellis, R. F. (2003). *Scale development: Theory and applications.* Thousand Oaks, CA: Sage.

DeVon, H. A., Block, M. E., Moyle-Wright, P., Ernst, D. M., Hayden, S. J., Lazzara, D. J., Savoy, S. M., & Dostas-Plston, E. (2007). A psychometric toolbox for testing validity and reliability. *Journal of Nursing Scholarship, 39,* 155–164.

Diers, D. (2005). Am I a nurse? *American Journal of Nursing, 105*(10), 39.

Dilthey, W. (1961). *Pattern and meaning in history: Thoughts on history and society* (H. P. Rickman, Ed., Trans.). New York: Harper and Row.

Donaldson, S. K., & Crowley, D. M. (1978). The discipline of nursing. *Nursing Outlook, 26,* 113–120.

Donly, K. J., Henson, T., Jamison, D., & Gerlach, R. W. (2006). Pediatric dentistry. Clinical trial evaluating two peroxide whitening strips used by teenagers. *General Dentistry, 54*, 110–112.

Dono, J. (2005). Introducing companion animals into nursing homes. *Nursing and Residential Care, 7*, 265–268.

Doornbos, M. M. (1995). Using King's systems framework to explore family health in the families of the young chronically mentally ill. In M. A. Frey & C. L. Sieloff (Eds.), *Advancing King's systems framework and theory of nursing* (pp. 192–205). Thousand Oaks, CA: Sage.

Doornbos, M. M. (2000). King's systems framework and family health: The derivation and testing of a theory. *Journal of Theory Construction and Testing, 4*, 20–26.

Doornbos, M. M. (2002). Predicting family health in families of young adults with severe mental illness. *Journal of Family Nursing, 8*, 241–263.

Downs, F. S. (1984). *A sourcebook of nursing research* (3rd ed.). Philadelphia: F. A. Davis.

Driever, M. J. (2002). Are evidence-based practice and best practice the same? *Western Journal of Nursing Research, 24*, 591–597.

Duffy, M., & Muhlenkamp, A. F. (1974). A framework for theory analysis. *Nursing Outlook, 22*, 570–574.

Du Mont, P. M. (1998). The effects of early menarche on health risk behaviors. *Dissertation Abstracts International, 60*, 3200B.

Dunn, K. S. (2004). Toward a middle-range theory of adaptation to chronic pain. *Nursing Science Quarterly, 17*, 78–84.

Dzurec, L. C. (1998). Certainty, leaps of faith, and tradition: Rethinking clinical interventions. *Advances in Nursing Science, 21*(2), 52–61.

Eakes, G. G., Burke, M. L., & Hainsworth, M. A. (1998). Middle range theory of chronic sorrow. *Image: Journal of Nursing Scholarship, 30*, 179–184.

Ehrenberger, H. E. (2000). Testing a theory of decision making derived from King's systems framework in women eligible for a cancer clinical trial. *Dissertation Abstracts International, 60*, 3201B.

Ehrenberger, H. E., Alligood, M. R., Thomas, S. P., Wallace, D. C., & Licavoli, C. M. (2002). Testing a theory of decision-making derived from King's systems framework in women eligible for a cancer clinical trial. *Nursing Science Quarterly, 15*, 156–163.

Ellis, R. (1968). Characteristics of significant theories. *Nursing Research, 17*, 217–222.

Erikson, E. H. (1963). *Childhood and society* (2nd ed.). New York: Norton.

Faber, M. J., Bosscher, R. J., & van Wieringen, P. C. W. (2006). Clinimetric properties of the Performance-Oriented Mobility Assessment. *Physical Therapy, 86*, 944–954.

Fain, J. A. (2004). *Reading, understanding, and applying nursing research: A text and workbook* (2nd ed.). Philadelphia: F. A. Davis.

Family Educational Rights and Privacy Act. (1974). 20 U.S.C. 1232g; 34 CFR Part 99.

Farrell, M. P. (2006). Living evidence: Translating research into practice. In K. Malloch & T. Porter-O'Grady (Eds.), *Introduction to evidence-based practice in nursing and health care* (pp. 107–123). Boston: Jones and Bartlett.

Fathima, L. (2004). The effect of information booklet provided to caregivers of patients undergoing haemodialysis on knowledge of home care management. *Nursing Journal of India, 95*(4), 81–82.

Fawcett, J. (1981). Needs of cesarean birth parents. *Journal of Obstetric, Gynecologic, and Neonatal Nursing, 10*, 372–376.

Fawcett, J. (1996). Putting the conceptual model into the research report. *Nurse Author and Editor, 6*(2), 1–4.

Fawcett, J. (1998). Reporting research results: Let's not forget clinical significance. *Nurse Author and Editor, 8*(4), 1–4.

Fawcett, J. (1999). *The relationship of theory and research* (3rd ed.). Philadelphia: F. A. Davis.

Fawcett, J. (2002). On science and human science: A conversation with Marilyn M. Rawnsley. *Nursing Science Quarterly, 15,* 41–45.

Fawcett, J. (2005a). Appendix N-2: Conceptual models and theories of nursing. In *Taber's cyclopedic medical dictionary* (20th ed., pp 2588–2618). Philadelphia: F. A. Davis.

Fawcett, J. (2005b). *Contemporary nursing knowledge: Analysis and evaluation of nursing models and theories* (2nd ed.). Philadelphia: F. A. Davis.

Fawcett, J. (2006). The Roy Adaptation Model and content analysis. *Aquichan, 6*(1), 34–37.

Fawcett, J., Aber, C., & Weiss, M. (2003). Teaching, practice, and research: An integrative approach benefiting students and faculty. *Journal of Professional Nursing, 19,* 17–21.

Fawcett, J., Aber, C., Weiss, M., Haussler, S., Myers, S.T., King, C., Newton, J., & Silva, V. (2005). Adaptation to cesarean birth: Implementation of an international multisite study. *Nursing Science Quarterly, 18,* 204–210.

Fawcett, J., & Buhle, E. L., Jr. (1995). Using the Internet for data collection: An innovative electronic strategy. *Computers in Nursing 13,* 273–279.

Fawcett, J., & Burritt, J. (1985). An exploratory study of antenatal preparation for cesarean birth. *Journal of Obstetric, Gynecologic, and Neonatal Nursing, 14,* 224–230.

Fawcett, J., Myers, S. T., Hall, J. L., & Waters, L. (2007). *Women's adaptation to cesarean birth: Oklahoma site.* Unpublished data.

Fawcett, J., Pollio, N., & Tully, A. (1992). Women's perceptions of cesarean and vaginal delivery: Another look. *Research in Nursing and Health, 15,* 439–446.

Fawcett, J., Pollio, N., Tully, A., Baron, M., Henklein, J. C., & Jones, R. C. (1993). Effects of information on adaptation to cesarean birth. *Nursing Research, 42,* 49–53.

Fawcett, J., & Russell, G. (2001). A conceptual model of nursing and health policy. *Policy, Politics, and Nursing Practice, 2,* 108–116.

Fawcett, J., Schutt, R. K., Gall, G. B., Riley–Cruz, E., & Woodford, M. L. (2007). The work of nurse case managers in a cancer and cardiovascular disease risk screening program. *Professional Case Management: The Leader in Evidence-Based Practice* (formerly, *Lippincott's Case Management), 12,* 93–105.

Fawcett, J., Tulman, L., & Spedden, J. P. (1994). Responses to vaginal birth after cesarean (VBAC). *Journal of Obstetric, Gynecologic, and Neonatal Nursing, 23,* 253–259.

Fawcett, J., Watson, J., Neuman, B., Hinton-Walker, P., & Fitzpatrick, J. J. (2001). On theories and evidence. *Journal of Nursing Scholarship, 33,* 115–119.

Fawcett, J., & Weiss, M. E. (1993). Cross-cultural adaptation to cesarean birth. *Western Journal of Nursing Research, 15,* 282–297.

Feinstein, A. R. (1987). *Clinimetrics.* New Haven, CT: Yale University Press.

Feldt, K. S. (2000). The Checklist of Nonverbal Pain Indicators (CNPI). *Pain Management Nursing, 1,* 13–21.

Ference, H. M. (1986). The relationship of time experience, creativity traits, differentiation, and human field motion. In V. M. Malinski (Ed.), *Explorations on Martha Rogers' science of unitary human beings* (pp. 95–106). Norwalk, CT: Appleton-Century-CroftsFerence.

Fessenden, C. C. (2003). Adoption of testicular self-examination. *Dissertation Abstracts International, 63,* 5157B.

Finfgeld, D. (2003). Metasynthesis: The state of the art—so far. *Qualitative Health Research, 13,* 893–904.

Fishbein, M., & Ajzen, I. (1975). *Belief, attitude, intention, and behavior.* New York: Wiley.

Fisher, R. A. (1925). *Statistical methods for research workers.* London: Oliver and Boyd.

Fisher, R. A. (1935). *The design of experiments.* London: Oliver and Boyd.

Fitzpatrick, J. J., & Wallace, M. (Eds.). (2006). *Encyclopedia of nursing research* (2nd ed.). New York: Springer.

Fitzpatrick, J. J., & Whall, A. L. (2005). *Conceptual models of nursing: Analysis and application* (4th ed.). Upper Saddle River, NJ: Pearson/Prentice Hall.

Flaherty, J. A., Gaviria, F. M., Pathak, D., Mitchell, T., Wintrob, R., Richman, J. A., & Birz, S. (1988). Developing instruments for cross-cultural psychiatric research. *Journal of Nervous and Mental Diseases, 176,* 257–263.

Flood, M. (2005). A mid–range nursing theory of successful aging. *Journal of Theory Construction & Testing, 9,* 35–39.

Ford-Gilboe, M., Campbell, J., & Berman, H. (1995). Stories and numbers: Coexistence without compromise. *Advances in Nursing Science, 18*(1), 14–26.

Fowler, F. J., Jr. (1993). *Survey research methods* (2nd ed.). Newbury Park, CA: Sage.

Frankl, V. E. (1984). *Man's search for meaning: An introduction to logotherapy.* Boston: Beacon.

Freire, P. (1972). *Pedagogy of the oppressed.* London: Sheed and Ward.

Frey, M. A. (1989). Social support and health: A theoretical formulation derived from King's conceptual framework. *Nursing Science Quarterly, 2,* 138–148.

Frey, M. A. (1995). Toward a theory of families, children, and chronic illness. In M. A. Frey & C. L. Sieloff (Eds.), *Advancing King's systems framework and theory of nursing* (pp. 109–125). Thousand Oaks, CA: Sage.

Frey, M. A., Sieloff, C. L., & Norris, D. M. (2002). King's conceptual system and theory of goal attainment: Past, present, and future. *Nursing Science Quarterly, 15,* 107–112.

Fries, J. E. (1998). Health and social support of older adults. *Dissertation Abstracts International, 59,* 6262B.

Froman, R. D. (2000). Measuring our words on measurement. [Editorial]. *Research in Nursing and Health, 23,* 421–422.

Fry, S. (1991). Ethics in health care delivery. In J. L. Creasia & B. Parker (Eds.). *Conceptual foundations of professional nursing practice,* (pp. 149–164). St. Louis: Mosby.

Fulk, G. D. (2004). Locomotor training with body weight support after stroke: The effect of different training parameters. *Journal of Neurologic Physical Therapy, 28,* 20–28.

Funk, S. G., Tornquist, E. M., & Champagne, M. T. (1995). Barriers and facilitators of research utilization. *Nursing Clinics of North America, 30,* 395–407.

Gadamer, H. G. (1976). *Philosophical hermeneutics* (D. E. Linge, Ed., Trans.). Berkeley: University of California Press.

Gadamer, H. G. (1989). *Truth and method* (2nd rev. ed.). (Translation revised by J. Weinsheimer & D. G. Marshall.) New York: Crossroad. [Original work published 1960.]

Gagliardi, B. A., Frederickson, K., & Shanley, D. A. (2002). Living with multiple sclerosis: A Roy adaptation model–based study. *Nursing Science Quarterly, 15,* 230–236.

Garity, J. (1999). Gender differences in learning style of Alzheimer family caregivers. *Home Healthcare Nurse, 17*(1), 37–44.

Garity, J. (2000). Cultural competence in patient education. *Caring Magazine, 19*(3), 18–20.

Garity, J. (2006). Caring for a family member with Alzheimer's disease: Coping with caregiver burden post-nursing home placement. *Journal of Gerontological Nursing, 32*(6), 39–48.

George, J. B. (2002). *Nursing theories: The base for professional nursing practice* (5th ed.). Upper Saddle River, NJ: Prentice Hall.

Geraci, E. P. (2004). Planned change. In S. J. Peterson & T. S. Bredow (Eds.), *Middle range theories: Application to nursing research* (pp. 323–340). Philadelphia: Lippincott Williams and Wilkins.

Gerrish, K., Ashworth, P., Lacy, A., Bailey, J., Cooke, J., Kendall, S., & McNeilly, E. (2007). Factors influencing the development of evidence-based practice: A research tool. *Journal of Advanced Nursing, 57,* 328–338.

Giger, J. N., & Davidhizar, R. E. (1999). *Transcultural nursing: Assessment and intervention* (3rd ed.). St. Louis: Mosby.

Gigliotti, E. (1997). Use of Neuman's lines of defense and resistance in nursing research: Conceptual and empirical considerations. *Nursing Science Quarterly, 10,* 136–143.

Gigliotti, E. (1999). Women's multiple role stress: Testing Neuman's flexible line of defense. *Nursing Science Quarterly, 12,* 36–44.

Gigliotti, E. (2002). A theory–based CNS practice exemplar using Neuman's systems model and nursing's taxonomies. *Clinical Nurse Specialist: The Journal of Advanced Practice Nursing, 16,* 10–21.

Gigliotti, E. (2004). Etiology of maternal–student role stress. *Nursing Science Quarterly, 17,* 156–164.

Giorgi, A. (1985). *Phenomenology and psychological research.* Pittsburgh: Duquesne University Press.

Giuliano, K. K., Tyer-Viola, L., & Lopez, R. P. (2005). Unity of knowledge in the advancement of knowledge. *Nursing Science Quarterly, 18,* 243–248.

Glanz, K. (2002). Perspectives on using theory. In K. Glanz, B. K. Rimer, & F. M. Lewis (Eds.), *Health behavior and health education: Theory, research, and practice* (3rd ed., pp. 545–558). San Francisco: Jossey-Bass.

Glaser, B. G. (2005). *The grounded theory perspective III: Theoretical coding.* Mill Valley, CA: Sociology Press.

Glaser, B. G., & Strauss, A. L. (1967). *The discovery of grounded theory: Strategies for qualitative research.* Chicago: Aldine.

Good, M. (2004). Pain: A balance between analgesia and side effects. In S. J. Peterson & T. S. Bredow (Eds.), *Middle range theories: Application to nursing research* (pp. 59–77). Philadelphia: Lippincott Williams and Wilkins.

Gous, A., & Roos, V. (2005). Ghosts in the nursery: A case study of the maternal representations of a woman who killed her baby. *Health SA Gesonheid, 10*(3), 3–13.

Grinnell, F. (1992). Theories without thought? *Nursing Times, 88*(22), 57.

Grubbs, J. (1974). An interpretation of the Johnson Behavioral System Model. In J. P. Riehl & C. Roy (Eds.), *Conceptual models for nursing practice* (pp. 160–197). New York: Appleton-Century-Crofts.

Haase, J. E., Leidy, N. K., Coward, D. D., Britt, T., & Penn, P. E. (2000). Simultaneous concept analysis: A strategy for developing multiple interrelated concepts. In B. L. Rodgers & K. A. Knafl (Eds.), *Concept development in nursing: Foundations, techniques, and applications* (2nd ed., pp. 209–229). Philadelphia: Saunders.

Haber, J. (2006). Sampling. In G. LoBiondo-Wood & J. Haber, *Nursing research: Methods and critical appraisal for evidence-based practice* (6th ed., pp. 260–288). St. Louis: Mosby Elsevier.

Hallberg, I. R. (2003). Guest Editorial. Evidence-based nursing, interventions, and family nursing: Methodological obstacles and possibilities. *Journal of Family Nursing, 9,* 3–22.

Hardin, S. R., & Kaplow, R. (2005). *Synergy for clinical excellence: The AACN synergy model for patient care.* Boston: Jones and Bartlett.

Harris, T. (1969). *I'm ok—You're ok: A practical guide to transactional analysis.* New York: Harper and Row.

Hasnain, M., Sinacore, J. M., Mensah, E. K., & Levy, J. A. (2005). Influence of religiosity on HIV risk behaviors in active injection drug users. *AIDS Care, 17,* 892–901.

Hasseler, M. (2006). Evidence-based nursing for practice and science. In H. S. Kim & I. Kollak (Eds.), *Nursing theories: Conceptual and philosophical foundations* (2nd ed., pp. 215–235). New York: Springer.

Hastings-Tolsma, M. (2006). Toward a theory of diversity of human field pattern. *Visions: The Journal of Rogerian Nursing Science, 14*(2), 34–47.

Headley, J. A., Ownby, K. K., & John, L. D. (2004). The effect of seated exercise on fatigue and quality of life in women with advanced breast cancer. *Oncology Nursing Forum, 31,* 977–983.

Health Insurance Portability and Accountability Act. (1996). Kennedy Kassebaum Act. Public Law 104–191.

Heaman, M., Chalmers, K., Woodgate, R., & Brown, J. (2006). Early childhood home visiting programme: Factors contributing to success. *Journal of Advanced Nursing, 55,* 291–300.

Heidegger, M. (1962). *Being and time* (J. Macquarrie & E. Robinson, Trans.). New York: Harper & Row. (Original work published 1927.)

Henderson, A. (2005). The value of integrating interpretive research approaches in the exposition of healthcare context. *Journal of Advanced Nursing, 52,* 554–560.

Hewitt, J., & Coffey, M. (2005). Therapeutic working relationships with people with schizophrenia: Literature review. *Journal of Advanced Nursing, 52*, 561–570.

Higgins, P. A., & Staub, A. J. (2006). Understanding the error of our ways: Mapping the concepts of validity and reliability. *Nursing Outlook, 54*, 23–29.

Higgs, J., & Jones, M. (2000). Clinical reasoning in the health professions. In J. Higgs & M. Jones (Eds.), *Clinical reasoning in the health professions* (2nd ed., pp. 3–14). Boston: Butterworth-Heinemann.

Hill, P. D., Aldag, J. C., Hekel, B., Riner, G., & Bloomfield, P. (2006). Maternal Postpartum Quality of Life Questionnaire. *Journal of Nursing Measurement, 14*, 205–220.

Hills, R. G. S., & Hanchett, E. (2001). Human change and individuation in pivotal life situations: Development and testing the theory of enlightenment. *Visions: The Journal of Rogerian Nursing Science, 9*, 6–19.

Holaday, B. (2006). Dorothy Johnson's behavioral system model and its applications. In M. E. Parker (Ed.), *Nursing theories and nursing practice* (2nd ed., pp. 79–93). Philadelphia: F. A. Davis.

Holaday, B., Turner-Henson, A., & Swan, J. (1996). The Johnson behavioral system model: Explaining activities of chronically ill children. In P. Hinton Walker & B. Neuman (Eds.), *Blueprint for use of nursing models* (pp. 33–63). New York: NLN Press.

Holden, L. M. (2005). Complex adaptive systems: Concept analysis. *Journal of Advanced Nursing, 52*, 651–657.

Holtzclaw, B. J., & Hanneman, S. K. (2002). Use of non-human biobehavioral models in crucial care nursing research. *Critical Care Nursing Quarterly, 24*(4), 30–40.

Horsley, J. A., Crane, J., Crabtree, M. K., & Wood, D. J. (1983). *Using research to improve nursing practice: A guide. CURN [Conduct and Utilization of Research in Nursing] project.* New York: Grune and Stratton.

Horsley, J. A., Crane, J., & Haller, K. B. (1981a). *Intravenous cannula change. CURN [Conduct and Utilization of Research in Nursing] project.* New York: Grune and Stratton.

Horsley, J. A., Crane, J., & Haller, K. B. (1981b). *Reducing diarrhea in tube-fed patients. CURN [Conduct and Utilization of Research in Nursing] project.* New York: Grune and Stratton.

Horsley, J. A., Crane, J., Haller, K. B., & Bingle, J. D. (1981a). *Closed urinary drainage systems. CURN [Conduct and Utilization of Research in Nursing] project.* New York: Grune and Stratton.

Horsley, J. A., Crane, J., Haller, K. B., & Bingle, J. D. (1981b). *Preventing decubitus ulcers. CURN [Conduct and Utilization of Research in Nursing] project.* New York: Grune and Stratton.

Horsley, J. A., Crane, J., & Reynolds, M. A. (1982a). *Clean intermittent catheterization. Deliberative nursing interventions. CURN [Conduct and Utilization of Research in Nursing] project.* New York: Grune and Stratton.

Horsley, J. A., Crane, J., & Reynolds, M. A. (1982b). *Pain: Deliberative nursing interventions. CURN [Conduct and Utilization of Research in Nursing] project.* New York: Grune and Stratton.

Horsley, J. A., Crane, J., Reynolds, M. A., & Bingle, J. D. (1981). *Structured preoperative teaching. CURN [Conduct and Utilization of Research in Nursing] project.* New York: Grune and Stratton

Horsley, J. A., Crane, J., Reynolds, M. A., & Haller, K. B. (1981a). *Distress reduction through sensory preparation. CURN [Conduct and Utilization of Research in Nursing] project.* New York: Grune and Stratton.

Horsley, J. A., Crane, J., Reynolds, M. A., & Haller, K. B. (1981b). *Preoperative sensory preparation to promote recovery. CURN [Conduct and Utilization of Research in Nursing] project.* New York: Grune and Stratton.

Horsley, J. A., Crane, J., Reynolds, M. A., & Haller, K. B. (1982). *Mutual goal setting in patient care. CURN [Conduct and Utilization of Research in Nursing] project.* New York: Grune and Stratton.

Howe, J. A., Innes, E. L., Venturini, A., Williams, J. I., & Verrier, M. C. (2006). The Community Balance and Mobility Scale—A balance measure for individuals with traumatic brain injury. *Clinical Rehabilitation, 20*, 885–895.

Hoyle, R. H., Harris, M. J., & Judd, C. M. (2002). *Research methods in social relations* (7th ed.). Fort Worth, TX: Wadsworth.

Huch, M. H., & Bournes, D. A. (2003). Community dwellers' perspectives on the experience of feeling very tired. *Nursing Science Quarterly, 16,* 334–339.

Hung, C.-H. (2005). Measuring postpartum stress. *Journal of Advanced Nursing, 50,* 417–424.

Hunt, J. (1981). Indicators for nursing practice: The use of research findings. *Journal of Advanced Nursing, 6,* 189–194.

Hurst, C., Montgomery, A. J., Davis, B. L., Killion, C., & Baker, S. (2005). The relationship between social support, self-care agency, and self-care practices of African-American women who are HIV-positive. *Journal of Multicultural Nursing and Health, 11*(3), 11–22.

Husserl, E. (1931). *Ideas: General introduction to pure phenomenology* (W. R. Boyce Gibson, Trans.). New York: Collins.

Husted, G. L., & Husted, J. H. (2001). Ethical decision making in nursing and healthcare: The symphonological approach (3rd ed.). New York: Springer.

Im, E.–O., & Chee, W. (2003). Feminist issues in e-mail group discussion among cancer patients. *Advances in Nursing Science, 26,* 287–298.

International Council of Nurses. (2007). *Nursing research: A tool for action.* Retrieved July 1, 2007, from http://www.icn.ch/matters_research.htm

Ip, W.-Y., Chan, D., & Chien, W.-T. (2005). Chinese version of the Childbirth Self-efficacy Inventory. *Journal of Advanced Nursing, 51,* 625–633.

Ingersoll, G. L. (2000). Evidence-based nursing: What it is and what it isn't. *Nursing Outlook, 48,* 151–152.

Jairath, N., & Fain, J. A. (1999). A strategy for converting clinical data into research databases. *Nursing Research, 48,* 340–344.

Jansen, I. H. M., Olde Rikkert, M. G. M., Hulsbos, H. A. J., & Hoefnagels, W. H. L. (2001). Toward individualized evidence-based medicine: Five "N of 1" trials of methylphenidate for geriatric patients. *Journal of the American Geriatrics Society, 49,* 474–476.

Janz, N. K., Champion, V. L., & Strecher, V. J. (2002). The health belief model. In K. Glanz, B. K. Rimer, & F. M. Lewis (Eds.), *Health behavior and health education: Theory, research, and practice* (3rd ed., pp. 45–66). San Francisco: Jossey-Bass.

Jirovec, M. M., Jenkins, J., Isenberg, M., & Bairdi, J. (1999). Urine control theory derived from Roy's conceptual framework. *Nursing Science Quarterly, 12,* 251–255.

Johnson, D. E. (1974). Development of theory: A requisite for nursing as a primary health profession. *Nursing Research, 23,* 372–377.

Jones, J. H. (1981). *Bad blood: The Tuskegee syphilis experiment.* New York: Free Press.

Kaewthummanukul, T., Brown, K. C., Weaver, M. T., & Thomas, R. R. (2006). Predictors of exercise participation in female hospital nurses. *Journal of Advanced Nursing, 54,* 663–675.

Kearney, M. H. (2001). Levels and applications of qualitative research evidence. *Research in Nursing and Health, 24,* 145–153.

Kearney, M. H. (2002). Evidence-based thinking: Make it a habit. [Editorial] *Journal of Obstetric, Gynecologic, and Neonatal Nursing, 31,* 499.

Kearney, M. H. (2007). Going deeper versus wider in qualitative sampling. *Journal of Obstetric, Gynecologic, and Neonatal Nursing, 36,* 299.

Keefe, M. R. (1988). Irritable infant syndrome: Theoretical perspectives and practice implications. *Advances in Nursing Science, 10*(3), 70–78.

Keefe, M. R., Barbosa, G. A., Froese-Fretz, A., Kotzer, A. M., & Lobo, M. (2005). An intervention program for families with irritable infants. *MCN: The American Journal of Maternal Child Nursing, 30,* 230–236.

Keeney, S., Hasson, F., & McKenna, H. (2006). Consulting the oracle: Ten lessons from using the Dephi technique in nursing research. *Journal of Advanced Nursing, 53,* 205–212.

Kelley, C. G., Daly, B. J., Anthony, M. K., Zauszniewski, J. A., & Strange, K. C. (2002). Nurse practitioners and preventive screening in the hospital. *Clinical Nursing Research, 11,* 433–449.

Kerlinger, F. N. (1979). *Behavioral research: A conceptual approach.* New York: Holt, Rinehart and Winston.

Kerlinger, F. N., & Lee, H. B. (2000). *Foundations of behavioral research* (4th ed.). Stamford, CT: Wadsworth/Thompson Learning.

King, I. M. (1981). *A theory for nursing: Systems, concepts, process.* New York: Wiley. [Reissued 1990. Albany, NY: Delmar.]

King, I. M. (1989). Theories and hypotheses for nursing administration. In B. Henry, M. Di Vincenti, C. Arndt, & A. Marriner (Eds.), *Dimensions of nursing administration. Theory, research, education, and practice* (pp. 35–45). Boston: Blackwell Scientific.

King, I. M. (1995). The theory of goal attainment. In M. A. Frey & C. L. Sieloff (Eds.), *Advancing King's systems framework and theory of nursing* (pp. 23–32). Thousand Oaks, CA: Sage.

King, I. M. (1997). King's theory of goal attainment in practice. *Nursing Science Quarterly, 10,* 180–185.

King, I. M. (2006). Part One: Imogene M. King's theory of goal attainment. In M. E. Parker (Ed.), *Nursing theories and nursing practice* (2nd ed., pp. 235–243). Philadelphia: F. A. Davis.

King, K. M. (2001). The problem of under-powering in nursing research. *Western Journal of Nursing Research, 23,* 334–335.

Kline, R. B. (2005). *Principles and practice of structural equation modeling* (2nd ed.). New York: Guilford Press.

Knapp, T. R. (1985). Validity, reliability, and neither. *Nursing Research, 34,* 189–192.

Knapp, T. R. (1991). Coefficient alpha: Conceptualizations and anomalies. *Research in Nursing and Health, 14,* 457–460.

Knipp, D. K. (2006). Teens' perceptions about attention deficit/hyperactivity disorder and medications. *Journal of School Nursing, 22,* 120–125.

Kolcaba, K. (2003). *Comfort theory and practice: A vision for holistic health care and research.* New York: Springer.

Kruszewski, A. Z. (1999). Psychosocial adaptation to termination of pregnancy for fetal anomaly. *Dissertation Abstracts International, 61,* 194B.

Lackey, N. R. (2000). Concept clarification: Using the Norris method in clinical research. In B. L. Rodgers & K. A. Knafl (Eds.), *Concept development in nursing: Foundations, techniques, and applications* (2nd ed., pp. 193–208). Philadelphia: Saunders.

Lancaster, D. R. (2004). Development and psychometric testing of the Coping with Breast Cancer Threat instrument. *Journal of Nursing Measurement, 12,* 33–46.

LaPierre, E., Ritchey, K., & Newhouse, R. (2004). Barriers to research use in the PACU. *Journal of PeriAnesthesia Nursing, 19,* 78–83. Online full text version retrieved from *ScienceDirect,* March 17, 2005, nine pages.

Laudan, L. (1981). A problem-solving approach to scientific progress. In I. Hacking (Ed.), *Scientific revolutions* (pp. 144–155). Fair Lawn, NJ: Oxford University Press.

Lazarus, R. S., & Folkman, S. (1984). *Stress, appraisal and coping.* New York: Springer.

Leddy, S. K. (1995). Measuring mutual process: Development and psychometric testing of the Person-Environment Participation Scale. *Visions: The Journal of Rogerian Nursing Science, 3,* 20–31.

Leddy, S. K. (2003). A unitary energy-based nursing practice theory: Theory and application. *Visions: The Journal of Rogerian Nursing Science, 11,* 21–28.

Leddy, S. K. (2006). *Health promotion: Mobilizing strengths to enhance health, wellness, and well-being.* Philadelphia: F. A. Davis.

Leeman, J., Baernholdt, M., & Sandelowski, M. (2007). Developing a theory-based taxonomy of methods for implementating change in practice. *Journal of Advanced Nursing, 58,* 191–200.

Leeman, J., Jackson, B., & Sandelowski, M. (2006). An evaluation of how well research reports facilitate the use of findings in practice. *Journal of Nursing Scholarship, 38,* 171–177.

Leerar, P. J., & Miller, E. W. (2002). Concurrent validity of distance-walks and timed-walks in the well-elderly. *Journal of Geriatric Physical Therapy, 25,* 3–7.

Legault, F., & Ferguson-Paré, M. (1999). Advancing nursing practice: An evaluation study of Parse's theory of human becoming. *Canadian Journal of Nursing Leadership, 12*(1), 30–35.

Leininger, M. M. (Ed.). (1985a). *Qualitative research methods in nursing.* New York: Grune and Stratton.

Leininger, M. M. (1985b). Transcultural care diversity and universality: A theory of nursing. *Nursing and Health Care, 6,* 208–212.

Leininger, M. M. (1991). Ethnonursing: A research method with enablers to study the theory of culture care. In M. M. Leininger (Ed.), *Culture care diversity and universality: A theory of nursing* (pp. 73–117). New York: National League for Nursing.

Leininger, M. M. (2006a). Ethnonursing research method and enablers. In M. M. Leininger & M. R. McFarland (Eds.), *Culture care diversity and universality: A worldwide nursing theory* (2nd ed., pp. 43–82). Boston: Jones and Bartlett.

Leininger, M. M. (2006b). Selected culture care findings of diverse cultures using culture care theory and ethnomethods. In M. M. Leininger & M. R. McFarland (Eds.), *Culture care diversity and universality: A worldwide nursing theory* (2nd ed., pp. 281–305). Boston: Jones and Bartlett.

Leininger, M. M., & McFarlane, M. R. (2006). *Culture care diversity and universality: A worldwide nursing theory.* Boston: Jones and Barlett.

Lenth, R. V. (2001). Some practical guidelines for effective sample size determination. *The American Statistician, 55,* 187–193.

Lenz, E. R., Pugh, L. C., Milligan, R., Gift, A., & Suppe. F. (1997). The middle-range theory of unpleasant symptoms: An update. *Advances in Nursing Science, 19*(3), 14–27.

Lerner, B. H. (2007). Hope or false hope: What stories about celebrities and their illnesses mean to the rest of us. *The Pennsylvania Gazette,* May/June, 16–17.

Levine, M. E. (1988). Myra Levine. In T. M. Schorr & A. Zimmerman (Eds.), *Making choices. Taking chances. Nurse leaders tell their stories* (pp. 215–228). St. Louis: Mosby.

Levine, R. J. (1981). *Ethics and regulation of clinical research.* Baltimore: Urban and Schwarzenberg.

Lewandowski, W. A. (2004). Patterning of pain and power with guided imagery. *Nursing Science Quarterly, 17,* 233–241.

Lewandowski, W., Good, M., & Draucker, C. B. (2005). Changes in the meaning of pain with the use of guided imagery. *Pain Management Nursing, 6*(2), 58–67.

Lewin, K. (1938). Experiments in autocratic and democratic principles. *Social Frontier, 4,* 316–319.

Lewin, K. (1946). Action research and minority problems. *Journal of Social Issues, 2*(4), 34–46.

Lewin, K. (1951). Psychological ecology. In D. Cartwright (Ed.). *Field theory in social science: Selected theoretical papers by Kurt Lewin* (pp. 170–187). New York: Harper and Brothers.

Li, M-F., & Wang, R-H. (2006). Factors related to avoidance of environmental tobacco smoke among adolescents in southern Taiwan. *Journal of Nursing Research, 14,* 103–112.

Liehr, P. R., & LoBiondo-Wood, G. (2006). Qualitative approaches to research. In G. LoBiondo-Wood & J. Haber (Eds.), *Nursing research: Methods and critical appraisal for evidence-based practice* (6th ed., pp. 148–175). St. Louis: Mosby Elsevier.

Liehr, P., & Smith, M. J. (2006). Theoretical framework. In G. LoBiondo-Wood & J. Haber (Eds.), *Nursing research: Methods and critical appraisal for evidence-based practice* (6th ed., pp. 111–125). St. Louis: Mosby Elsevier.

Lin, L-C., Kao, C-C., Tzeng, Y-L., & Lin, Y-J. (2007) Equivalence of Chinese version of the Cohen-Mansfield Agitation Inventory. *Journal of Advanced Nursing, 59,* 178–185.

Lin, P-F., Hsu, M-Y., & Tasy, S-L. (2003). Teaching clinical judgment in Taiwan. *Journal of Nursing Research, 11,* 159–166.

Lincoln, Y. S., & Guba, E. G. (1985). *Naturalistic inquiry.* Beverly Hills, CA: Sage.

Liu, H. E. (2006). Fatigue and associated factors in hemodialysis patients in Taiwan. *Research in Nursing and Health, 29,* 40–50.

LoBiondo-Wood, G. (2006). Introduction to quantitative research. In G. LoBiondo-Wood & J. Haber (Eds.), *Nursing research: Methods and critical appraisal for evidence-based practice* (6th ed., pp. 201–219). St. Louis: Mosby Elsevier.

LoBiondo-Wood, G., & Haber, J. (2006). Nonexperimental designs. In G. LoBiondo-Wood & J. Haber (Eds.), *Nursing research: Methods and critical appraisal for evidence-based practice* (6th ed., pp. 238–259). St. Louis: Mosby Elsevier.

Lobo, M. (2005). Descriptive research is the bench science of nursing. *Western Journal of Nursing Research, 27,* 5–6.

Lou, M.-F., & Dai, Y.-T. (2002). Nurses' experience of caring for delirious patients. *Journal of Nursing Research, 10,* 270–289.

Ludomirski-Kalmanson, B. (1984). The relationship between the environmental energy wave frequency pattern manifest in red light and blue light and human field motion in adult individuals with visual sensory perception and those with total blindness. *Dissertation Abstracts International, 45,* 2094B.

Lynn, M. R. (1986). Determination and quantification of content validity. *Nursing Research, 36,* 382–385.

MacGuire, J. M. (1989/2006). Putting nursing research findings into practice: Research utilization as an aspect of the management of change. *Journal of Advanced Nursing, 15,* 614–621. [Reprinted in *Journal of Advanced Nursing, 53,* 65–74, 2006.]

Macnee, C. L. (2004). *Understanding nursing research: Reading and using research in practice.* Philadelphia: Lippincott Williams and Wilkins.

Macnee, C. L., & McCabe, S. (2008). *Understanding nursing research: Reading and using research in evidence-based practice.* Philadelphia: Wolters Kluwer/Lippincott Williams and Wilkins.

Mahon, N. E., Yarcheski, A., & Yarcheski, T. J. (2004). Social support and positive health practices in early adolescents: A test of mediating variables. *Clinical Nursing Research, 13,* 216–236.

Mahoney, J. S. (2001). An ethnographic approach to understanding the illness experience of patients with congestive heart failure and their family members. *Heart and Lung, 30,* 429–436.

Maldonado, N., Callahan, K., & Efinger, J. (2003). Spiritual reflections concerning end of life caring decisions: A qualitative case study. *International Journal for Human Caring, 7*(2), 13–26.

Malinowksi, B. (1922). *Argonauts of the Western Pacific.* London: Routledge and Kegan Paul.

Malinski, V. M. (1994). Spirituality: A pattern manifestation of the human/environment mutual process. *Visions: The Journal of Rogerian Nursing Science, 2,* 12–18.

Malinski, V. M. (2006). Part One: Martha E. Rogers' science of unitary human beings. In M. E. Parker (Ed.), *Nursing theories and nursing practice* (2nd ed., pp. 160–167). Philadelphia: F. A. Davis.

Marcellus, L. (2003). Critical social and medical constructions of perinatal substance misuse: Truth in the making. *Journal of Family Nursing, 9,* 438–452.

Marriner Tomey, A., & Alligood, M. R. (2006). *Nursing theorists and their work* (6th ed.). St. Louis: Mosby Elsevier.

Masson, V. (2001). Negative conditioning. *American Journal of Nursing, 101*(5), 47.

Maxwell, J. A. (2005). *Qualitative research design: An interactive approach* (2nd ed.). Thousand Oaks, CA: Sage.

May, B. A. (2000). Relationships among basic empathy, self-awareness, and learning styles of baccalaureate pre-nursing students within King's person system. *Dissertation Abstracts International, 61,* 2991B.

Mayo, E. (1953). *The human problems of an industrialized civilization.* New York: McGraw-Hill.

McCaffery, M., & Arnstein, P. (2006). The debate over placebos in pain management. *American Journal of Nursing, 106*(2), 62–66.

McCaffrey, R., & Freeman, E. (2003). Effect of music on chronic osteoarthritis pain in older people. *Journal of Advanced Nursing, 44,* 517–524.

McCorkle, R. (2006). A program of research on patient and family caregiver outcomes: Three phases of evolution. *Oncology Nursing Forum, 33,* 25–31.

McDonald, D. D., & Nicholson, N. R. (2006). Dietary supplement information and intention to continue and recommend supplements. *International Journal of Nursing Studies, 43,* 51–57.

McGahee, T. W., & Tingen, M. S. (2000). The effects of a smoking prevention curriculum on fifth-grade children's attitudes, subjective norms and refusal skills. *Southern Online Journal of Nursing Research, 1*(2), 1–28.

McKenna, H. (1994). *Nursing theories and quality of care.* Brookfield, VT: Ashgate.

McCubbin, H. I., & Patterson, J. M. (1983). The family stress process: The double ABCX model of adjustment and adaptation. *Marriage and Family Review, 6,* 7–37.

Mefford, L. C. (2004). A theory of health promotion for preterm infants based on Levine's conservation model of nursing. *Nursing Science Quarterly, 17,* 260–266.

Meighan, M. M. (2000). Testing a nursing intervention to enhance paternal-infant interaction and promote paternal role assumption. *Dissertation Abstracts International, 60,* 3204B.

Meisenhelder, J. B. (2006). An example of personal knowledge: Spirituality. In L. C. Andrist, P. K. Nicholas, & K. A. Wolf (Eds.), *A history of nursing ideas* (pp. 151–155). Boston: Jones and Bartlett.

Melancon, B., & Miller, L. H. (2005). Massage therapy versus traditional therapy for low back pain relief: Implications for holistic nursing practice. *Holistic Nursing Practice, 19,* 116–121.

Melnyk, B. M., & Fineout-Overholt, E. (2004). *Evidence-based practice in nursing and healthcare: A guide to best practice.* Philadelphia: Lippincott Williams and Wilkins.

Merleau-Ponty, M. (1962). *Phenomenology of perception* (C. Smith, Trans.). New York: Humanities Press.

Merton, R. K. (1968). *Social theory and social structure.* New York: The Free Press.

Messmer, P. R. (2006). Professional model of care: Using King's theory of goal attainment. *Nursing Science Quarterly, 19,* 227–229.

Mirowsky, J., & Ross, C. E. (2001). Age and the effect of economic hardship on depression. *Journal of Health and Social Behavior, 42,* 132–150.

Mishel, M. H. (1988). Uncertainty in illness. *Image: Journal of Nursing Scholarship, 20,* 225–231.

Mishel, M. H. (1990). Reconceptualization of the Uncertainty in Illness Theory. *Image: Journal of Nursing Scholarship, 22,* 256–262.

Mitchell, P., Ferketich, S., Jennings, B., & the American Academy of Nursing Expert Panel on Quality Healthcare. (1998). Quality health outcomes model. *Image: Journal of Nursing Scholarship, 30,* 43–46.

Mitchell, S., Beck, S. L., & Erickson, J. M. (2007). Fatigue during and following cancer and its treatment: A qualitative metasynthesis. *Oncology Nursing Forum, 34,* 197. [Abstract]

Mock, V., Dow, K. H., Meares, C. J., Grimm, P. M., Dienemann, J. A., Chakravarthy, A., & Gage, I. (1997). Effects of exercise on fatigue, physical functioning, and emotional distress during radiation therapy for breast cancer. *Oncology Nursing Forum, 24,* 991–1000.

Mock, V., Frangakis, C., Davidson, N. E., Ropka, M. E., Pickett, M., Poniatowski, B., Steward, K. J., Cameron, L., Zawacki, K., Podewils, L. J., Cohen, G., & McCorkle, R. (2005). Exercise manages fatigue during breast cancer treatment: A randomized controlled trial. *Psycho-Oncology, 14,* 464–477.

Mock, V., Picket, M., Ropka, M. E., Lin, E. M., Stewart, K. J., Rhodes, V. A., McDaniel, R., Grimm, P. M., Krumm, S., & McCorkle, R. (2001). Fatigue and quality of life outcomes of exercise during cancer treatment. *Cancer Practice, 9,* 119–127.

Montgomery, P., Tompkins, C., Forchuk, C., & French, S. (2006). Keeping close: Mothering with serious mental illness. *Journal of Advanced Nursing, 54,* 20–28.

Mooney, M., & Nolan, L. (2006). A critique of Freire's perspective on critical social theory in nursing education. *Nurse Education Today, 26,* 240–244.

Morse, J. M. (2000). Exploring pragmatic utility: Concept analysis by critically appraising the literature. In B. L. Rodgers & K. A. Knafl (Eds.), *Concept development in nursing: Foundations, techniques, and applications* (2nd ed., pp. 333–352). Philadelphia: Saunders.

Muecke, M. A. (1994). On the evaluation of ethnographies. In J. M. Morse (Ed.), *Critical issues in qualitative research methods* (pp. 187–209). Thousand Oaks, CA: Sage.

Munro, B. H. (2005). *Statistical methods for health care research* (5th ed.). Philadelphia: Lippincott Williams and Wilkins.

National Commission for the Protection of Human Subjects of Biomedical and Behavioral Research. (1978). *Belmont report: Ethical principles and guidelines for research involving human subjects*. Washington, DC: U.S. Government Printing Office. Retrieved February 21, 2007, from http://www.hhs.gov/ohrp/humansubjects/guidance/belmont.htm

Neill, J. (2005). Health as expanding consciousness: Seven women living with multiple sclerosis or rheumatoid arthritis. *Nursing Science Quarterly, 18,* 334–343.

Neuman, B. (2002). The Neuman systems model. In B. Neuman & J. Fawcett (Eds.), *The Neuman systems model* (4th ed., pp. 3–33). Upper Saddle River, NJ: Prentice Hall.

Neuman, B., & Fawcett, J. (Eds.). (2002). *The Neuman systems model* (4th ed.). Upper Saddle River, NJ: Prentice Hall.

Newman, D. M. L. (2005). Functional status, personal health, and self-esteem of caregivers of children in a body cast. *Orthopaedic Nursing, 24,* 416–423.

Newman, M. A. (1992). Window on health as expanding consciousness. In M. O'Toole (Ed.), *Miller-Keane encyclopedia and dictionary of medicine, nursing, and allied health* (5th ed., p. 650). Philadelphia: Saunders.

Newman, M. A. (1994). *Health as expanding consciousness* (2nd ed.). New York: National League for Nursing. [Reprinted 2000. Boston: Jones and Bartlett.]

Newman, M. A. (1997). Evolution of the theory of health as expanding consciousness. *Nursing Science Quarterly, 10,* 22–25.

Ngondi, J., Onsarigo, A., Adamu, L., Matende, I., Baba, S., Reacher, M., Emerson, P., & Zingeser, J. (2005). The epidemiology of trachoma in Eastern Equatoria and Upper Nile States, southern Sudan. *Bulletin of the World Health Organization, 83,* 804–912.

Nieswiadomy, R. M. (2008). *Foundations of nursing research* (5th ed.). Upper Saddle River, NJ: Prentice Hall.

Nir, Z., Zolotogorsky, Z., & Sugarman, H. (2004). Structured nursing intervention versus routine rehabilitation after stroke. *American Journal of Physical Medicine and Rehabilitation, 83,* 522–529.

Niska, K. J. (2001). Mexican American family survival, continuity, and growth: The parental perspective. *Nursing Science Quarterly, 14,* 322–329.

Norris, A. E. (2005). Structural equation modeling. In B. H. Munro, *Statistical methods for health care research* (5th ed., pp. 405–434). Philadelphia: Lippincott Williams and Wilkins.

Nuamah, I. F., Cooley, M. E., Fawcett, J., & McCorkle, R. (1999). Testing a theory for health-related quality of life in cancer patients: A structural equation approach. *Research in Nursing and Health, 22,* 231–242.

Nunnally, J. C., & Bernstein, I. H. (1994). *Psychometric theory* (3rd ed.). New York: McGraw-Hill.

Oddi, L. F., & Cassidy, V. R. (1990). Nursing research in the United States: The protection of human subjects. *International Journal of Nursing Studies, 27,* 21–34.

Office of Portfolio Analysis and Strategic Initiatives. (2007). *NIH roadmap for medical research: Re-engineering the clinical research enterprise*. Retrieved January 9, 2007, from http://nihroadmap.nih.gov/clinicalresearch/overview-translational.asp

Orem, D. E. (2001). *Nursing: Concepts of practice* (6th ed.). St. Louis: Mosby.

Orlando, I. J. (1961). *The dynamic nurse-patient relationship. Function, process and principles.* New York: G. P. Putnam's Sons.

Ortiz, M. R. (2003). Lingering presence: A study using the human becoming hermeneutic method. *Nursing Science Quarterly, 16,* 146–154.

Osborne, J. W., & Costello, A. B. (2004). Sample size and subject to item ratio in principal components analysis. *Practice Assessment, Research, and Evaluation, 9*(11), 14 pages. Retrieved August 29, 2006, from http://PAREonline.net/getvn.asp?v=9&n=11

Osgood, C. E., Suci, G. J., & Tannenbaum, P. H. (1957). *The measurement of meaning.* Chicago: University of Illinois Press.

Oxford English Dictionary. (2005). Definitions retrieved September 19 from http://dictionary.oed.com.eresources.lib.umb.edu/cgi

Oxford English Dictionary. (2007). Definition retrieved May 9 from http://dictionary.oed.com.eresources.lib.umb.edu

Padgett, D. K. (1998). *Qualitative methods in social work research: Challenges and rewards.* Thousand Oaks, CA: Sage.

Paley, J. (1996). How not to clarify concepts. *Journal of Advanced Nursing, 24,* 572–578.

Parahoo, K. (2006). *Nursing research: Principles, process and issues* (2nd ed.). New York: Palgrave Macmillan.

Parker, K. P. (1989). The theory of sentience evolution: A practice-level theory of sleeping, waking, and beyond waking patterns based on the science of unitary human beings. *Rogerian Nursing Science News, 2*(1), 4–6.

Parker, M. E. (2006). *Nursing theories and nursing practice* (2nd ed.). Philadelphia: F. A. Davis.

Parse, R. R. (1997). Concept inventing: Unitary creations. *Nursing Science Quarterly, 10,* 63–64.

Parse, R. R. (1998). *The human becoming school of thought: A perspective for nurses and other health professionals.* Thousand Oaks, CA: Sage.

Parse, R. R. (2001). *Qualitative inquiry: The path of sciencing.* Boston: Jones and Bartlett.

Parse, R. R. (2005). Parse's criteria for evaluation of theory with a comparison of Fawcett's and Parse's approaches. *Nursing Science Quarterly, 18,* 135–137.

Parse, R. R. (2006). Concept inventing: Continuing clarification. *Nursing Science Quarterly, 19,* 289.

Patterson, G. J., & Zderad, L. T. (1976). *Humanistic nursing.* New York: Wiley.

Payton, O. D. (1994). *Research: The validation of clinical practice* (3rd ed.). Philadelphia: F. A. Davis.

Pearson, A., Wiechula, R., Court, A., & Lockwood, C. (2007). A re-consideration of what constitutes "evidence" in the healthcare professions. *Nursing Science Quarterly, 20,* 85–88.

Pedhazur, E. (1982). *Multiple regression in behavioral research: Explanation and prediction* (2nd ed.). New York: Holt, Rinehart and Winston.

Pender, N., Murdaugh, C., & Parsons, M. (2992). *Health promotion in nursing practice* (4th ed.). Upper Saddle River, NJ: Prentice Hall.

Peplau, H. E. (1952). *Interpersonal relations in nursing.* New York: G. P. Putnam's Sons.

Peplau, H. E. (1997). Peplau's theory of interpersonal relations. *Nursing Science Quarterly, 10,* 162–167.

Perkins, E. (2001). Johns Hopkins tragedy: Could librarians have prevented a death? *Information Today, 18,* 51, 54. Retrieved February 21, 2007, from http://newsbreaks.infotoday.com/nbreader.asp?ArticleID=17534

Persily, C. A., & Hildebrandt, E. (2003). The theory of community empowerment. In M. J. Smith & P. R. Liehr (Eds.), *Middle range theory for nursing* (pp. 111–123). New York: Springer.

Peterson, S. J., & Bredow, T. S. (2004). *Middle range theories: Application to nursing research.* Philadelphia: Lippincott Williams and Wilkins.

Phillips, D. C. (1987). *Philosophy, science and social inquiry: Contemporary methodological controversies in social science and related applied fields of research.* New York: Pergamon Press.

Pilkington, F. B. (2005). Grieving a loss: The lived experience for elders residing in an institution. *Nursing Science Quarterly, 18,* 233–242.

Piper, B. F., Dibble, S. L., Dodd, M. J., Weiss, M. C., Slaughter, R. E., & Paul, S. M. (1998). The revised Piper Fatigue Scale: Psychometric evaluation in women with breast cancer. *Oncology Nursing Forum, 25,* 677–684.

Platt, J. R. (1964). Strong inference. *Science, 146,* 347–353.

Poirier, P. (2005). Policy implications of the relationship of sick leave benefits, individual characteristics, and fatigue to employment during radiation therapy for cancer. *Policy, Politics, and Nursing Practice, 6,* 305–318.

Polit, D. F., & Beck, C. T. (2004). *Nursing research: Principles and methods* (7th ed.). Philadelphia: Lippincott Williams and Wilkins.

Polit, D. F., & Beck, C. T. (2006). *Essentials of nursing research: Methods, appraisal, and utilization* (6th ed.). Philadelphia: Lippincott Williams and Wilkins.

Polit, D. F., & Beck, C. T. (2008). *Nursing research: Generating and assessing evidence for nursing practice* (8th ed.). Philadelphia: Wolters Kluwer/Lippincott Williams and Wilkins.

Polit, D. F., & Hungler, B. P. (1999). *Nursing research: Principles and methods* (6th ed.). Philadelphia: Lippincott.

Popham, W. J. (1978). *Criterion referenced measurement.* Englewood Cliffs, NJ: Prentice –Hall.

Popper, K. R. (1965). *Conjectures and refutations: The growth of scientific knowledge.* New York: Harper and Row.

Porter-O'Grady, T. (2006). A new age for practice: Creating the framework for evidence. In K. Malloch & T. Porter-O'Grady (Eds.), *Introduction to evidence-based practice in nursing and health care* (pp. 1–29). Boston: Jones and Bartlett.

Powel, L. L., & Clark, J. A. (2005). The value of the marginalia as an adjunct to structured questionnaires: Experiences of men after prostate cancer surgery. *Quality of Life Research, 14,* 827–835.

Powers, B. A., & Knapp, T. R. (2006). *Dictionary of nursing theory and research* (3rd ed.). New York: Springer.

Pravikoff, D. S., Tanner, A. B., & Pierce, S. T. (2005). Readiness of U.S. nurses for evidence-based practice. *American Journal of Nursing, 105*(5), 40–52.

Prescott, P. A., & Soeken, K. L. (1989). The potential uses of pilot work. *Nursing Research, 38,* 60–62.

Prochaska, J., DiClemente, C., & Norcross, J. (1992). In search of how people change: Applications to addictive behaviors. *American Psychologist, 47,* 1102–1114.

Racher, F. E., & Annis, R. C. (2005). Community partnerships: Translating research for community development. *Canadian Journal of Nursing Research, 37,* 169–175.

Radcliffe-Brown, A. R. (1952). *Structure and function in primitive society.* London: Oxford University Press.

Radwin, L. (2000). Oncology patients' perceptions of quality nursing care. *Research in Nursing and Health, 23,* 179–190.

Radwin, L., & Alster, K. (1999). Outcomes of perceived quality nursing care reported by oncology patients. *Scholarly Inquiry for Nursing Practice: An International Journal, 13,* 327–343.

Radwin, L., & Fawcett, J. (2002). A conceptual model based programme of nursing research: Retrospective and prospective applications. *Journal of Advanced Nursing, 40,* 355–360.

Radwin, L. E., Washko, M., Suchy, K. A., & Tyman, K. (2005). Development and pilot testing of four desired health outcomes scales. *Oncology Nursing Forum, 32,* 92–96.

Ravesloot, C., Seekins, T., & White, G. (2005). Living well with a disability health promotion intervention: Improved health status for consumers and lower costs for health care policymakers. *Rehabilitation Psychology, 50,* 239–245.

Reed, P. G. (1991). Toward a theory of self-transcendence: Deductive reformulation using developmental theories. *Advances in Nursing Science, 13*(4), 64–77.

Reed, P. G. (2003). Theory of self-transcendence. In M. J. Smith & P. R. Liehr (Eds.), *Middle range theory for nursing* (pp. 145–165). New York: Springer.

Reed, P. G. (2006). Commentary on neomodernism and evidence-based nursing: Implications for the production of nursing knowledge. *Nursing Outlook, 54,* 36–38.

Reich, W. T. (Ed.). (1995). *Encyclopedia of bioethics.* New York: Simon and Schuster.

Reichert, J. A., Baron, M., & Fawcett, J. (1993). Changes in attitudes toward cesarean birth. *Journal of Obstetric, Gynecologic, and Neonatal Nursing, 22,* 159–167.

Rempher, K. J. (2006). Putting theory into practice: Six steps to success. *American Nurse Today, 1*(2), 41–42.

Rempher, K. J., & Urquico, K. (2007). The *P* value: What it really means. *American Nurse Today, 2*(5), 13–15.

Renker, P. R. (2006). Perinatal violence assessment: Teenagers' rationale for denying violence when asked. *Journal of Obstetric, Gynecologic, and Neonatal Nursing, 35,* 56–67.

Rew, L. (2003). A theory of taking care of oneself grounded in experiences of homeless youth. *Nursing Research, 52,* 234–241.

Rex–Smith, A. (2007). Using the synergy model to study spirituality in intermediate care: Report of a pilot study. [Abstract]. *American Journal of Critical Care, 16,* 314–315.

Rhodes, V. A., Watson, P. M., & Johnson, M. H. (1984). Development of a reliable and valid measure of nausea and vomiting. *Cancer Nursing, 7,* 33–41.

Ricoeur, P. (1976). *Interpretation theory: Discourse and the surplus of meaning.* Fort Worth, TX: Texas Christian University Press.

Richmond, T., Tang, S. T., Tulman, L., Fawcett, J., & McCorkle, R. (2004). Measuring function. In M. Frank-Stromborg & S. J. Olsen (Eds.), *Instruments for clinical health-care research* (3rd ed., pp. 83–99). Boston: Jones and Bartlett.

Ritzer, G. (1980). *Sociology: A multiple paradigm science* (rev. ed.). Boston: Allyn and Bacon.

Rodgers, B. L. (2000). Concept analysis: An evolutionary view. In B. L. Rodgers & K. A. Knafl (Eds.), *Concept development in nursing: Foundations, techniques, and applications* (2nd ed., pp. 77–102). Philadelphia: Saunders.

Rodgers, B. L., & Knafl, K. A. (2000). *Concept development in nursing: Foundations, techniques, and applications* (2nd ed.). Philadelphia: Saunders.

Rodriguez, C. M. (1981). Cesarean family care: Hospital policies and future trends. In C. F. Kehoe (Ed.), *The cesarean experience: Theoretical and clinical perspectives for nurses* (pp. 251–267). New York: Appleton-Century-Crofts.

Roelands, M., Van Oost, P., Depoorter, A. M., Buysse, A., & Stevens, V. (2006). Introduction of assistive devices: Home nurses' practices and beliefs. *Journal of Advanced Nursing, 54,* 180–188.

Rogers, E. M. (2003). *Diffusion of innovations* (5th ed.). New York: Free Press.

Rolfe, G. (2006). Nursing praxis and the science of the unique. *Nursing Science Quarterly, 19,* 39–43.

Rosenberg, M. (1965). *Society and the adolescent self-image.* Princeton, NJ: Princeton University Press.

Rosenberg, M. (1968). *The logic of survey analysis.* New York: Basic Books.

Rosenthal, R. (1991). *Meta-analytic procedures for social research* (rev. ed.). Newbury Park, CA: Sage.

Roy, C. (1988). Altered cognition: An information processing approach. In P. H. Mitchell, L. C. Hodges, M. Muwaswes, & C. A. Walleck (Eds.), *AANN's neuroscience nursing: Phenomenon and practice: Human responses to neurological health problems* (pp. 185–211). Norwalk, CT: Appleton and Lange.

Roy, C., & Roberts, S. L. (1981). *Theory construction in nursing. An adaptation model.* Englewood Cliffs, NJ: Prentice–Hall.

Roy, C., & Andrews, H. A. (1999). *The Roy adaptation model* (2nd ed.). Stamford, CT: Appleton and Lange.

Rujkorakarn, D., & Sukmak, V. (2002). Meaning of health and self-care in married men and women. *Thai Journal of Nursing Research, 6,* 69–75.

Russell, G. E., & Fawcett, J. (2005). The conceptual model for nursing and health policy revisited. *Policy, Politics, and Nursing Practice, 6,* 319–326.

Rutter, M. (1987). Psychosocial resilience and protective mechanisms. *American Journal of Orthopsychiatry, 57,* 316–331.

Saburi, G. L., Mapanga, K. G., & Mapanga, M. B. (2006). Perceived family reactions and quality of life of adults with epilepsy. *Journal of Neurological Nursing, 38,* 156–165.

Salamonson, Y., & Andrew, S. (2006). Academic performance in nursing students: Influence of part-time employment, age and ethnicity. *Journal of Advanced Nursing, 55,* 342–351.

Salsberry, P. (1994). A philosophy of nursing: What is it? What is it not? In J. F. Kikuchi & H. Simmons (Eds.), *Developing a philosophy of nursing* (pp. 11–19). Thousand Oaks, CA: Sage.

Samarel, N., Fawcett, J., & Tulman, L. (1997). Effects of support groups with coaching on adaptation to breast cancer. *Research in Nursing and Health, 20,* 15–26.

Samarel, N., Tulman, L., & Fawcett, J. (2002). Effects of two types of social support and education on adaptation to early stage breast cancer. *Research in Nursing and Health, 25,* 459–470.

Sanares, D. C., & Heliker, D. (2006). A framework for nursing clinical inquiry: Pathway toward evidence-based nursing practice. In K. Malloch & T. Porter-O-Grady (Eds.), *Introduction to evidence-based practice in nursing* (pp. 31–64). Boston: Jones and Bartlett.

Sanday, P. R. (1983). The ethnographic paradigm(s). In J. Van Maannen (Ed.)., *Qualitative methodology* (pp. 19–36). Beverly Hills, CA: Sage.

Sandelowski, M. (1986). The problem of rigor in qualitative research. *Advances in Nursing Science, 8*(3), 27–37.

Sandelowski, M. (1993). Rigor or rigor mortis: The problem of rigor in qualitative research revisited. *Advances in Nursing Science, 16*(2), 1–8.

Sandelowski, M. (1995). Sample size in qualitative research. *Research in Nursing and Health, 18,* 179–183.

Sandelowski, M. (2000). Combining qualitative and quantitative sampling, data collection, and analysis techniques in mixed-method studies. *Research in Nursing and Health, 23,* 246–255.

Sandelowski, M. (2006). "Meta-jeopardy": The crisis of representation in qualitative metasynthesis. *Nursing Outlook, 54,* 10–16.

Sandelowski, M., Barroso, J., & Voils, C. I. (2007). Using qualitative metasummary to synthesize qualitative and quantitative descriptive findings. *Research in Nursing and Health, 30,* 99–111.

Scharer, K., & Jones, D. S. (2004). Child psychiatric hospitalization: The last resort. *Issues in Mental Health Nursing, 25,* 79–101.

Schaefer, K. M. (2006). Myra Levine's conservation model and its applications. In M. E. Parker (Ed.), *Nursing theories and nursing practice* (2nd ed., pp. 94–112). Philadelphia: F. A. Davis.

Schaefer, K. M., & Pond, J. B. (Eds.). (1991). *Levine's conservation model: A framework for nursing practice.* Philadelphia: F. A. Davis.

Schaffer, M. A. (2004). Social support. In S. J. Peterson & T. S. Bredow (Eds.), *Middle range theories: Application to nursing research* (pp. 179–202). Philadelphia: Lippincott Williams and Wilkins.

Schlotfeldt, R. M. (1975). The need for a conceptual framework. In P. J. Verhonick (Ed.), *Nursing research I* (pp. 3–24). Boston: Little, Brown.

Schmieding, N. J. (2006). Ida Jean Orlando (Pelletier): Nursing process theory. In A. Marriner Tomey & M. R. Alligood, *Nursing theorists and their work* (6th ed., pp. 4311–451). St. Louis: Mosby Elsevier.

Schneider, S. M., Prince-Paul, M., Allen, M. J., Silverman, P., & Talaba, D. (2004). Virtual reality as a distraction intervention for women receiving chemotherapy. *Oncology Nursing Forum, 31,* 81–88.

Scholastic Aptitude Test. (2007). SAT reasoning test. Retrieved February 25, 2007, from http://www.collegeboard.com/student/testing/sat/about/SATI.html

Schumacher, K. L., & Gortner, S. R. (1992). (Mis)conceptions and reconceptions about traditional science. *Advances in Nursing Science, 14*(4), 1–11.

Schwarz, T. (2001). Family presence? *Not* mine. *American Journal of Nursing, 101*(5), 11.

Schwartz-Barcott, D., & Kim, H. S. (2000). An expansion and elaboration of the hybrid model of concept development. In B. L. Rodgers & K. A. Knafl (Eds.), *Concept development in nursing: Foundations, techniques, and applications* (2nd ed., pp. 129–159). Philadelphia: Saunders.

Scordo, K. A. (2007). Medication use and symptoms in individuals with mitral valve prolapse syndrome. *Clinical Nursing Research, 16,* 58–71.

Scott-Findlay, S. (2005). Keeping your practice cutting edge: Why using research in practice matters. *AWHONN Lifelines, 9,* 43–45.

Scott-Findlay, S. (2007). Fostering evidence-based practice. *Nursing for Women's Health, 11,* 250–252.

Scottish Intercollegiate Guidelines Network (SIGN) (2003, July). *Cutaneous melanoma. A national clinical guideline.* Edinburgh: Author (SIGN Publication No. 72). Retrieved July 14, 2007, from http://www.guideline.gov/summary/summary.aspx?doc_id=3877&nbr=003086&string=cutaneous+AND+melanoma

Sechrist, K., & Pravikoff, D. (2002). Solomon four-group design. *Cinahl Information Systems.* Retrieved May 29, 2006, from http://www.cinahl.com

Serlin, R. C. (1987). Hypothesis testing, theory building, and the philosophy of science. *Journal of Counseling Psychology, 34,* 365–371.

Siegel, S. (1956). *Nonparametric statistics for the behavioral sciences.* New York: McGraw-Hill.

Sieloff, C. L. (2006). Imogene King: Interacting systems framework and middle range theory of goal attainment. In A. Marriner Tomey & M. R. Alligood, *Nursing theorists and their work* (6th ed., pp. 297–317). St. Louis: Mosby Elsevier.

Sieloff, C. L. (1995). Development of a theory of departmental power. In M. A. Frey & C. L. Sieloff (Eds.), *Advancing King's systems framework and theory of nursing* (pp. 46–65). Thousand Oaks, CA: Sage.

Sieloff, C. L. (2004). Leadership behaviors that foster nursing group power. *Journal of Nursing Management, 12,* 246–251.

Silva, M. C. (1987). Conceptual models of nursing. In J. J. Fitzpatrick & R. L. Tauton (Eds.), *Annual review of nursing research* (Vol. 5, pp. 229–246). New York: Springer.

Silva, M. C., & Rothbart, D. (1984). An analysis of changing trends in philosophies of science on nursing theory development and testing. *Advances in Nursing Science, 6*(2), 1–13.

Sinding, C., Wiernikowski, J., & Aronson, J. (2005). Cancer care from the perspectives of older women. *Oncology Nursing Forum, 32,* 1169–1175.

Sitzman, K., & Eichelberger, L. W. (2004). *Understanding the work of nurse theorists: A creative beginning.* Boston: Jones and Bartlett.

Skalski, C. A., DiGerolamo, L., & Gigliotti, E. (2006). Stressors in five client populations: Neuman systems model–based literature review. *Journal of Advanced Nursing, 56,* 69–78.

Slakter, M. J., Wu, Y.-W. B., & Suzuki-Slakter, N. S. (1991). *, **, and ***; Statistical nonsense at the .00000 level. *Nursing Research, 40,* 248–249.

Smith, D. W. (1994). Toward developing a theory of spirituality. *Visions: The Journal of Rogerian Nursing Science, 2,* 35–43.

Smith, L. S. (2001). Evaluation of an educational intervention to increase cultural competence among registered nurses. *Journal of Cultural Diversity, 8,* 50–63.

Smith, M. H. (2007). What you must know about minors and informed consent. *American Nurse Today, 2*(5), 49–50.

Smith, M. J., & Liehr, P. R. (Eds.). (2003). *Middle range theory for nursing.* New York: Springer.

Sousa, V. D., & Zauszniewski, J. A. (2005). Toward a theory of diabetes self-care management. *Journal of Theory Construction & Testing, 9,* 61–67.

Speziale, H. J. S., & Carpenter, D. R. (2003). *Qualitative research in nursing: Advancing the humanistic imperative* (3rd ed.). Philadelphia: Lippincott Williams and Wilkins.

Steele, N. M., French, J., Gatherer-Boyles, J., Newman, S., & Leclaire, S. (2001). Effect of acupressure by Sea-Bands on nausea and vomiting of pregnancy. *Journal of Obstetric, Gynecologic, and Neonatal Nursing, 30,* 61–70.

Stepans, M. B. F., & Knight, J. R. (2002). Application of Neuman's framework: Infant exposure to environmental tobacco smoke. *Nursing Science Quarterly, 15,* 327–334.

Stepans, M. B. F., Wilhelm, S. L., & Dolence, K. (2006). Smoking hygiene: Reducing infant exposure to tobacco. *Biological Research for Nursing, 8,* 104–114.

Stetler, C. B. (2001a). To the editor. *Nursing Outlook, 49,* 286.

Stetler, C. B. (2001b). Updating the Stetler model of research utilization to facilitate evidence-based practice. *Nursing Outlook, 49,* 272–279.

Stevens, S. S. (1946). On the theory of scales of measurement. *Science, 102,* 677–680.

Stevens, S. S. (1951). Mathematics, measurement, and psychophysics. In S. S. Stevens (Ed.), *Handbook of experimental psychology* (pp. 1–49). New York: Wiley.

Stewart, D. W., & Shamdasani, P. N. (1990). *Focus groups: Theory and practice.* Newbury Park, CA: Sage.

Stolberg, S. G. (1999, November 28). The biotech death of Jesse Gelsinger. *The New York Times Magazine.* Retrieved May 28, 2007, from
http://www.nytimes.com/library/magazine/home/19991128mag-stolberg.html

Streubert, H. J. (1991). Phenomenological research as a theoretic initiative in community health nursing. *Public Health Nursing, 8,* 119–123.

Stringer, E., & Genat, W. (2004). *Action research in health.* Upper Saddle River, NJ: Pearson Merrill Prentice Hall.

Swanson, K. M. (1991). Empirical development of a middle range theory of caring. *Nursing Research, 40,* 161–166.

Tabachnick, B. G., & Fidell, L. S. (2001). *Using multivariate statistics* (4th ed.). Boston: Allyn and Bacon.

Thomas, K. (1976). Conflict and conflict management. In M. D. Dunnette (Ed.), *Handbook of industrial and organizational psychology* (pp. 889–935). Chicago: Rand-McNally.

Thomas, L., & Juanes, F. (1996). The importance of statistical power analysis: An example from *Animal Behaviour. Animal Behaviour, 52,* 856–859.

Thomas–Hawkins, C. (2000). Symptom distress and day-to-day changes in functional status in chronic hemodialysis patients. *Nephrology Nursing Journal, 27,* 369–379.

Thomas–Hawkins, C. (2005). Assessing role activities of individuals receiving long-term hemodialysis: Psychometric testing of the revised Inventory of Functional Status–Dialysis. *International Journal of Nursing Studies, 42,* 687–694.

Thompson, C., McCaughan, D., Cullum, N., Sheldon, T., & Raynor, P. (2005). Barriers to evidence-based practice in primary care nursing—Why viewing decision–making as context is helpful. *Journal of Advanced Nursing, 52,* 432–444.

Thompson, G., McClement, S., & Daeninck, P. (2006). Nurses' perceptions of quality end–of–life care on an acute medical ward. *Journal of Advanced Nursing, 53,* 169–177.

Tomlinson, M., & Gibson, G. J. (2006). Obstructive sleep apnoea syndrome: A nurse-led domiciliary service. *Journal of Advanced Nursing, 55,* 391–397.

Tsai, P.–F. (1999). Development of a middle–range theory of caregiver stress from the Roy adaptation model. *Dissertation Abstracts International, 60,* 133B.

Tsai, P.–F. (2003). A middle–range theory of caregiver stress. *Nursing Science Quarterly, 16,* 137–145.

Tsai, P. (2005). Predictors of distress and depression in elders with arthritic pain. *Journal of Advanced Nursing, 51,* 158–165.

Tsai, P., Tak, S., Moore, C., & Palencia, I. (2003). Testing a theory of chronic pain. *Journal of Advanced Nursing, 43,* 158–169.

Tsai, S.–L., & Chai, S.–K. (2005). Developing and validating a nursing website evaluation questionnaire. *Journal of Advanced Nursing, 49,* 406–413.

Tulman, L., Higgins, K., Fawcett, J., Nunno, C., Vansickel, C., Haas, M. B., & Speca, M. M. (1991). The Inventory of Functional Status–Antepartum Period: Development and testing. *Journal of Nurse-Midwifery, 36,* 117–123.

Tulman, L., & Fawcett, J. (2003). *Women's health during and after pregnancy: A theory-based study of adaptation to change.* New York: Springer.

Tyberg, K., & Chlan, L. (2006). Interrater agreement of the Checklist of Nonverbal Pain Indicators in intubated and sedated patients in surgical intensive care units. [Abstract]. *American Journal of Critical Care, 15,* 326.

United States Department of Health and Human Services. (2005, June 23). Protection of human subjects. Code of Federal Regulations, Title 45 Public Welfare, Part 46 Protection of Human Subjects. [Originally published June 18, 1991]. Retrieved February 21, 2007, from http://www.hhs.gov/ohrp/humansubjects/guidance/45cfr46.htm#subparta

United States Food and Drug Administration. (2006, April 1). Code of Federal Regulations, Title 21 Food and Drugs, Part 50 Protection of human subjects. Retrieved May 28, 2007, from http://www.accessdata.fda.gov/scripts/cdrh/cfdocs/cfcfr/CFRSearch.cfm?CFRPart=50

United States vs. Stanley, 107 S. CT. 3054 (1987).

Van de Ven, A. H. (1989). Nothing is quite so practical as a good theory. *Academy of Management Review, 14,* 486–489.

Vanderwee, K., Grypdonck, M. H. F., De Bacquer, D., & Defloor, T. (2006). The reliability of two observation methods of nonblanchable erythema, Grade 1 pressure ulcer. *Applied Nursing Research, 19,* 156–162.

Van Horn, E. (2005). An exploration of recurrent injury prevention in patients with trauma. *Orthopaedic Nursing, 24,* 249–258.

van Kaam, A. (1959). A phenomenological analysis exemplified by the feeling of being really understood. *Individual Psychology, 15,* 66–72.

van Kaam, A. L. (1966). Application of the phenomenological method. In A. L. van Kaam, *Existential foundations of psychology* (pp. 294–329). Pittsburgh: Duquesne University Press.

van Manen, M. (1984). Practicing phenomenological writing. *Phenomenology and Pedagogy, 2*(1), 36–69.

Varricchio, C. G. (2004). Measurement issues concerning linguistic translations. In F. Frank-Stromborg & S. J. Olsen (Eds.), *Instruments for clinical health-care research* (3rd ed., pp. 56–64). Boston: Jones and Bartlett.

Veatch, R. M., & Fry, S. (2006). *Case studies in nursing ethics* (3rd ed.). Boston: Jones and Bartlett.

Villarruel, A. M. (1995). Mexican–American cultural meanings, expressions, self–care and dependent–care actions associated with experiences of pain. *Research in Nursing and Health, 18,* 427–436.

Villarruel, A. M., Bishop, T. L., Simpson, E. M., Jemmott, L. S., & Fawcett, J. (2001). Borrowed theories, shared theories, and the advancement of nursing knowledge. *Nursing Science Quarterly, 14,* 158–163.

Visser-Meily, J. M. A., Post, M. W. M., Riphagan, I. I., & Lindeman, E. (2004). Measures used to assess burden among caregivers of stroke patients: A review. *Clinical Rehabilitation, 18,* 601–623.

Walker, L. O., & Avant, K. C. (2005). *Strategies for theory construction in nursing* (4th ed.). Upper Saddle River, NJ: Prentice Hall.

Wallin, L. (2005). Clinical practice guidelines in nursing. *AWHONN Lifelines, 9,* 248–251.

Waltz, C. F., Strickland, O. L., & Lenz, E. R. (2005). *Measurement in nursing and health research* (3rd ed.). New York: Springer.

Watson, J. (1985). *Nursing: Human science and human care.* Norwalk, CT: Appleton-Century-Crofts.

Watson, J. (2006). Jean Watson's theory of human caring. In M. E. Parker (Ed.), *Nursing theories and nursing practice* (2nd ed., pp. 295–302). Philadelphia: F. A. Davis.

Weaver, K., & Olson, J. K. (2006). Understanding paradigms used for nursing research. *Journal of Advanced Nursing, 53,* 459–469.

Weber, R. P. (1990). *Basic content analysis* (2nd ed.). Newbury Park, CA: Sage.

Weiss, M., Aber, C., & Fawcett, J. (2006–2009). *Readiness for hospital discharge and adaptation following childbirth.* Research in progress.

West, S., King, V., Carey, T. S., Lohr, K. N., McKoy, N., Sutton, S. F., & Lux, L. (2002). *Systems to rate the strength of scientific evidence.* Evidence Report/Technology Assessment No. 47 (Prepared by the Research Triangle Institute–University of North Carolina Evidence-based Practice Center under Contract No. 290-97-0011). AHRQ Publication No. 02-E016. Rockville, MD: Agency for Healthcare Research and Quality. (Available online at http://www.ncbi.nlm.nih.gov/books/bv.fcgi?rid=hstaat1.chapter.70996)

Westra, B. L., & Rodgers, B. L. (1991). The concept of integration: A foundation for evaluating outcomes of nursing care. *Journal of Professional Nursing, 7,* 277–282.

Wewers, M. E., Sarna, L., & Rice, V. H. (2006). Nursing research and treatment of tobacco dependence: State of the science. *Nursing Research, 55*(4S), S11–S15.

Whall, A. L. (2005). The structure of nursing knowledge: Analysis and evaluation of practice, middle range and grand theory. In J. J. Fitzpatrick & A. L. Whall, *Conceptual models of nursing: Analysis and application* (4th ed., pp. 5–20). Upper Saddle River, NJ: Pearson/Prentice Hall.

White, J. (1995). Patterns of knowing: Review, critique, and update. *Advances in Nursing Science, 17*(4), 73–86.

Whittemore, R. (2005). Analysis of integration in nursing science and practice. *Journal of Nursing Scholarship, 37,* 261–267.

Whittemore, R., & Grey, M. (2002). The systematic development of nursing interventions. *Journal of Nursing Scholarship, 34,* 115–120.

Whittemore, R., & Grey, M. (2006). Experimental and quasiexperimental designs. In G. LoBiondo-Wood & J. Haber (Eds.), *Nursing research: Methods and critical appraisal for evidence-based practice* (6th ed., pp. 220–237). St. Louis: Mosby Elsevier.

Whittemore, R., & Roy, C. (2002). Adapting to diabetes mellitus: A theory synthesis. *Nursing Science Quarterly, 15,* 311–317.

Wicks, M. N. (1995). Family health as derived from King's framework. In M. A. Frey & C. L. Sieloff (Eds.), *Advancing King's systems framework and theory of nursing* (pp. 97–108). Thousand Oaks, CA: Sage.

Wicks, M. N. (1997). A test of the Wicks family health model in families coping with chronic obstructive pulmonary disease. *Journal of Family Nursing, 3,* 189–212.

Williams, B. (1978). *A sampler on sampling.* New York: Wiley.

Williams, J. K., Schutte, D. L., Evers, C., & Holkup, P. A. (2000). Redefinition: Coping with normal results from predictive gene testing for neurogenerative disorders. *Research in Nursing and Health, 23,* 260–269.

Williams, S. A., & Schreier, A. M. (2005). The role of education in managing fatigue, anxiety, and sleep disorders in women undergoing chemotherapy for breast cancer. *Applied Nursing Research, 18,* 138–147.

Winfield, C., Davis, S., Schwaner, S., Conaway, M., & Burns, S. (2007). Evidence: The first word in safe I.V. practice. *American Nurse Today, 2*(5), 31–33.

Winker, C. K. (1995). A systems view of health. In M. A. Frey & C. L. Sieloff (Eds.), *Advancing King's systems framework and theory of nursing* (pp. 35–45). Thousand Oaks, CA: Sage.

Winker, C. K. (1996). A descriptive study of the relationship of interaction disturbance to the organization health of a metropolitan general hospital. *Dissertation Abstracts International, 57,* 4306B.

World Medical Association. (1964–2004). World Medical Association Declaration of Helsinki: Ethical principles for medical research involving human subjects. Retrieved February 21, 2007, from http://www.wma.net/e/policy/b3.htm

Wuest, J. (1994). A feminist approach to concept analysis. *Western Journal of Nursing Research, 15,* 577–586.

Wuest, J. (2000). Concept development situated in the critical paradigm. In B. L. Rodgers & K. A. Knafl (Eds.), *Concept development in nursing: Foundations, techniques, and applications* (2nd ed., pp. 369–386). Philadelphia: Saunders.

Yarcheski, A., Mahon, N. E., & Yarcheski, T. J. (1997). Alternative models of positive health practices in adolescents. *Nursing Research, 46,* 85–92.

Zahourek, R. P. (2004). Intentionality forms the matrix of healing: A theory. *Alternative Therapies in Health and Medicine, 10*(6), 40–49.

Zahourek, R. P. (2005). Intentionality: Evolutionary development in healing: A ground theory study for holistic nursing. *Journal of Holistic Nursing, 23,* 89–109.

Ziegler, S. M (Ed.). (2005). *Theory–directed nursing practice* (2nd ed.). New York: Springer.

Index